Heart Failure

Pathophysiology, Molecular Biology
and Clinical Management

Heart Failure

Pathophysiology, Molecular Biology and Clinical Management

Arnold M. Katz, M.D., D.MED.(HON.), F.A.C.C., F.A.C.P.

Professor of Medicine
Cardiology Division, Chief Emeritus
University of Connecticut School of Medicine
Farmington, Connecticut;
Visiting Professor of Medicine,
Dartmouth Medical School,
Lebanon, New Hampshire

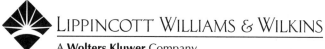

LIPPINCOTT WILLIAMS & WILKINS
A **Wolters Kluwer** Company
Philadelphia • Baltimore • New York • London
Buenos Aires • Hong Kong • Sydney • Tokyo

Acquisitions Editor: Ruth W. Weinberg
Developmental Editor: Michelle M. LaPlante
Production Editor: Frank Aversa
Manufacturing Manager: Kevin Watt
Cover Designer: Mark Lerner
Compositor: Lippincott Williams & Wilkins, Desktop Division
Printer: Edwards Brothers

© 2000 by Lippincott Williams & Wilkins
227 East Washington Square
Philadelphia, PA 19106-3780 USA
LWW.com

Printed in the USA

Library of Congress Cataloging-in-Publication Data

Katz, Arnold M.
  Heart failure: pathophysiology, molecular biology and clinical management.
    p.   cm.
  Includes bibliographical references and index.
  ISBN 0-7817-1549-0
  1. Heart Failure.   I. Title.
  [DNLM: 1. Heart Failure, Congestive—pathology.   WG 370 K195h 1999]
  RC685.C53K38 1999
  616.1′29—dc21
  DNLM/DLC
  for Library of Congress   99-34752
                                                                 CIP

Care has been taken to confirm the accuracy of the information presented and to describe generally accepted practices. However, the author and publisher are not responsible for errors or omissions or for any consequences from application of the information in this book and make no warranty, expressed or implied, with respect to the currency, completeness, or accuracy of the contents of the publication. Application of this information in a particular situation remains the professional responsibility of the practioner.

The author and publisher have exerted every effort to ensure that drug selection and dosage set forth in this text are in accordance with current recommendations and practice at the time of publication. However, in view of ongoing research, changes in government regulations, and the constant flow of information relating to drug therapy and drug reactions, the reader is urged to check the package insert for each drug for any change in indications and dosage and for added warnings and precautions. This is particularly important when the recommended agent is a new or infrequently employed drug.

Some drugs and medical devices presented in this publication have Food and Drug Administration (FDA) clearance for limited use in restricted research settings. It is the responsibility of the health care provider to ascertain the FDA status of each drug or device planned for use in their clinical practice.

10 9 8 7 6 5 4 3 2 1

For Phyllis

CONTENTS

FOREWORD

Despite the dramatic advances in the care of patients with cardiovascular diseases that have occurred in the second half of the twentieth century, these conditions remain by far the most common causes of death in developed nations. Moreover, the prevalence of cardiovascular diseases is now rising rapidly in developing nations as well. It has been projected that by 2020 cardiovascular disease will, for the first time in human history, be the most common cause of death worldwide.

Heart failure is the most frequent "final common pathway" to death in cardiovascular disease, and in the United States it is the most frequent primary hospital discharge diagnosis of Medicare patients. It is therefore mandatory that physicians involved in the care of patients with this common and serious condition understand its pathogenesis, its clinical features, and the mechanisms underlying various therapies. Of equal importance, investigators of heart failure, whether basic or clinical scientists, have a great need to understand the relation between abnormalities on the molecular, cellular, organ, and clinical levels.

Heart failure is a much more complex condition than it was thought to be as recently as twenty years ago. At that time, the pathophysiology of heart failure had been well described, but the responsible alterations in cellular biochemistry and biophysics were just being elucidated. The underlying genetic alterations were a total mystery.

Heart Failure provides important insights into this important condition. Single-authored, comprehensive medical texts on complex subjects are now a great rarity because few individuals possess the understanding and perspective to do justice to fields as enormous as heart failure. Dr. Arnold Katz has successfully tackled this Herculean task, and in this magnificent book he has not only reviewed all relevant aspects of this vast subject but has provided a "grand vision" of how molecular biology provides explanations of the abnormalities of myocardial contraction and relaxation, and how abnormalities of myocyte function affect the performance of the cardiac pump. The breadth and depth of understanding provided by the author, who uniquely spans the disciplines of molecular biology, cardiac biochemistry, cardiac physiology, and clinical cardiology, are matched by his extraordinary ability to relate these fields to one another, and to explain complex concepts clearly, both in words and in diagrams.

This book is truly a joy to study. It will be equally useful to clinicians, scientists, and their trainees. Coming at the junction of two millennia, it will surely stand as a landmark in the field.

Eugene Braunwald, M.D.
Boston, Massachusetts

PREFACE

Heart failure is defined in this text as a clinical syndrome in which heart disease reduces cardiac output, increases venous pressures, and is accompanied by molecular abnormalities that cause progressive deterioration of the failing heart and premature myocardial cell death. That heart failure is a syndrome, rather than a disease, is evidenced by its appearance when the myocardium is damaged by infarction, or when the heart is forced to contract against an excessive load, is infected by a virus, is poisoned by alcohol or anticancer therapy, contains a defective protein, has its blood supply chronically reduced, or is subjected to inappropriately rapid electrical stimuli.

The manifestations of heart failure in most patients are similar, so that at a clinical level, the disabilities in this syndrome appear simple. This is because, like any pump, the heart has but two ways to fail—reduced ejection of blood under pressure into the aorta and pulmonary artery ("forward failure"), and inadequate emptying of the venous reservoirs that carry blood to the heart ("backward failure"). The apparent simplicity of these hemodynamic concepts, however, is deceptive. In the first place, a heart that empties poorly cannot fill normally, and a heart that fills poorly will not be able to eject a normal stroke volume. Furthermore, the ability of so many pathogenic processes to cause this syndrome means that, even among patients whose clinical problems appear similar to one another, many different mechanisms can operate to damage the heart. Adding to this complexity are the many mechanisms that the body calls upon to compensate for the impaired pumping of blood. Virtually all of these compensatory mechanisms, while initially beneficial, have deleterious long-term consequences that often represent a major cause of the progression that is so important in this syndrome. These and many other mechanisms contribute to a molecular disorder in the failing heart muscle, a disorder that is so malignant that death usually follows within 5 years after the onset of symptoms. This reflects the fact that, although impaired pumping is responsible for the clinical manifestations, the major problem in most patients is progressive deterioration of overloaded myocardial cells, a process that I have called a "cardiomyopathy of overload."

Only recently has prognosis been recognized as an important problem in heart failure. The result has been a paradigm shift that has altered the goals of therapy, which now include prolongation of survival as well as relief of symptoms. Complicating this change in therapeutic objectives has been the realization that many drugs that improve symptoms over the short term worsen long-term prognosis, and conversely, that some drugs prolonging survival can temporarily worsen symptoms. These counterintuitive findings, in which short-term and long-term effects of therapy can be opposite to one another, make it increasingly important that those who treat heart failure understand the pathophysiology of this syndrome.

The fact that many clinical manifestations of heart failure are caused by compensatory mechanisms that are triggered by the impaired circulation adds to the challenges facing those who manage this syndrome. These neurohumoral responses include a hemodynamic defense reaction that attempts to maintain blood pressure and cardiac output, and an inflammatory response, in which the failing heart and other organs of the body seem to act as if they were attacked as foreign objects. Of even greater importance in understanding this syndrome are the maladaptive consequences of cardiac hypertrophy.

Although hypertrophy improves pump performance over the short term, this growth response appears to worsen long-term survival by accelerating the deterioration of myocardial cells.

A major stimulus that led me to write this book was the need for a relatively simple explanation of the molecular abnormalities in the failing heart. This text seeks to clarify the interplay among primary abnormalities that injure the heart; the resulting hemodynamic abnormalities; abnormalities in excitation-contraction coupling, contraction and relaxation; the neurohumoral responses; and the molecular mechanisms that damage the failing myocardium. My attempts to understand this interplay led me to review many new concepts in molecular biology. The result is a text that, in some ways, represents an overview of signal transduction and the regulation of growth and proliferation in the heart. Although it was not my original goal to write a book on the molecular biology of heart failure, the importance of these concepts became increasingly apparent as I sought to clarify the pathophysiology of heart failure and to explain the causes of the poor prognosis in this syndrome.

This book is intended to help both health care providers and research scientists navigate among the many mechanisms that operate in heart failure. The historical overview that begins this text reminds us of the terrible suffering once seen in these patients, as well as the remarkable insights of the 19th Century clinician-pathologists who understood both the adaptive and maladaptive nature of cardiac hypertrophy and the significance of the progressive dilatation we now call "remodeling." This history also reminds us that we remain fallible, and that we are not immune to errors such as were made by those who came before us. After all, as recently as a decade ago, the consensus in this field was that inotropic therapy was the best way to treat heart failure. Chapter 2 reviews the hemodynamics of heart failure, emphasizing the clinical manifestations caused by the molecular abnormalities discussed in later chapters. Chapter 3 moves to the mechanisms responsible for the contraction and relaxation abnormalities once thought to be at the root of the problem in these patients. Highlighted in Chapters 4 and 5 are the many clinical manifestations caused by the body's misguided efforts to "put things right." Striking differences between the short-term and long-term consequences of the compensatory response to a fall in cardiac output become clear when we examine the hemodynamic defense reaction and inflammatory response, two major aspects of the neurohumoral response that is triggered by heart failure.

Subsequent chapters explore the impact of the rapidly advancing fields of molecular biology on our understanding of the pathophysiology of heart failure. Chapter 6 reviews mechanisms that cause the failing heart to hypertrophy, describing how extracellular mediators of the neurohumoral response, supplemented by the actions of peptide growth factors and cell adhesion molecules, lead to maladaptive growth of the overloaded heart. This chapter also describes the terminally differentiated myocytes of the adult human heart, how the hypertrophic response of these cells differs from the proliferative response in the embryonic heart, and how the molecular signals that stimulate cell growth also cause apoptosis (programmed cell death), which has been called an "abortive attempt at mitosis." The intracellular signaling cascades that mediate these responses are detailed in Chapter 7 because these mechanisms appear likely to become targets for new therapies for heart failure. Chapter 8 builds on these concepts in presenting possible explanations for the "cardiomyopathy of overload," the maladaptive growth response seen in most failing hearts. This chapter also describes a growing number of familial cardiomyopathies that are emerging as a major cause of heart failure. The details in these chapters provide a foundation for the review of current strategies of therapy that is presented in Chapter 9.

The text ends with a brief chapter that discusses some practical means by which this material can be used to benefit the patient with heart failure.

My attempt to cover aspects of heart failure ranging from clinical manifestations and therapy to the underlying molecular mechanisms is, at one level, presumptuous because I am not expert in all of these fields. However, my primary goal is to provide an overview that can help the reader integrate the many diverse mechanisms that operate in this important clinical syndrome — to see the forest rather than the trees. This book should not be viewed as an encyclopedic and authoritative text that can substitute for the many large, multiauthored volumes that deal with this subject. The sections on therapy must not be read as instructions for patient management; instead, they set out what I view as important principles of therapy. Details of this therapy, which change from year to year, should be sought in more authoritative texts and chapters, and most importantly, in the many original articles on the treatment of heart failure.

Selecting and summarizing the bibliography was a daunting task. In preparing this text, I have referred to many more papers and reviews than I had originally intended. In compiling what I hope will be a useful bibliography, some key articles may have been left out; however, in the interest of meeting my publishing deadline, my literature search ended in early 1999. A frustrating task, since each week brought new articles of seminal importance in this field.

My major goal in preparing this text has been to use a single voice in providing a clear exposition of our current understanding of heart failure, and most important, to explain and integrate the many mechanisms that operate in patients suffering from this clinical syndrome. Like my other book, *Physiology of the Heart*, this discussion of heart failure tries to be a fluid, "user friendly" presentation that can be read from cover to cover. I hope the reader finds both the time and a comfortable chair in which to appreciate, and understand and integrate, the many important mechanisms that operate in the patient with heart failure.

Arnold M. Katz, M.D., D.MED.(HON.)

ACKNOWLEDGMENTS

Much of this text was written in Norwich, Vermont, during a writing sabbatical leave from the University of Connecticut. I could not have written this book without access to the Lyman Maynard Stowe Library of the University of Connecticut and the medical libraries of the Dartmouth Medical School. I thank the latter for appointing me a Visiting Professor of Medicine, and providing me with an internet link to the Dartmouth libraries.

A few chapters that I found most difficult were reviewed by my friends Criss Hartzell, Seigo Izumo, Doug Mann, and Achilles Pappano, whose help is gratefully acknowledged; however, I take full responsibility for any errors that may remain in this text. I am grateful to Reed Detar for help in preparing Figures 2-1 and 2-20. I also thank Ruth Weinberg, my Editor at Lippincott Williams & Wilkins, whose patience and gentle prodding helped me to meet at least a few deadlines.

This book could not have been written without the support of Phyllis, my wife of 40 years, who fostered the intellectually stimulating yet tranquil environment needed for this task. The patience and understanding of my children and their families when I disappeared during their visits to work on the *Heart Failure* book is also gratefully acknowledged. Finally, I thank Telemachus and Peisistratus ("Max" and "Pi"), our two Springer Spaniels, who took me away from my computer for many walks in the woods that restored my circulation and recharged my intellectual batteries.

Arnold M. Katz

End-Stage Heart Failure in the Mid-19th Century

The respiration, always short, becomes hurried and laborious on the slightest exertion or mental emotion. The effort of ascending a staircase is particularly distressing. The patient stops abruptly, grasps at the first object that presents itself and fixing the upper extremities in order to afford a fulcrum for the muscles of respiration, gasps with an aspect of extreme distress.

Incapable of lying down, he is seen for weeks, and even for months together, either reclining in the semi-erect posture supported by pillows, or sitting with the trunk bent forward and the elbows or forearms resting on the drawn-up knees. The latter position he assumes when attacked by a paroxysms of dyspnea—sometimes, however, extending the arms against the bed on either side, to afford a firmer fulcrum for the muscles of respiration. With eyes widely expanded and staring, eye-brows raised, nostrils dilated, a ghastly and haggard countenance, and the head thrown back at every inspiration, he casts around a hurried, distracted look of horror, of anguish, of supplication: now imploring, in plaintive moans, or quick broken accents, and half-stifled voice, the assistance already often lavished in vain: now upbraiding the impotency of medicine; and now in an agony of despair, drooping his head on his chest, and muttering a fervent invocation for death to put a period to his sufferings. For a few hours—perhaps only for a few minutes—he tastes an interval of delicious respite, which cheers him with the hope that the worst is over, and that his recovery is at hand. Soon that hope vanishes. From a slumber fraught with the horrors of a hideous dream, he starts up with a wild exclamation that "it is returning." At length, after reiterated recurrences of the same attacks, the muscles of respiration, subdued by the efforts of which the instinct of self-preservation alone renders them capable, participate in the general exhaustion, and refuse to perform their function. The patient gasps, sinks, and expires.

Hope, J. *A Treatise on the Diseases of the Heart and Great Vessels*
(Philadelphia: Haswell & Johnson, 1842; 381–382).

Acute Pulmonary Edema at the Beginning of the 20th Century

A physician receives an emergency call, and knows, if it is not a patient who has hysteria, that it is his duty to see the patient immediately. The friends of the patient all anxiously await the physician's arrival; front doors are often wide open, and the servants and the whole household are in a great state of excitement and anxiety. The position in which the patient will be found is that which he has learned gives him the greatest comfort. If the physician knows his patients, he will know how he will find him. He may be sitting up in bed; he may be standing, leaning over a chair; he may be sitting in a chair leaning over a table or leaning over the back of another chair; but he is using every auxiliary muscle he possesses to respire. He is generally bathed in cold perspiration; the extremities are often icy cold; he calls for air, and to stop fanning all in one breath; he wishes the perspiration wiped off his brow, and nearly goes frantic while it is being done; there is agony depicted on his face; his eyes stare; his expirations are often groaning. Sometimes there is even incontinence of urine and feces, often hiccup or short coughs, perhaps vomiting, and possibly sharp pangs of pain in the cardiac region. A patient with these symptoms may die at any moment, and the wonder is that so many times one lives through these paroxysms.

The patient can hardly be questioned, can certainly not be carefully examined; and herein lies the advantage of the family physician who knows the patient and his heart, and in whom the patient has confidence. In fact, this confidence which such a patient has in the physician who has more or less frequently aided him in weathering these terrible attacks is alone the greatest boon the patient can have.

Two factors may normally, without treatment, stop these paroxysms, and the "bad heart turn" may be cured spontaneously. The first of these is self control. If the patient does not lose his head, by an effort of the will he saves himself from becoming nervous or frightened and therefore escapes the result of mental excitement; the increased peripheral blood pressure from fear does not occur, and in a shorter or longer time the heart quiets down. The physician recognizes this power, and gives his patient immediate assurance that he will be all right; the patient who knows his physician immediately feels this assurance and is quickly improved.

The second factor in spontaneous cure of the heart attack is relaxation. The exhaustion from the respiratory muscular efforts, together with the drowsy condition caused by cerebral hyperemia and from the imperfectly aerated blood, causes finally a dulling of the mental activity, and the nervous excitement abates, which with the exhaustion, gives a relaxation of peripheral arterioles; the resistance to the flow of blood is removed, the surface of the body becomes warm, the heart quiets down by the equalization of the circulation, and the paroxysm is over.

Osborne, OT. *Disturbances of the Heart,* 2nd Ed.
(Chicago: The American Medical Association, 1916; 142–144).

1

Overview, Definition, Historical Aspects

OVERVIEW AND DEFINITION

In writing a book about heart failure, it is appropriate to begin by defining this condition. Yet this is not a simple task. Whereas the usual definitions of this clinical syndrome focus on failure of the heart *as a pump*, those who read through these pages will quickly learn that there is much more to heart failure than an impaired ability to pump blood from the veins to the arteries. This is true in part because heart failure patients are troubled by more than a low cardiac output and too much blood in their veins. Although these obvious hemodynamic disorders are important, abnormalities involving other organs often dominate the clinical picture in these patients. For example, accumulation of blood in the pulmonary circulation behind a failing left ventricle increases the work of breathing and so leads to shortness of breath, while the low cardiac output signals the kidneys to retain salt and water, which in heart failure represents a serious mistake because it worsens pulmonary congestion. The profound weakness in these patients, which is initiated by the low cardiac output, is due to a skeletal muscle myopathy whose causative mechanisms remain poorly understood. Despite the prominent abnormalities in the lungs, kidneys, skeletal muscle, and other organs, these are victims of this syndrome, whose cause obviously lies in the heart.

Another problem in defining heart failure is that this condition is not a disease but instead represents the final common pathway by which a number of disorders damage the heart so as to cause disability and premature death. These disorders include coronary disease, hypertension, valvular disorders, and a diverse group of heart muscle diseases referred to as the cardiomyopathies. Furthermore, because this syndrome establishes a number of vicious cycles, heart failure begets more heart failure.

There are many ways that one can define heart failure. At the level of organ physiology, heart failure can be defined as a hemodynamic disorder caused by an impaired muscular pump. However, there is much more to this clinical syndrome because myocardial cells are molecular machines in which calcium-regulated interactions between the contractile proteins give rise to the rhythmic contractions and relaxations that pump blood. Heart failure, regardless of etiology, is accompanied by abnormalities in both the contractile machinery and the membrane systems that regulate the cardiac cycle, so that this syndrome can also be defined in terms of the disordered biochemical and biophysical processes that impair myocardial contractility and relaxation. However, the molecular composition of the heart is also changed in most of these patients, so that even these biochemical definitions are inadequate. Furthermore, molecular abnormalities differ in different forms of heart failure, and change with time as this condition progresses. Some of these changes are compensatory, some are deleterious, and most are both compensatory and deleterious. For example, hypertrophy increases the mass of the failing heart, which improves ejection but, at the same time, impairs relaxation and probably shortens my-ocyte survival.

The failing heart is generally a dying heart because the growth response that leads to hypertrophy appears also to cause the premature death of cardiac myocytes. In the adult heart, myocyte death is a calamity because the cells that are lost cannot be replaced. It is largely for this reason that heart failure is a progressive condition, with a prognosis that is worse than that of most common malignancies. This fact is not widely appreciated, largely because death from heart failure is usually less cruel than that from lung or breast cancer. Because the 5-year survival rate, once heart failure becomes symptomatic, is less than 50% (Ho et al., 1993a), any definition of heart failure that does not consider the mol-ecular processes that accelerate myocardial cell death overlooks a major clinical feature in this syndrome.

Growth abnormalities in the failing heart have recently assumed a practical importance that equals that of the impaired pump performance. This is due in part to the fact that some drugs that alleviate the clinical manifestations caused by the failing pump worsen prognosis, whereas other drugs not only relieve suffering and improve well-being in these patients but also prolong survival. In many cases, therapy can reduce the cost of manag-ing this common syndrome, which in the industrialized world has become a major factor in escalating health care expenses. The importance of these developments has been am-plified by new technology that has made it possible to identify patients who are destined to die of heart failure, even before the initial appearance of symptoms. Together, these achievements have opened a new era of preventive medicine that has enormous potential benefits both for the patient and for society. However, understanding of these new ap-proaches requires a more complete and better focused definition for this condition.

One way to view the failing heart is to compare it with a defective gasoline-powered pump that moves water from a leaky basement to a garden. Failure of the pump can allow the basement to flood and, at the same time, fail to provide enough water to maintain the garden. In heart failure, these are analogous to abnormalities in organ physiology. How-ever, if the underlying problem in the defective pump were to lie somewhere in the gaso-line engine—a malfunctioning valve, worn pistons, a blocked fuel line, or a short circuit in the ignition system—this would be analogous to an abnormality in cell biochemistry in the patient with heart failure. To pursue this analogy, if the defective pump wears out rapidly and soon stops altogether, this would have a clear parallel in the patient with heart failure in whom, regardless of etiology, rapid worsening of the condition generally ends with early death.

Traditional definitions of heart failure highlight the clinical signs and symptoms that arise when the failing cardiac pump cannot satisfy the needs of the body. Although the resulting clinical manifestations can be traced to heart disease, the picture in most patients is dominated by the secondary abnormalities discussed earlier: in the lungs (shortness of breath), kidneys (salt and water retention), and skeletal muscle (fatigue). But these organs are the victims and not the initiators of this syndrome, so that defini-tions of heart failure that are based on clinical manifestations tend to draw attention away from the diseased heart, which is at the center of this syndrome.

Another difficulty with traditional definitions of heart failure that highlight the pump abnormality is that they often understate—and sometimes ignore—the progressive clini-cal course and poor prognosis. The importance of this oversight lies in evidence that drugs that improve symptoms over the short term often worsen prognosis, and, con-versely, that drugs that initially worsen symptoms can have remarkable long-term bene-fits both on well-being and survival. These counterintuitive findings, which have cost the pharmaceutical industry hundreds of millions—and probably billions—of dollars in wasted development costs and lost opportunities, highlight the importance of including the molecular factors responsible for the poor prognosis in defining heart failure. Heart failure, therefore, must be viewed not only in terms of the abnormal organ and cell function that impair its pumping but also in terms of the molecular abnormalities that determine prognosis.

The definition that follows, although imperfect, recognizes not only the impaired organ physiology and altered cell biochemistry but also the progressive changes that cause rapid deterioration of the heart. This definition views heart failure as *a clinical syndrome in which heart disease reduces cardiac output, increases venous pressures, and is accompanied by molecular abnormalities that cause progressive deterioration of the failing heart and premature myocardial cell death.* This definition, which expands our view beyond the traditional focus on impaired pump function and depressed myocardial contractility, highlights the molecular abnormalities that hold the key to explaining the shortened survival in these patients. Integration of the modern paradigm of molecular biology with the earlier paradigms of organ physiology and cell biochemistry is also essential in developing new therapeutic strategies that not only palliate the clinical, hemodynamic, and metabolic manifestations associated with impaired pump function but also slow the molecular processes responsible for the progressive downhill course in these patients.

HISTORICAL ASPECTS

The cardinal features of heart failure have been recognized since antiquity, although it is only recently that these signs and symptoms could be attributed to disorders of the cardiac pump. [An expanded version of this discussion is found in Katz (1997, 1998).] The most evident clinical manifestations of heart failure (Table 1-1), which are discussed at length in Chapter 2, depend on whether the underlying cause affects primarily the right

TABLE 1-1. *Common clinical manifestations of heart failure*

Right heart (backward) failure: accumulation of blood "behind" the right ventricle, elevated right atrial and systemic venous pressures.
  Edema: a painless "soft" swelling caused by fluid accumulation in the soft tissues, often referred to as "pitting edema," because an impression remains after a finger is slowly pressed into the swelling. This differs from edema caused by infection, which is generally painful, inflamed, and "hard." Cardiac edema is "dependent" and is most prominent in the legs, where gravity increases the pressure that forces fluid out of the capillaries into the soft tissues.
  Dropsy or anasarca: filling of the body with fluid. In addition to dependent edema, fluid accumulates in the body cavities, notably the peritoneal cavity (ascites), the spaces surrounding the lungs (pleural effusion), and occasionally the pericardium (pericardial effusion). This fluid is generally thin and colorless, and does not clot, in contrast to the purulent fluid found when these cavities are infected or the bloody fluid often found in malignant effusions.
Left heart (backward) failure: accumulation of blood "behind" the left ventricle, with elevated left atrial and pulmonary venous pressures causing the lungs to become stiff and fluid to leak into the pulmonary alveoli.
  Dyspnea: shortness of breath, characteristically worsened by effort.
  Orthopnea: shortness of breath that is worse when the patient lies down.
  Paroxysmal nocturnal dyspnea: episodes when shortness of breath occurs suddenly during sleep.
Low output (forward) failure: the state of low cardiac output caused when ejection of the heart's contents is reduced.
  Weakness and fatigue: symptoms associated with chronically reduced cardiac output caused by a skeletal muscle myopathy.
  "Shock": a marked decrease in cardiac output that lowers blood pressure, causes weakness, cool and sweaty skin, confusion, and kidney failure. When severe, can cause syncope (fainting).

or left ventricle. In patients with failure of the right heart, the principal clinical manifestations are caused by accumulation of blood "behind" the failing right ventricle, which elevates right atrial and systemic venous pressures. The result is edema that, because of the effects of gravity, initially accumulates mainly in the legs. Before the development of drugs that could eliminate salt and water from these patients, this fluid eventually filled the body cavities: in the peritoneal cavity as ascites, in the spaces surrounding the lungs as pleural effusions, and as pericardial effusion in the sac that surrounds the heart. These are the manifestations of the *"dropsy,"* or *"anasarca,"* caused by right heart failure, in which the body becomes filled with fluid. In left heart failure, inadequate emptying of the vessels behind a diseased left ventricle causes few obvious signs, simply because the fluid accumulates almost entirely within the lungs. Patients with left heart failure are, however, quite ill because the elevated left atrial pressure causes overfilling of the pulmonary capillaries and lymphatics. This stiffens the lungs, which increases the work of breathing, and impairs oxygen exchange across the alveolar membranes. Eventually, this fluid becomes transudated into the air spaces, which, when severe, causes pulmonary edema that can literally drown a patient. In milder cases, left heart failure causes shortness of breath (*dyspnea*) that is characteristically worsened by effort and by reclining (*orthopnea*). Common to both right and left heart failure is a decrease in cardiac output; however, the symptoms associated with impaired perfusion of the tissues—mainly weakness and fatigue—are rarely recognizable as symptoms of heart failure in older texts.

Edema, dropsy, anasarca, and dyspnea are mentioned frequently in ancient writings, but none are specific for heart failure. The soft, painless dependent edema seen in heart failure differs from that caused by infection, in which the swelling is hard (indurated) and accompanied by pain and redness; however, liver and kidney failure, along with malnutrition and anemia, also cause edema, dropsy, and anasarca that closely resemble the fluid retention seen in heart failure. Lung disease, notably pulmonary tuberculosis, was a common cause of dyspnea in the ancient world and, as already noted, the weakness and fatigue associated with low cardiac output are nonspecific. For these reasons, until clinical findings could be correlated with autopsy descriptions, it was generally impossible to attribute these clinical findings to disorders of the heart.

A useful way to understand this history is described by Thomas Kuhn (1970), who characterizes the development of scientific knowledge as a series of shifting paradigms, which he defines as "models from which spring particular coherent traditions of scientific research" that are "sufficiently unprecedented to attract an enduring group of adherents away from competing models of scientific theory," and "sufficiently open-ended to leave all sorts of problems for the redefined group of practitioners to resolve." Progress in science, according to Kuhn, occurs when growing awareness of the inability of an established paradigm to explain new knowledge leads to a "crisis" that is then resolved by a *paradigmatic shift*. The latter is viewed by Kuhn as a "revolutionary" change in which a new paradigm provides a radically new way to address an unresolved problem, while at the same time invalidating the earlier paradigm. As noted below, this view of scientific progress is not always appropriate in describing the history of discovery in heart failure.

The evolution of our understanding of heart failure since the Hippocratic descriptions of dyspnea and anasarca can be viewed in terms of the six paradigms listed in Table 1-2. [Readers may be familiar with the author's earlier reviews of this history, which describe only the three later paradigms—"organ," "cell," and "gene" (Katz, 1988). Those earlier reviews focused on the 20th century, whereas this discussion looks back much further, accounting for the expanded list.] In some cases, this progress occurred by paradigmatic shifts as described by Kuhn, for example, when Galen's concept that the heart's function

TABLE 1-2. *Six paradigms in the evolution of modern understanding of heart failure*

1. Clinical observation
   Case reports describing signs and symptoms
2. Anatomic pathology
   Autopsy correlations with clinical findings
   Microscopic pathology
3. Circulatory physiology
   Abnormalities in the circulation of the blood
4. Cardiac hemodynamics
   Pressure and flow abnormalities in the failing heart
5. Cell biochemistry and biophysics
   Abnormal contraction, relaxation, and energetics
6. Molecular biology
   Growth abnormalities

is to heat the blood was replaced with Harvey's description of the circulation. Another paradigmatic shift occurred when the modern understanding that shortness of breath can be caused when blood accumulates behind a failing left heart replaced the Hippocratic explanation that this symptom is due to cold phlegm descending from the brain to the chest. However, not all progress in understanding the nature of heart failure required that "an older paradigm [be] replaced in whole or in part by an incompatible new one" (Kuhn, 1970). The 20th century transitions from physiologic to biochemical explanations of heart failure, and more recently the application of concepts of molecular biology to the failing heart, in the words of Kuhn were "substantial and necessary for progress" and so can be viewed as paradigmatic shifts. However, each of these advances took place without the new knowledge invalidating earlier concepts (Katz, 1988; Katz and Katz, 1991), so that while the new paradigms were revolutionary, they are not "irreconcilable" with earlier paradigms.

Clinical observation, the first paradigm listed in Table 1-2, is seen in Hippocrates' meticulous descriptions written during the 6th century B.C.E. Attempts to define the causes of these syndromes, however, were off the mark because the Hippocratic physician lacked a scientific basis by which to explain his observations, and so was forced to rely on philosophical concepts that had just emerged from Greek mythology (Katz and Katz, 1995). More than 2,000 years were to pass before correlations of clinical observations with autopsy findings made it possible to use *anatomic pathology*, the second paradigm, in understanding the causes of heart failure. At almost the same time, William Harvey introduced the paradigm of *circulatory physiology*, which by overthrowing the Galenic view that the function of the heart is to generate and distribute heat throughout the body, made it possible to understand how a failing cardiac pump in patients with narrowed or leaky heart valves could cause dyspnea and edema. Harvey's discovery, as noted earlier, clearly exemplifies a Kuhnian paradigm shift.

The 19th century saw rapid developments in the first three paradigms listed in Table 1-2. Most important is an almost forgotten understanding of the anatomic pathology of heart failure, with its emphasis on different architectural patterns of cardiac enlargement seen in failing hearts. In the early years of the 20th century, when it became possible to relate the clinical valve disorders identified by anatomic pathologists hundreds of years earlier to pressure and flow abnormalities in animal models of heart disease (Wiggers, 1928, 1949), attention shifted rapidly to the fourth paradigm of *cardiac hemodynamics*. The introduction of cardiac catheterization in the 1940s integrated this hemodynamic physiology with clinical cardiology, thereby altering the clinical approach to cardiac patients. As a result, by the 1960s the hemodynamic physiology that for almost 50 years had been viewed as arcane "basic science" provided the foundation for advances in cardiac surgery that, for the first time, provided effective treatment for many forms of valvular and congenital heart disease. Recognition that changes in myocardial contractility, as well as altered end-diastolic volume (the Frank-Starling relationship) play an important role in regulating the performance of the heart, led in the 1950s to clinical applications of the fifth paradigm, *cell biochemistry and biophysics*. New understanding of the chemistry of muscular contraction, notably the role of calcium in initiating and regulating cardiac contraction, led to the recognition that contractility was depressed in heart failure (Spann et al., 1967). This, in turn, stimulated the search for drugs that could improve the depressed myocardial contractility seen in these patients. The introduction of noninvasive methods to measure wall motion in the 1970s was soon followed by the recognition that heart failure could be caused not only by weakness of the myocardium, but also by relaxation abnormalities.

The increasing pace of discovery has, over the past decade, identified the paradigm of altered gene expression, commonly referred to as *molecular biology*, as being of major importance in the progressive deterioration seen in most patients with heart failure. This most recent paradigmatic shift appears to hold the key to developing new means to slow the rapid deterioration of the failing heart.

The remainder of this historical section highlights two key discoveries involving the first three paradigms listed in Table 1-2. These are the role of impaired cardiac pumping in causing the clinical syndrome that is currently recognized as heart failure, and the clinical implications of the different patterns of hypertrophy and dilatation seen in these patients. The final three paradigms in Table 1-2 are the central focus of the remainder of this text.

Clinical Observations: From Hippocrates to the Middle Ages

The writings attributed to Hippocrates (*c*460–370 B.C.E.) (Fig. 1-1) include dozens of clinical case histories, some of which probably represent descriptions of heart disease (Katz and Katz, 1962). These books contain examples of dyspnea that could represent left heart failure and of dropsy that could represent right heart failure. It is likely, however, that in many cases, these were manifestations of other diseases such as pneumonia or tuberculosis (dyspnea) and liver failure, kidney failure, or cellulitis (dropsy). Hippocrates viewed dyspnea as the result of "phlegm" (the cold humor) passing from the brain to the heart, stating that "when the phlegm descends cold to the lungs and heart the blood is chilled; and the veins . . . beat forcefully against the lungs and heart, and the heart palpates, so that under this compulsion difficulty of breathing and orthopnea result" (*The Sacred Disease IX*, translation by Jones, 1923–1931). He also appears to have encountered the heart failure seen in the second trimester of pregnancy in a woman with rheumatic mitral valve disease when he described a patient who:

> in the fourth or fifth month of her pregnancy, had watery swellings in her legs, swellings in the hollows of her eyes, and her whole body puffed up. Besides these she had a dry cough, sometimes orthopnea, dyspnea and suffocation. Sometimes she was so near suffocation that that she was obliged to sit up in bed without being able to lie down; and if she tried to sleep it was in a sitting position. Yet there was not much fever. (Epidemics VII, from Littré, 1839–1861)

These symptoms improved after the woman delivered her child.

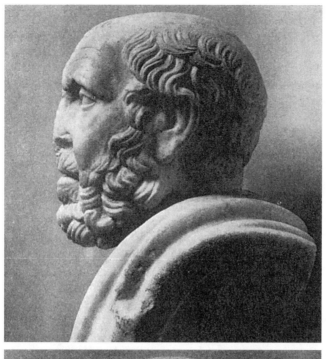

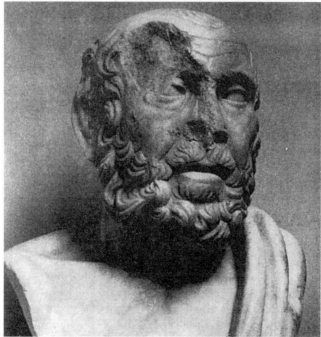

FIG. 1-1. Roman copy of a Greek bust, presumed to be of Hippocrates.

Hippocrates distinguished between the soft pitting edema of the legs seen in chronic heart failure (as well as hepatic and renal failure) and the indurated edema in acute cellulitis:

> Swellings that are painful . . . and hard indicate a danger of death in the near future; such as are soft and painless, yielding to the pressure of the finger, are of a more chronic character. (*Prognostics VII*, trans. Jones, 1923–1932)

Hippocrates also provided an important description of the wasting of the body (*cachexia*) in patients with dropsy:

> Dropsy is usually produced when the patient remains for a long time with impurities of the body following a long illness. The flesh is consumed and becomes water . . . the abdomen fills with water, the feet and legs swell, the shoulders, clavicles, chest and thighs melt away. (*Affections XXII*, translation by the author from Littré, 1839–1861)

While the context of this description is that of a patient suffering from malaria or nephritis, and not heart disease, this passage has been included here because of growing awareness that the mechanisms responsible for this wasting reaction to chronic illness also play an important role in patients with chronic heart failure.

Later Roman observers, many of whom were not trained in medicine, describe what might be heart failure. The poet Horace (65–8 B.C.E.) equated the effects of the consumption of water in dropsy to the demands of a life of luxury in a man who "carried elaborate opulence almost to the point of decadence":

> Dire dropsy swells by feeding, and thirst
> is not quenched until the disease's cause
> has fled from the veins and watery dullness
> from the pallid flesh.
>   (*Odes*, Book II, 2, translation by Shepherd, 1983)

Even though it does not provide a link to heart failure, this ode does suggest that Horace understood that dropsy is caused when fluid leaves the blood vessels. A generation later, the Roman aristocrat Celsus (25 B.C.E.–50 C.E.) compiled a medical text that appears to describe cardiac dyspnea:

> When moderate and without any choking, [difficulty in breathing] is called dyspnoea; when more severe, so that the patient cannot breathe without making a noise and gasping, asthma; but when in addition the patient can hardly draw in his breath unless with the neck outstretched, orthopnoea. Of these the first can last a long while, the two following are as a rule acute. . . . Blood-letting is the remedy unless anything prohibits it. Nor is that enough, but also the bowels are to be relaxed by milk, the stool being rendered liquid, at times even a clyster is given; as the body becomes depleted by these measures the patients begins to draw his breath more readily. Moreover, even in bed the head is to be kept raised. . . . (*De Medicina*, IV. 8, trans. Spencer, 1938)

Galen (130– *c*200 C.E.), who attempted to organize all of the medical knowledge of his time, recognized the muscular nature of the heart, noting that contraction of fibers in its walls causes ventricular volume to decrease during systole. He also described ventricular "suction" during diastole and understood the function of the heart's valves, whose purpose he says is

> to prevent matter from flowing backward, each [valve] in its own fashion, two of them [aortic and pulmonary valves] to prevent any of the contents of the heart which are going outwards from returning back into it, and two, those in the mouths of the vessels bringing matter in [mitral and tricuspid valves], to prevent matter from flowing back out of it. (*De usupartium,* II, K. iii, trans. Harris, 1973)

Galen also highlighted palpation of the arterial pulse, which he used for an elaborate system of prognostication, and describes "complete irregularity or unevenness [of the pulse], both in the single beat and in the succession of beats" that probably represents atrial fibrillation. In light of his recognition of the muscular nature of the heart, its systole and diastole, the function of the valves, the fact that the heart is responsible for the arterial pulse, and that arteries contain blood and not air, it is surprising that Galen failed to appreciate that the heart pumps blood through the body. This puzzling error may have been due in part to Galen's demonstration that ligating a small hollow tube within an artery, while allowing the continued flow of blood, abolishes the distal pulsations—an observation that led him to conclude that the pulse is transmitted along the walls of the arteries rather than by movement of the blood contained within these vessels (Furley and Wilkie, 1984). Whatever the reason, Galen failed to recognize the circulation of the blood, instead describing the heart's function as to generate and distribute the vital spirit (*pneuma*) and heat throughout the body. This view effectively forestalled any understanding of the role of heart failure in causing dyspnea, edema, and dropsy until Harvey's description of the circulation, coupled with the widespread practice of autopsy more than 1,500 years later.

Aretæus of Cappadocia, a contemporary of Galen, noted the effects of gravity on the distribution of edema fluid:

> When in an erect posture, then [the patients] become swollen in their feet and legs, but when reclining, in the parts they lay upon; and if they change their position, the swelling changes accordingly, and the course of the cold humor [edema] is determined by its weight. (Adams, 1856)

Almost 1,000 years later, the effect of posture on dyspnea was noted by Avicenna (980–1037). This Arab physician, who looked to the Greeks and Romans as well as the Persian compilers and Hindu systems for the roots of medical learning, may have been referring to heart failure in his description of

> pernicious suffocation [that] hastens to stop the breathing; when the patient lies down, his breathing is hindered completely, and when he is not recumbent his breathing is difficult also. In addition, he himself keeps extending his neck in contriving to breathe. He is restless and wants to stand erect and cannot lie down. (*Cannon of Medicine*, iii. II, trans. Jarcho, 1980)

Although Avicenna had no idea of the pathophysiologic connection between heart disease and dyspnea, he seems to have been aware of the ability of pericardial tamponade to impair ventricular filling:

> For fluids are very often found between [the bulk of the heart and its membrane]. And it is known that when they are abundant they restrain the heart from diastole. (Jarcho, 1980)

Clinical Observations before Harvey's Description of the Circulation

The Fasciculus Medicinae of Johannes de Ketham, published in 1491 shortly after Gutenberg's invention of movable type, represents a medical guide that combined "various rules, graphic diagrams and schemes that were in actual daily use by medical men (Singer, 1988) (Fig. 1-2). The author/compiler Johannes de Ketham (Johan von Kircheim, active 1455–1470) defined dropsy as "an error of the nutritive faculty" and for treatment recommends that the physician

> take scabwort and grind and squeeze its juice through a cloth, collect in an eggshell and temper with honeycomb; give the patient daily a full shell of the juice, do this for eleven days when the moon is waning because also man wanes in his abdomen. (Singer, 1988)

His description of carditis, defined as "the disease by which the heart palpitates," reflects Galen's view of the heart as the source of the body's heat in proposing that this condition is caused "from great warmth and from overabundant blood." For carditis, de Ketham's treatment centers on aromatic ointments made of roses, violets, and flax, or from cinnamon, clove-gilly flowers, cubeb, aloe wood, and the bone of stag's heart along with anise and violets, along with phlebotomy from the left hand. Lest we be tempted to laugh at these treatments, it should be remembered that the medieval physician had no knowledge of the pathology and pathophysiology of heart disease. We should also be humble because it was not until the early 1990s that we realized that inotropic therapy for heart failure can do much more harm than Johannes de Ketham's perfumed ointments.

Hieronymus Capivaccius, a professor at the University of Padua who died in 1589, less than 40 years before Harvey's discovery of the circulation, accepted Galen's teachings that the heart is the source of the body's warmth. He did, however, recognize the importance of the heart in generating the pulse, writing that "in syncope anyone recognizes that the pulse is removed and disappears, and these things certainly have to do with the pulsific force or motor force of the heart" (*Opera Omnia*, 2.9, trans. Jarcho, 1980). Capivaccius provided an excellent description of the neurohumoral response to a decrease in cardiac output:

> In general this disease is recognized by the fact that the pulse becomes small and weak in all dimensions. . . . It is recognized also by the fact that the face is pale because the spirit, and with the spirit the blood, is recalled to the heart; for the same reason the external structures are cold. It is recognized also by sweat and dewy moisture, especially in the forehead . . . and the skin is cold because the heat has been recalled. (Jarcho, 1980)

Galen's influence is seen in Capivaccius' statement that the extremities are cold because they are deprived of heat, that this syndrome "is nothing else than the vital spirit collected, and violently in the heart, and that dropsy is caused by cooling of the liver. . . ." (*Opera Omnia*, 3.2, trans. Jarcho, 1980). The errors forced by adherence to the teachings of Galen are also found in the works of the Spanish physician Ludovicus Mercatus (Luiz Mercado, *c*1520–*c*1606). Although Mercatus recognized the relationship between dyspnea and dropsy, in describing the origins of the transudate in pleural effusion, he follows earlier views that can be traced back to Hippocrates when he referred to the "thin, serous fluid, which either rushes down copiously by reason of its thinness from the brain through the trachea and lungs, or from the rest of the body or from the abdominal

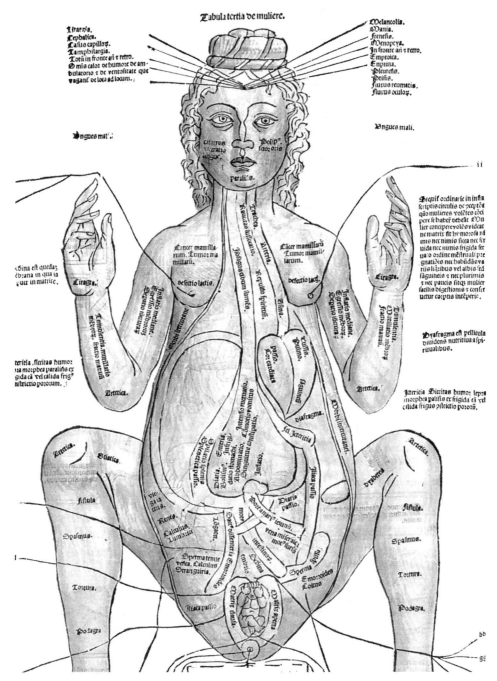

FIG. 1-2. Detail of a drawing of the anatomy of a pregnant woman showing the heart in the left chest giving rise to a single vessel that connects to the throat. The words in the left heart are "cough of lung" and "sanguineness." Those in the right heart are "cardiac ailment." At the base of the "aorta" is written "asthma." [From Singer (1988), with permission.]

cavity in dropsical persons, and reaches there through hidden ducts" (*De internorum morborum curatione*, 2.4, trans. Jarcho, 1980).

The beginning appreciation of the role of fluid retention in heart failure is seen in the writings of Carolus Piso (Charles le Pois, 1563–1633), who studied at the University of Padua about 15 years before Harvey. Piso provides an elegant description of paroxysmal nocturnal dyspnea complicating what is likely to be progressive left ventricular failure seen in a nobleman "somewhat more than eighty years old" who

> gradually began to be oppressed by severe difficulty in breathing, which manifested itself especially at night. After he had first fallen asleep as usual, a suffocation would suddenly excite the old man and interrupt his sleep, so that against his will he was obliged to get out of bed and rush at once to the windows of his bedroom in order to breathe fresh air through dilated nostrils. The old man could be seen, with inflamed face, drawing breath deeply, and with his shoulders trembling. He could not remain quietly in one place and especially could not stand the fireplace but exposed himself even in a severe winter. Gradually and inevitably as the day advanced he would be relieved of his oppression, especially in the afternoon, but during the next sleep the affection returned and troubled the old man again....

> Having carefully observed the gasping and having reflected for hours on the causes of such obstinate oppression, which made a daily cycle, I concluded finally that the fluid which was occupying his bronchi and the lung itself, or which more probably was stagnating in the middle of his chest, was of the kind that at the time of sleep through return of the vital spirit flowing back into the precordia received a certain new fervor, so that while bubbling in this way it could not be kept within its own space as formerly and it would necessarily compress the lungs and block their free motion. However, when this fervor gradually became spontaneously quiescent and the spirit flowed again out of the precordia into the body generally, as is the case of persons who are awake, then the lungs could more freely regain their space and the patient could breathe without such great oppression. (*Selectiorum observationum et consiliorum de praetervisis hactenus morbis affectibusque praeter naturam, ab aqua seu serosa colluvie et diluvie ortis,* 214–216, trans. Jarcho, 1980)

Piso confirmed his diagnosis of dropsy of the thorax (hydrothorax) when the patient's surgeon "who was bolder in dissecting the dead patient than in striking and opening him while he was alive, found the lung and precordia floating in a large amount of water which was enclosed within the walls of the thorax." This passage not only documents Piso's recognition that fluid accumulation in the lungs caused the patient's progressive dyspnea, but also his appreciation of the role of gravity in removing fluid from the central circulation during the day, when because the patient was erect this fluid "flowed again out of the precordia into the body generally." However, Piso did not understand the circulation or how the heart pumped blood from the lung into the periphery, so that he was unable to draw the connection between "dropsy of the thorax" and heart failure.

HARVEY'S DISCOVERY OF THE CIRCULATION

William Harvey (1578–1657) (Fig. 1-3), whose *De Motu Cordis* (*Movement of the Heart*) was published in 1628, provided the first clear description of the circulation in a proof that included a mathematical calculation that showed that the amount of blood flowing from the heart greatly exceeded the amount that could be derived from foodstuffs metabolized in the liver. Harvey's conclusion was stated forcefully and succinctly:

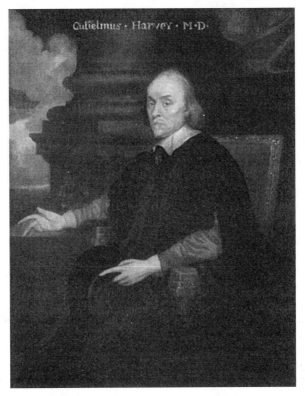

FIG. 1-3. Harvey. State portrait at the Royal College of Physicians, painted *c*1655 when Harvey was 68 years old.

> I am obliged to conclude that in animals the blood is driven round a circuit with an unceasing, circular sort of movement, that this is an activity or function of the heart which it carries out by virtue of its pulsation, and that in sum it constitutes the sole reason for that heart's pulsatile movement. (Franklin, 1957)

The validity of this statement, which demolished Galen's view that the function of the heart is to heat the blood, provides a clear example of a paradigm shift as described by Kuhn (see earlier discussion).

Harvey was aware that obstruction of venous return to the heart causes edema, and he described the swelling that follows application of a ligature sufficiently tight to obstruct venous but not arterial flow. He also appears to have recognized that heart failure, by causing blood to accumulate in the lungs, leads to dyspnea when he described a "fever" that:

> making first for the heart, lingers around that organ and the lungs and brings about shortness of breath [ahelosos = puffing], difficulty in breathing [suspiriosus = breathing deeply, with difficulty], and disinclination for exertion in those affected. For the vital principle is oppressed, and the blood is forced into the lungs, becomes inspissated, and does not get through those organs. (I speak with experience on this point through my dissections of subjects who have died at the beginning of attacks). At this time the pulsations are always rapid and small in amplitude, and now and then irregular. (Franklin, 1957)

Harvey's discovery of the circulation was made possible not only by his own genius but also by the extraordinary time during which he lived. As is common in scientific discovery, others were on the verge of describing the circulation. These include Michael Servetus, who in 1553 had described the pulmonary circulation; however, his contribution was lost for almost 150 years (and his books—along with Servetus himself—were burned for theological reasons). Realdus Columbus, Vesalius' successor at the University of Padua, found blood and not air when he opened the pulmonary artery, and so suggested in 1559 that "blood is carried by the [pulmonary artery] to the lungs, and being made thin is brought back thence together with air by the [pulmonary veins] to the left ventricle of the heart" (Cournand, 1964). Andrea Cesalpino, in a book published in 1606, also came close to describing the circulation (Arcieri, 1945), and Fabricius of Aquapendente, who was Harvey's teacher at Padua, provided a description of the function of the venous valves, which Harvey cites as evidence that the veins returned blood to the heart (Fig. 1-4).

Many of the physician-scientists associated with the discovery of the circulation were teachers or students at the University of Padua, which a generation before Harvey had included Galileo as well as Vesalius. This central role reflects the fact that Padua, which was one of a handful of European universities that admitted and awarded degrees to protestant and Jewish students, and was the first to award a doctoral degree to a woman, maintained considerable independence in the Republic of Venice during the period of turmoil and religious intolerance that followed the Reformation (Hamilton, 1997).

Although Harvey's concepts would, within a century, provide the basis for an accurate understanding of the hemodynamics in heart failure, Galenic views persisted long after the appearance of *De Motu Cordis*. For example, Melchior Sebezius Jr., in a text published in 1661, dismisses the possibility that pleural effusions arose by "drip[ping] from

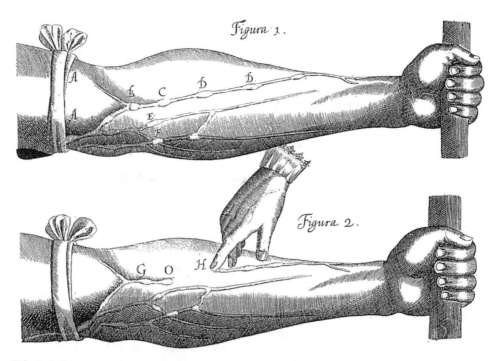

FIG. 1-4. Illustration of the function of the venous valves from Harvey's *De Motu Cordis*. A similar figure was published by Harvey's teacher, Fabricius.

the heart and its pericardium into the thorax," stating "it is improbable that so great a quantity of fluid can be held in the heart or pericardium as to produce dropsy" (*Manualis, sive speculi medicinae practici* 3.1.815-818, trans. Jarcho, 1980). Like Galen, Sebezius attributed hydrothorax to lung disease, stating:

> In some patients the water of dropsy travels through imperceptible and hidden channels into the thoracic cavity and then into the bronchi of the lungs, even though these channels are unknown to us. . . . For when the lung is strongly chilled by food, drink, medicine, air and other causes, it is likely that it can produce a large amount of serum and water, and this is properly regarded as a cause of dropsy. . . . (*Manualis, sive speculi medicinae practici* 3.1.815-818, trans. Jarcho, 1980)

Correlations Between Anatomic Pathology and a Disordered Circulation

The coupling of Harvey's physiology with early autopsy examinations led rapidly to an understanding of the causes of fluid accumulation in patients with heart disease. In describing a patient who died in 1646, 18 years after publication of *De Motu Cordis*, Lazare Rivière (1589–1655), who introduced the study of chemistry into the medical curriculum and was an early advocate of Harvey's view of the circulation (Major, 1954), understood the consequences of impaired blood flow through the lungs when he described a patient with bacterial endocarditis involving the aortic valve ("carbuncles in the heart"). After an illness that began with "palpitation of the heart," the patient "began to suffer from difficulty in breathing & his legs appeared swollen"; his condition steadily worsened until "no pulse appeared at the wrist, and when the hand was applied over the heart, a most rapid, weak, and irregular palpitation was felt" (Major, 1945, p 458). After the appearance of bloodstained sputum, the patient died and, at autopsy: "in the left ventricle of the heart round carbuncles were found. . . the larger of which resembled a cluster of hazelnuts & filled up the opening of the aorta, which I judged caused the failure of pulsations in the arteries" (Major, 1945, p 459). Referring to the consequences of obstruction to left ventricular ejection, Rivière observed:

> The ventricle was filled with a blood mass and the whole lung was filled with much blood from which the suffocation of the natural beat spread to each part. . . . For the blood ascending continually by the vena cava not coming freely to the heart overflowed in the lung and filled it up. (Major, 1945, p 459)

This description, while demonstrating an appreciation of the hemodynamic consequences of impaired left ventricular ejection, echoes Galen's view of the heart as a furnace. This is seen when Rivière speculates that the carbuncles "were caused by the excessive blood which the marked heat of the ventricle hardened & in this manner changed its substance" (Major, 1945, p 459). Yet this elegant description of the consequences of aortic valve obstruction also describes the hemodynamics of left ventricular failure.

Marcello Malpighi (1628–1694), who completed the description of the circulation with his discovery of the capillaries, was a physician as well as an experimentalist. Malpighi viewed dyspnea as arising when "particles" impeded the passage of blood through the lungs, and edema as occurring when "the veins were not resorbing the fluid pushed forth by the arteries." This is documented in the following analysis of the causes of dyspnea in the King of Poland:

> When blood reaches the heart and lungs, the dregs [assumed here to have been caused by the inclusion of "acid particles" arising from poorly digested food] with which the

ends of the veins are supplied alter the entry of blood into the heart. As a result the respiration and pulse are changed, for when blood in the lungs has been delayed, their weight is increased. This causes dyspnea. (*Marcelli Malpighi, et Jo: Marie Lancisii consultationum medicarum.* Consultation 2, trans. Jarcho, 1980)

The increasing pace of medical discovery during the 18th century is seen in a description of acute pulmonary edema, caused when the rapid appearance of left heart failure literally drowns a patient, published in a text by Georgio Baglevi (1668–1706) 68 years after *De Motu Cordis*:

> Next is to be considered a dangerous disease of the lungs, which is called suffocative catarrh. It is caused chiefly by stagnation and sudden coagulation of blood in the lungs and about the precordium.... In this kind of catarrh the patient has a cold, and pain in the chest, and difficulty in breathing; also interrupted speech, anxiety, cough, stertor, a widely spaced slow pulse, foam at the mouth, and the like....
>
> The foam at the mouth is caused by impaired circulation of blood about the lungs and consequent circulation of the lymph in the upper parts of the body near the face; hence this [kind of] catarrh comes from sudden stagnation of blood in the vicinity of the heart and lungs, and not from phlegm running down from the head as the ancients believed to be the condition in this disease.
>
> An instant remedy for this disease during the paroxysm is repeated bloodletting.....The disease is very precipitous; unless phlebotomy is done immediately the blood coagulates more and stagnates. Thus the opportunity for cure is lost. (*De praxi medica,* trans. Jarcho, 1980)

Even though virtually every physician of the time practiced phlebotomy, the urgency of Baglevi's recommendation suggests that he may have appreciated the need to reduce blood volume in pulmonary edema.

Additional pathophysiologic explanations of the clinical manifestations of impaired left ventricular ejection were provided by Giovanni Maria Lancisi (1654–1720), who discussed the mechanism by which heart failure caused dyspnea in a young man who died suddenly after experiencing shortness of breath and a "buried strangling over the precordia" for about a year. At autopsy, the patient was found to have a huge heart, which Lancisi assumed had compressed the descending aorta so as to impair ejection of blood into the aorta. Although this pathophysiologic mechanism is most improbable, it did lead Lancisi to consider the consequences of obstruction to left ventricular ejection:

> And through the blood that remained, of course, abundantly [in the left side of the heart], a new resistance was continually being built up both to the movements of the heart itself as well as to the waves of liquids flowing in from the lung.
>
> Through this is brought to light the principal cause of that hidden oppression and of that heaviness of the precordia from which the patient ultimately died.... the left ventricle, on account of the lessened force because of the dilatation, was prevented from propelling readily the larger amount of blood into the obstructed aorta. This delay of blood, to be sure, brought about the oppression of the precordia and ultimately the deadly suffocation and syncope. (*De subitaneis mortibus* 185-195, trans. Jarcho, 1980)

It was Raymond Vieussens (*c*1635–1715) (Fig. 1-5), however, who provided the clearest discussion of the pathophysiology of dyspnea. His long and colorful description of the final years in a young man who died of mitral stenosis not only described the clinical his-

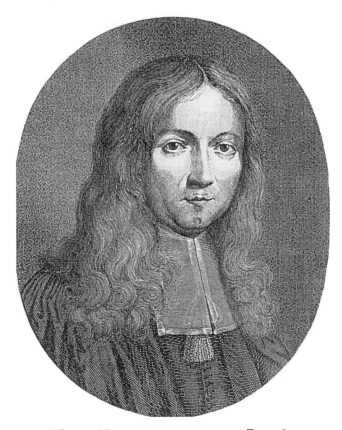

FIG. 1-5. Vieussens as a young man. Engraving.

tory and autopsy findings but also correctly explained why the patient was short of breath and why a large pleural effusion was found at autopsy. Vieussens described the initial symptoms of dependent edema and breathlessness, which were then followed by orthopnea and atrial fibrillation:

> He was lying in bed with his head very high. It seemed to me that his breathing was very difficult. His heart was burdened by a violent palpitation. His pulse seemed very small, weak and altogether irregular. His lips had the color of lead, his eyes showed great dejection, and his legs and thighs were swollen and were cold instead of warm. (*Traité nouveau de la structure et des causes du movement naturel du coeur.* 103, trans. Jarcho, 1980)

A week later the patient died, and when his body was opened (in the presence of several medical students), the entire thoracic cavity was found to be filled with yellowish serum. The heart was huge, approaching in size that of an ox heart. The key to the patient's symptoms was severe mitral stenosis (Fig. 1-6):

> The entrance of the left ventricle appeared to be extremely small and . . . in looking for the cause of such a surprising fact I discovered that the [mitral valve leaflets] were truly bony...that the [mitral valve] had shrunk greatly.

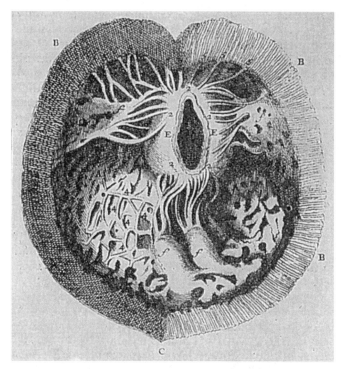

FIG. 1-6. Vieussens' illustration of the stenotic mitral valve, viewed from below, illustrating the typical "fish mouth" appearance.

The entry of the left ventricle having become greatly contracted and its margin having lost all its natural suppleness, the blood could not pass freely and as abundantly as it should into the cavity of this ventricle. As soon as the circulation became impeded by this, it began to expand to an extraordinary extent the trunk of the pulmonary vein, because the blood remained there too long and accumulated there in too large an amount. The blood had no sooner begun to stay too long in the trunk of this vein than it delayed the course of the blood in all the blood vessels of the lung, so that the branches of the pulmonary artery and vein, spread by all the tissue of this organ, were always too full of blood and hence so dilated that they compressed the ventricles enough to prevent the air from entering freely and leaving just as freely. This is why the patient always breathed with great difficulty. Since the blood in the lung thickened considerably during its long sojourn in the blood vessels, part of its serum separated little by little and fell into the thoracic cavity. (Traité nouveau de la structure et des causes du movement naturel du coeur. 105-106, trans. Jarcho, 1980)

Vieussens' perceptive analysis continued with the observation that the small pulse was "caused by the excessive smallness of the amount of blood that the left ventricle furnished to the aorta...."

The first effective pharmacologic treatment of heart failure was published in 1783 by William Withering (1741–1799), who identified digitalis as the active ingredient in the herbal remedy prescribed by "an old woman of Shropshire" for the treatment of dropsy. Withering recognized that digitalis "has a power over the motion of the heart, to a degree yet unobserved in any other medicine, and that this power may be converted to salutary ends," but did not appreciate that this therapeutic value reflected the ability of digitalis to slow the heart and increase myocardial contractility. Instead, he viewed digitalis primarily as a diuretic. Among the cases in which Withering used digitalis was in a woman in whom dyspnea and fluid retention developed between ages 40 and 50 years. Withering's description of his first encounter describes a patient

> nearly in a state of suffocation; her pulse extremely weak and irregular, her breath very short and laborious, her countenance sunk, her arms of a leaden colour, clammy and cold. She could not lye down in bed, and had neither strength nor appetite but was extremely thirsty. Her stomach, legs and thighs were greatly swollen; her urine very small in quantity, not more than a spoonful at a time, and that very seldom. It had been proposed to scarify her legs, but the proposition was not acceded to...[Administration of five doses of digitalis] made her very sick, and acted very powerful upon the kidneys, for within the first twenty-four hours she made upwards of eight quarts of water. The sense of fullness and oppression across her stomach was greatly diminished, her breath was eased, her pulse became more full and regular, and the swellings in her legs subsided. (Major, 1945, p 442).

This case, which according to Withering "gave rise to a very widespread use of [digitalis] in that part of Shropshire," clearly demonstrates the value of diuresis in patients with heart failure.

ARCHITECTURAL CHANGES IN THE FAILING HEART

A generally forgotten chapter in the history of cardiology began at the end of the 18th century, when emphasis in autopsy studies of heart failure, in addition to identifying the valve abnormalities that, because of the high incidence of rheumatic heart disease, were common in the 19th century, included studies of the architecture of the failing heart. As a result, postmortem examinations, which were generally performed by the same physician who cared for the patient in an effort to discover the causes of the fatal outcome, began to focus on the size and shape of the diseased heart in an effort to understand the connections between clinical signs and symptoms, circulatory abnormalities, and pathologic anatomy.

Many 17th and 18th century descriptions note enlargement of the failing heart. John Mayow (1634–1679), who was among several at Oxford who continued the experimental tradition established by William Harvey, states that dilatation of the heart could be caused by distending forces that develop when blood accumulates behind an obstructed mitral valve:

> For as the blood could not, on account of the obstruction, pass into the left ventricle of the heart, the pulmonary vessels and also the right ventricle were necessarily distended with blood. (*Tractus Quinque*, trans. East, 1958)

A more systematic discussion of cardiac enlargement is found in Lancisi's *Aneurysmatibus*, published in 1745, which provides a detailed discourse on the causes of aneurysms (dilatation) of the arteries and the heart. Lancisi divides these into two types. One he calls "genuine," which refers to disorders that arise in the walls of the arteries and heart, for example, following wounds or contusions. The other type, which he calls "spurious," is due to increased force of the impetus . . . that propels the blood that is too much for the natural and normal resistance of the arteries and heart. (*Aneurysmatibus* Proposition V, trans. by Wright, 1952)

Lancisi is generally viewed as the first to distinguish between dilatation [*dilatatione*] and hypertrophy [*augmento molis*], a distinction he makes in his discussion of the causes of aneurysm:

So varied and so serious are the maladies of the heart that we often discover that it has suffered from an increase of its own bulk [*molis*], combined with aneurysm [*aneurysmate*]. Nor do I mean here by increase of bulk dilatation [*dilatationem*] of the cavities only, but thickening of the fibers and increase of density [which] makes the base of the heart larger and heavier than is normal. (*Aneurysmatibus,* Proposition XLVIII, trans. Wright, 1952)

Jean-Baptiste de Sénac (1693–1770), who shortly after Lancisi's death commented on the clinical significance of changes in the size of the heart, distinguishes between dilatation and atrophy. Sénac was educated in France and in 1752 was appointed physician to Louis XV. His masterpiece "Treatise on the Structure of the Heart," published in 1749, includes the following discussion of changes in the size and shape of the failing heart:

The volume of the heart can be contracted or it can dilate; this diminution and expansion present two illnesses that are not equally felt, but can be equally fearsome: we will examine their causes, their variations, their outcomes and their treatment.

To judge the volume of the heart only in terms of the action of this organ, one would not believe that it could become smaller. Its fluid-filled cavities ought to dilate. If its minute vesicles fill little by little; if their dilatation often becomes extraordinary, even though the substance responsible for this dilatation only enters drop by drop into these tiny vesicles, must not the blood that enters the ventricles of the heart distend their walls? Is not this movement a force that hinders its drawing back together? Yet exact observations teach us that the tissues of the heart contract and harden; that its cavities become smaller; or that they can become almost completely obliterated. (Sénac, 1749. Book IV, Chapter VIII, I, translation by the author)

Sénac's distinction between dilatation and contraction of the cavities of the heart, and his recognition that less force is developed by the walls of diseased hearts, identifies processes that have become central to modern efforts to characterize the molecular abnormalities in the failing myocardium.

It appears that Giovanni Battista Morgagni (1682–1771) (Fig. 1-7) was the first to describe the adaptive nature of overload-induced cardiac hypertrophy. Morgagni's observations, published in 1761 as a series of letters entitled *De sedibus et causes morborum*, describe 640 autopsies that include not only his own cases but also reports by others and unpublished work of his teacher and colleague Antonio Maria Valsalva. In referring to Vieussens' case of mitral stenosis (see earlier discussion), Morgagni highlighted the consequences of the obstruction of blood flow from the left atrium to the left ventricle:

Both the auricles, with their adjoining [veins] . . . and the trunk of the pulmonary artery, and the right ventricle, were much distended, and the columnae and fibers of the same ventricle, were become very thick; which might happen because . . . a greater thickness of the muscles is the consequence of their more frequent and

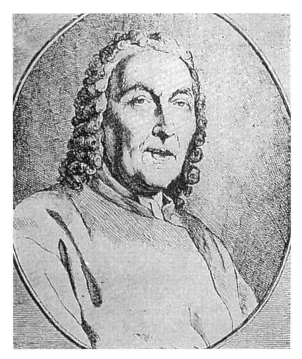

FIG. 1-7. Morgagni. Engraving by Angela Kauffman.

stronger actions. (*The Seats and Causes of Diseases*, Letter XVII, Article 13. trans. Alexander, 1769)

In addition to this description of compensatory (adaptive) hypertrophy of the heart, Morgagni noted left ventricular enlargement in a 33-year-old shoemaker who died after suffering from dyspnea for several years. The cause of this condition was found in the aortic valve leaflets, which were "very lank, and contracted into themselves, somewhat rigid also, and a little hard." Morgagni postulated a causal relationship between cardiac chamber dilatation and the obstruction to ejection which,

by resisting the heart, and by retaining the blood therein, (which, as it was in greater quantity, would more irritate the fibres, and at the same time give more resistance to the increased efforts of the heart), could by degrees more and more distract, and dilate the heart. (*The Seats and Causes of Diseases*, Letter XVIII, Article 4. trans. Alexander)

In another case, Morgagni described the hemodynamic consequences of "indurated valve leaflets" that caused both stenosis and insufficiency:

[Because they were] less yielding to the blood, they might increase the obstacles to its exit, and, on the other hand, not sufficiently prevent its return, when soon after, repuls'd by the contraction of the [aorta]; so that as some portion of it return'd into the left ventricle of the heart, when this ventricle ought to receive the blood that was coming in from the lungs. Which circumstance, finally, could not but overload both the lungs and the heart.... (*The Seats and Causes of Diseases*, Letter XXIII, Article 9. trans. Alexander)

These and other observations demonstrate Morgagni's recognition that overload caused the heart to enlarge.

Remarkable insights regarding the architecture of the failing heart were provided by Jean Nicolas Corvisart (1755–1821) (Fig. 1-8), who studied medicine in Paris at the time of the French Revolution and became physician to Napoleon Bonaparte. The terms *aneurism* (enlargement) and *parietes* (the wall of a cardiac chamber) are preserved in the following passages, taken from Gates' translation of Corvisart's 1801 text *Essai sur les maladies et les lésions organiques du coeur* (*Essai*). In distinguishing between "active" and "passive" aneurism—what came later to be called hypertrophy and dilatation (Table 1-3), Corvisart noted:

The real existence of these two species is proved to the physician by symptoms different and appropriate to each; to the anatomist by constant and repeated observation of two very distinct states in which the heart is found when it has been the seat of the disease.... In the first species (active aneurism) the heart is dilated, its parietes thickened, the energy of its action increased.... In the second (passive aneurism) there is likewise a dilatation, but an attenuation [thinning] of the parietes, and diminution of energy in the action of the organ. (*Essai*. Second Class, Article I. trans. Gates)

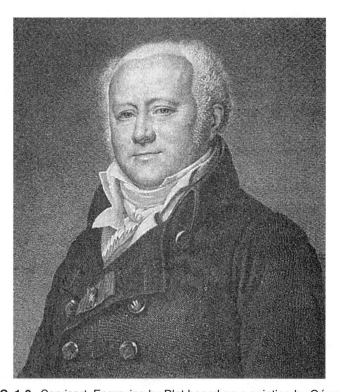

FIG. 1-8. Corvisart. Engraving by Blot based on a painting by Gérard.

TABLE 1-3. *Classification of cardiac enlargement*

Corvisart
  Active aneurism: dilated cavities, thickened walls, increased energy of action.
  Passive aneurism: dilated cavities, thinned walls, diminished energy of action.
Bertin
  Simple hypertrophy: increased wall thickness without change in cavity size.
  Eccentric hypertrophy: increased wall thickness with cavity dilatation.
  Concentric hypertrophy: increased wall thickness with "contracted" cavities.
Latham
  Hypertrophy versus atrophy: augmentation or diminution of the heart's bulk.
  Dilatation versus contraction: increased or decreased capacity of the heart's cavities.
Virchow
  Hypertrophy (simple hypertrophy): cell enlargement without increased cell number.
  Hyperplasia (numerical hypertrophy): formation of new cells.
Bramwell
  Hypertrophy
    Simple hypertrophy: cavities of normal size
    Concentric hypertrophy: decreased cavity size
    Eccentric hypertrophy: increased cavity size
  Dilatation
    Simple dilatation: no change in cardiac mass.
    Dilatation with hypertrophy: "active dilatation"
    Dilatation with thinning: "passive dilatation"
Osler
  Hypertrophy
    Simple hypertrophy: cavities of normal size
    Hypertrophy with dilatation: enlarged cavities with thickened walls (eccentric hypertrophy)
  Dilatation
    Dilatation with thickening (corresponds to Hypertrophy with dilatation, above)
    Dilatation with thinning
Vaquez
  Essential hypertrophy: hypertrophy of growth, of exercise, of pregnancy.
  Symptomatic hypertrophy: hypertrophy caused by heart disease, renal disease.
  Dilatation: heart failure, myocarditis.

Corvisart equated *active aneurism* to the "extraordinary evolution of the muscle of the body," noting that the walls of the heart become thickened in this form of enlargement. In explaining the mechanism by which obstruction to emptying causes active aneurism, he stated:

[The first effect is] to determine the extension and elongation of the fibres of the heart; the second to obtain a longer residence of blood in the cavities of this organ, and consequently a longer impression of its stimulus. In fine, the coronary arteries, as well as the capillaries of the heart, continuing in a permanent state of engorgement, will furnish more nutritive fluid to the fleshy substance of this organ. Hence the dilatation of the cavities, the elongation of the fibres, the thickening of their masses, the more vigorous the action of the organ. (*Essai.* Second Class, Ch. I, Article II. trans. Gates)

This passage highlights Corvisart's view of active aneurism as dilatation and thickening of the walls of the heart in response to outflow obstruction, most often in the left ventricle of patients with aortic stenosis, as well as the 19th century view that hypertrophy is caused by "overnutrition" of the heart. In attempting to discern the clinical significance of *passive aneurism* and how this differs from active aneurism, Corvisart wrote:

[passive aneurism] involves both thinning of its parietes, and debilitated action of the heart, [and] pursues in its formation, a course totally different from that of active aneurism.... The heart, in [active aneurism], seems to become the centre of a more active circulation and nutrition. In that of [passive aneurism], this organ, on the contrary, is distended in the same manner as the bladder in cases of retention of urine ... The heart, which in [active aneurism] seems to employ... its own action to augment the organic lesion already existing, is, in [passive aneurism] an organ as passive as it appears to be active in the first. (*Essai.* Second Class, Ch. II, Article I. trans. Gates)

Corvisart thus viewed active aneurism (hypertrophy) as a response to pressure load in conditions such as aortic stenosis, whereas passive aneurism (dilatation) represents a response to volume load seen in aortic and mitral regurgitation. In noting these different patterns of cardiac enlargement, Corvisart anticipated by almost 200 years the concept that cardiac phenotype is altered in the hypertrophied heart (see Chapter 6).

The common occurrence of simultaneous discovery in medicine is seen in a book written by John Bell (1763–1820), a contemporary of Corvisart, who studied at the University of Edinburgh. Bell, like Corvisart, sought to understand the clinical implications of cardiac enlargement:

But the heart may be too big for its system, is a melancholy fact; for when it becomes relaxed, it enlarges, and as it grows in bulk loses its power. ... While the heart gradually enlarges, the system changes, and accommodates itself to its powers. There is little distress; often we find a heart enlarged to a degree such as we never could have suspected before death. But slowly there is formed such an accumulation of ill oxydated blood as oppresses the vital powers, and chokes the motions of the heart, and draws after it those other disorders. (Bell, 1802, p 223)

Bell also described concentric hypertrophy in patients without evident valvular disease:

The heart, which is so often dilated by weakness, is sometimes reduced in size by an increase in strength and action. It becomes dense, firm, thick in substance, but small in its cavity; it appears to be dilated without, but is, in fact, contracted within. This thickening of the wall of the ventricles is what I cannot understand, though I have cut many such hearts with the utmost care. There is no ossification of the valves, no straightening of the aorta, nor any other obstruction to excite the heart. (Bell, 1802, pp 231–232)

Although this pathologic picture is consistent with a hypertrophic cardiomyopathy, as discussed later, the cause was much more likely to be renovascular hypertension (Bright's disease).

Réné-Joseph-Hyacinthe Bertin (1767–1828), who served as a surgeon in Napoleon's army before becoming professor of hygiene at the Cochin Hospital in Paris, replaced Corvisart's term "aneurism" with "hypertrophy," and provided a classification of hypertrophy (see Table 1-3) that, in distinguishing between concentric and eccentric growth patterns, set the stage for derivative classifications that are found in a number of 19th century texts. He provided an elegant description of the consequences of loading when he wrote:

When from any cause the blood is obstructed in its course, it accumulates in the cavities of the heart and distends them: it enters in too great a quantity, and reverts upon the coronary arteries. The heart, irritated by the presence of this increased quantity of fluid, redoubles its energies, struggles, as it were, with all its powers against the resistance which it meets with: but these violent exertions themselves have the effect to solicit a new afflux of blood into the texture of the organ; so that the effect soon begins to take part with the cause. Stimulated beyond measure, the heart augments in bulk and thickness, and acquires an energy of contraction proportioned to the development of its hypertrophy. (Bertin, 1833, p 342)

Bertin also noted the maladaptive nature of dilatation:

Now it is very evident, that, considered in the abstract, the dilatation of the heart has the effect to weaken the contractile power of the muscular substance of that organ, in consequence of the distention to which it is subjected. The muscular fibres lose in strength what they acquire in extent. (Bertin, 1833, p 380)

Bertin, like Corvisart, viewed hypertrophy as increasing the "energy" of the heart's contraction whereas dilatation diminishes this energy, and echoed Corvisart's postulate that hyperemia and hypernutrition provide the stimuli that lead to hypertrophy. This was restated by Francois Aran (1817–1861), who in describing the adaptive nature of cardiac hypertrophy, noted:

Every time that a muscle takes on increased action, it receives an increased flow of blood; and consequently a proportional increase in nutrition results. What is seen in the arm of blacksmiths, in the legs of dancers, is also seen in the heart.... In proportion as the walls are thickened, its contractile power augments. (Aran, 1843, pp 100–101)

Aran also provided an early description of the progressive nature of remodeling, noting that:

If the dilatation...[has] reached a certain degree, and so far as to induce a morbid dyspnoea, the disease has a marked tendency to increase, unless the circulation be maintained in a state of complete repose. We may consider the tendency of dropsy to be reproduced immediately after its disappearance under proper treatment, as a fatal sign. (Aran, 1843, p 117)

By the middle of the 19th century, most high-quality textbooks of medicine and cardiology provided classifications of cardiac enlargement. One of the simplest is that of Peter Mere Latham (1789–1875), who based his classification simply on heart weight and cavity size (see Table 1-3). Although Latham emphasized that hypertrophy is generally the result of the valvular disease that was then prevalent, like Bell he observed "hypertrophy which is independent of valvular injury" (Latham, 1845). His description of atherosclerotic arteries whose " natural calibre is altered" in these cases led him to suggest the relationship between kidney disease and cardiac hypertrophy that, as discussed later, came to be recognized as Bright's disease (renovascular hypertension). The different morphologic responses to systolic stress (pressure overload, seen in hypertension and aortic stenosis) and diastolic stretch (volume overload, seen in mitral and aortic insufficiency) are clearly described by John Milner Fothergill (1841–1888), who noted the role of diastolic stretch in causing the heart to dilate:

With increase in the distending force [aortic insufficiency], hypertrophy is always combined with dilatation of the cardiac chambers; in obstruction to be overcome, without any increase in the distending force, as in aortic stenosis, there is pure hypertrophy, usually without dilatation.... (Fothergill, 1879, p 113)

Fothergill also recognized that hypertrophy, by "adding to the heart's power...tends to maintain itself, while dilatation tends downwards" (Fothergill, 1879, pp 133–134). In attempting to explain the harmful effects of left ventricular dilatation caused by severe aortic regurgitation, he wrote:

[Because of] escape of the blood backwards past the coronary orifices, the nutrition of the heart walls soon becomes impaired, and the hypertrophy, though massive, is not durable; muscular degeneration soon leads to further and uncontrollable dilatation, ending commonly by cessation of the action of the ventricle in diastole.... (Fothergill, 1879, p 135)

A more elaborate classification of hypertrophy that is typical of those found in late 19th century texts was published by Byrom Bramwell (1884, see Table 1-3). While observing that hypertrophy is a "compensatory and beneficial condition, in fact, nature's effort to meet a difficulty," he also noted the deleterious effects of dilatation, which he said is "the direct opposite of hypertrophy, inasmuch as it impairs the efficiency of the cardiac pump." Bramwell did recognize that dilatation is an essential element of the heart's response to chronic volume overload, noting that although dilatation is "usually bad":

In regurgitant valvular lesions dilatation of the cavity which is situated behind the affected orifice is beneficial, providing that it is just sufficient to accommodate the blood which is regurgitated at each systole.... (Bramwell, 1884)

Valvular Disease and Hypertrophy: Cause-Effect or Effect-Cause?

As noted in the preceding section, by the early 19th century, the causal relationships between abnormalities of the heart's valves and changes in its muscular walls had become controversial. Bertin is said by Vaquez (1924) to have believed that valve abnormalities found in patients with heart failure were secondary and largely irrelevant to the clinical picture. Bouillard in 1835 returned to Morgagni's view that cardiac enlargement in patients with valvular heart disease was caused when the deformed valve imposed a circulatory overload; according to Vaquez (1924), "this conception was soon accepted universally; then its importance was exaggerated and for a long time it was thought that there could be no hypertrophy without lesion of the valves." However, Bright's report that patients with kidney disease commonly had hypertrophied hearts, which was soon followed by observations that patients with "Bright's disease" had elevated blood pressure, established the modern view that hypertrophy is a response of the heart to overload.

Richard Bright (1789–1858), who noted that both cardiac hypertrophy and dropsy were common in patients with renal disease, suggested:

The obvious structural changes in the heart [in patients with shrunken kidneys] have consisted chiefly of hypertrophy with or without valvular disease; and, what is most striking, out of 52 cases of hypertrophy, no valvular disease whatsoever could be detected in 34.... This naturally leads us to look for some less local cause for the unusual efforts to which the heart has been impelled; and the two most ready solutions appear to be either that the altered quality of the blood affords irregular and unwonted stimulus to the organ immediately, or that it so affects the minute and capillary circulation as to render greater action necessary to force the blood through distant subdivisions of the vascular system. (Bright, 1836)

Twenty years later, Traube, who found the heart to be hypertrophied in more than 90% of patients with shrunken kidneys, by then called Bright's disease, proposed that cardiac hypertrophy occurred when capillary obstruction in the atrophied kidneys elevated arterial blood pressure (Traube, 1856). However, according to Vaquez (1924), Traube wavered in this interpretation because he realized that obstruction to the renal circulation was not likely to increase arterial pressure enough to cause cardiac hypertrophy. When, after small peripheral arteries were observed to be thickened and narrowed in Bright's disease (Johnson, 1868), a process later called "aterio-capillary fibrosis" (Gull and Sutton, 1872), Traube returned to the view that left ventricular hypertrophy occurs when arteriolar narrowing increases aortic pressure (Traube, 1878). This hypothesis found critical support in 1863 when Marey, using an instrument that compresses the radial artery to provide an index of intrarterial pressure, found that arterial pressure was increased in patients with Bright's disease. Mahomed, using a modification of Marey's device to obtain quantitative pressure data, documented the correlation between hypertension, heart failure, and "chronic Bright's disease without albuminuria" (Mahomed, 1881). As a result, within 10 years, Osler was able to write that cardiac hypertrophy could be caused by

all states of increased arterial tension induced by the contraction of the smaller arteries under the influence of certain toxic substances, which act, as Bright suggested, by affecting "the minute capillary circulation, to render greater action necessary to send the blood through distant subdivisions of the vascular system. (Osler, 1892, p 629)

Introduction of the sphygmomanometer as a simple means by which to measure brachial artery pressure at the end of the 19th century (Riva-Rocci 1896, 1897) established the pathophysiologic correlations between pressure overload, ventricular hypertrophy, and heart failure (Mancia, 1997). However, controversies as to whether heart failure in patients with valvular disease was due to worsening of the structural abnormality or deterioration of the myocardium continued well into the 20th century.

HYPERTROPHY AND HYPERPLASIA

Improvements in the compound microscope led, in the middle of the 19th century, to a major advance in understanding the pathophysiology of heart failure. Because of its importance, histopathology could be listed as a separate paradigm in Table 1-1; however, because microscopic anatomy reflects more an advance in technology than in approach, it is considered as part of the paradigm of anatomic pathology. Rudolph Virchow (1821–1902), often viewed as "the father of pathology," described an inflammatory response in some failing hearts (myocarditis) that probably caused some of Corvisart's cases of passive aneurism. Another major contribution was his distinction between two different types of cardiac enlargement (see Table 1-2): hypertrophy (increased cell size) and hyperplasia (increased cell number):

Hypertrophy, according to the meaning which I attach to the word, designates those cases in which the individual elements of structure take up a considerable amount of matter, and thereby become larger; and in which, in consequence of the simultaneous enlargement of a number of elements, at last the whole of the organ may become swollen. When a muscle becomes thicker, all its primitive fasciculi become thicker.... Essentially different from this process are the cases in which an enlargement takes place in consequence of an *increase in the number of the elements*. (Virchow, 1860, p 65)

ADAPTIVE AND MALADAPTIVE HYPERTROPHY

As already discussed, observers as early as Morgagni had recognized that overload caused the heart to hypertrophy and, in the early years of the 19th century, Aran had noted the similarity between the hypertrophic response of the heart to a circulatory overload and the enlargement of a skeletal muscle following athletic activity. This relationship was elegantly stated by Austin Flint (1812–1886), who was professor of medicine at the University of Louisville in the middle of the 19th century:

[Overload] excites a more forcible ventricular action which for a time enables the ventricles to expel their contents. Meanwhile, hypernutrition follows, and hypertrophy is produced. The increased muscular growth for a certain period protects against the occurrence of dilatation. At length, the hypertrophy reaches a point beyond which it cannot advance; for the muscles of the heart, like other muscles, cannot increase indefinitely. There is a limit to the hypertrophic enlargement, and this limit varies in different persons just as the voluntary muscles in different persons attain, by the same efforts, to different degrees of development. The causes, however, persist and perhaps become more and more operative after the utmost degree of hypertrophy which is possible has taken place. These causes then can produce only dilatation, and from this period the progressive enlargement is due to augmentation of the cavities. This view is not only rational, but sustained by the facts derived from clinical experience.... According to this view, hypertrophy becomes an important conservative provision, first, against over-accumulation of blood, and second, against the more serious form of enlargement, viz., dilatation. (Flint, 1870, p 33)

It was not until the late 20th century, however, that rediscovery of the applicability of the Law of Laplace to the heart (Burch et al., 1952; Burton, 1957) allowed wall stress to be determined in the living human heart. These calculations confirmed Flint's intuition that, in its initial (adaptive) phase, the hypertrophic response of the overloaded heart returned wall stress virtually to normal (Sandler and Dodge, 1963; Hood et al., 1968; Grossman et al., 1975).

The poor prognosis in patients with cardiac hypertrophy was recognized in 1876 by Leopold Schroetter, who wrote in Ziemssen's *Practice of Medicine*:

Hypertrophy always occurs wherever a portion of the heart has been called upon to perform work beyond its normal capacity, either to overcome mechanical obstacles or in consequence of increased innervation.... Hypertrophy may exist for many years, and the individual still continue to have relatively good health, but in the end it certainly leads to a so-called catastrophe through some of its sequels, at all events by fatty degeneration and subsequent dilatation to disturbances of the circulation, which are of themselves full of danger to the patient. (Schroetter, 1876, pp 191 and 217)

The poor prognosis in patients with cardiac hypertrophy was also noted by Constantin Paul in 1884, when he wrote:

It has frequently been said that the heart hypertrophies in order to establish a sort of compensation, and this process has been called providential. This view would be correct if the hypertrophy remained stationary; but experience has shown that the excess of work imposed upon the heart finally deteriorates its fibres, which become changed either by fatty degeneration* or by the process of irritation of the connective tissue, which develops excessively and finally strangulates the muscular fibres. (Paul, 1884, p 319)

Paul's passage documents the growing realization that hypertrophy, while initially compensatory, eventually leads to myocardial deterioration, but it was Osler who most clearly stated that hypertrophy can be both adaptive and maladaptive.

William Osler (1849–1917), in the first (1892) edition of *The Principles and Practice of Medicine*, presents a remarkably modern view of hypertrophy when he notes that, while enlargement of the overloaded heart is initially beneficial, with time maladaptive features of this growth response cause the overloaded myocardium to deteriorate:

The course of any case of cardiac hypertrophy may be divided into three stages:

(a) The period of development, which varies with the nature of the primary lesion. For example, in rupture of an aortic valve . . . it may require months before the hypertrophy becomes fully developed; or indeed, it may never do so and death may follow from an uncompensated dilatation. On the other hand, in sclerotic affections of the valves, with stenosis or incompetency, the hypertrophy develops step by step with the lesion, and may continue to counterbalance the progressive and increasing impairment of the valve.

(b) The period of full compensation—the latent stage—during which the heart's vigor meets the requirements of the circulation. This period has an indefinite time and the patient may never be made aware by any symptoms that he has a valvular lesion.

(c) The period of broken compensation, which may come on suddenly during very severe exertion. Death may result from acute dilatation; but more commonly takes place slowly and results from degeneration and weakening of the heart muscle. (Osler, 1892, p 634)

Osler classifies cardiac enlargement as *hypertrophy*, with and without wall thickening, and *dilatation*, again with and without wall thickening (see Table 1-3). (The first and last of these, which represent eccentric hypertrophy, are similar.) This classification omits concentric hypertrophy, which he defines as "diminution in the size of the cavity with thickening of the walls"; like Bramwell, Osler considers this to be a postmortem change.

Osler's open mind and ability to follow the changing trends in medicine is seen in the 8th edition of his textbook, published in 1918, in which this analysis of hypertrophy is replaced with a discussion of cardiac hemodynamics, which was developing rapidly at that time. As already noted, this shift in focus from pathology to physiology attests to the excitement that followed Starling's announcement of the "Law of the Heart" (Starling, 1918).

An elegant description of compensatory hypertrophy is also found in a text written by Broadbent and Broadbent a few years after publication of Osler's first edition. These au-

---

*The term *fatty degeneration,* which appears commonly in older texts, is often used imprecisely; this appears to have been used by many to describe dying or dead cells.

thors relate how hypertrophy of the overloaded heart relieves symptoms of heart failure when they describe a boy

> who is allowed to go about immediately after he has contracted a valvular lesion of some severity and is suffering, say, from aortic incompetence, will be extremely short of breath, and incapable of walking any distance, will have attacks of severe pain in the precordium, and perhaps fainting fits, one of which may prove fatal; whereas if the same patient, if he is kept at rest till the compensatory changes have had time to develop, will be able to take moderate exercise comfortably and go about his work free from pain or respiratory distress, though he may be incapable of any prolonged or violent exertion. (Broadbent and Broadbent, 1898, p 47)

ROLE OF THE MYOCARDIUM IN HEART FAILURE

The earlier controversy regarding the relative importance of valve abnormalities and myocardial dysfunction in producing the syndrome of heart failure was revived by James Mackenzie (1853–1925), who in the first (1908) edition of his *Diseases of the Heart*, highlights the importance of myocardial abnormalities in causing the clinical syndrome of heart failure. He notes that because "the heart muscle supplies the force which maintains the circulation," valve abnormalities produce no clinical manifestations of heart failure "so long as the heart can overcome the impediment" by means of normal adjustments. This reasoning led Mackenzie to state that

> heart failure is simply inability of the heart muscle to maintain the circulation, and . . . this failure of the heart muscle is due to disturbance of the normal adjustment of the various factors concerned in the circulation. (Mackenzie, 1908, p 2)

The role of heart muscle, he says, is "of such prime importance in what we call heart failure, that a close and intimate study of its properties is essential." He seeks to assess this role using the concept of the *reserve force* of the heart, stating:

> The more I study the symptoms of heart failure, and the more I reflect on the part played by the heart muscle, the more convinced am I that the explanation of heart failure can be summed up in the general statement that heart failure is due to the exhaustion of the reserve force of the heart muscle as a whole, or of one or more of its functions. This statement may seem so self-evident as scarcely to need amplification, but as a matter of fact, this, the essential principle on which diagnosis, prognosis and treatment should be based, is often practically ignored. (Mackenzie, 1908, p 2)

If this seems so self-evident as to be unworthy of note, it should be remembered that as recently as the late 1950s, the clinical manifestations of heart failure were considered to be due largely to disordered renal function that led to salt and water accumulation.

Attempts to distinguish different forms of cardiac enlargement continued into the mid-1920s, as seen in Henri Vaquez' (1860–1936) 1924 classification of the causes of cardiac hypertrophy, which illustrates problems caused by incomplete understanding of physiology (see Table 1-3). His "essential hypertrophy" (associated with growth, exercise, and pregnancy) represents what currently would be referred to as physiologic hypertrophy, but the distinction between "symptomatic hypertrophy" and "dilatation" fails to appreciate the differences between pressure overload, volume overload, and myocardial weakness. Indeed, Vaquez echoes the earlier view of Bertin (see earlier discussion) when he emphasizes the role of dilatation in producing valve leaks, rather than the other way around. This causal mechanism certainly exists, for example, when tricuspid insufficiency develops in patients with chronic atrial fibrillation, or mitral insufficiency occurs when a markedly dilated left ventricle stretches the mitral annulus. However, in Vaquez' time, when the major cause of heart failure was rheumatic valvular disease, it was far more common for the leaky valve to cause a volume overload that dilates the heart's chambers, rather than the other way around.

CHANGING CAUSES OF HEART FAILURE

The history reviewed earlier comes from a time when rheumatic heart disease was almost certainly the most common cause of heart failure. As the ability to diagnose heart failure improved with the technologic advances in the 20th century, however, the diseases causing heart failure changed. In the early years of this century, structural abnormalities were by far the most important causes of heart failure; for example, Coombs (1927) reported that about three-fourths of patients hospitalized for heart disease in England had structural abnormalities (51% rheumatic heart disease, 11% subacute bacterial endocarditis, 9% cardiovascular syphilis, and 2% congenital heart disease). It is difficult currently to conceive of the impact of rheumatic heart disease, which is rarely seen in people born in the United States. Yet in the 1920s, rheumatic heart disease was responsible for as many as 60% to 80% of the cases of heart disease seen in adults (Cohn, 1927; Paul, 1930; Wilson, 1940). Much less common though far more dramatic was congenital heart disease, which at the end of the first half of the 20th century affected about 0.1% of children (MacMahon et al., 1953). Because there was no cardiac surgery to alleviate the structural abnormalities at that time, the clinical course of heart disease depended mainly on the natural history of the underlying valve abnormalities.

The public health importance of heart failure is apparent in the United States, where between 2 and 4 million Americans, more than 1% of the population, suffer from heart failure. This condition has been estimated each year to account for between 750,000 and 1,000,000 hospital admissions, adding more than $8,000,000,000 annually to health care costs (Garg et al., 1993; Ho et al., 1993b, NHLBI Report, 1994). Owing largely to aging of the population and dramatic advances in delaying death from the cardiac diseases that lead to heart failure, almost 400,000 new cases are seen annually. Each year, heart failure develops in more than 1% of men and women older than age 75 years in the United States, and in those older than 85 years, the annual incidence is about 3%. It is for these reasons that heart failure has recently become the most frequent discharge diagnosis in patients insured by Medicare in Connecticut (Hennen et al., 1995).

BIBLIOGRAPHY

Adams F (1856). *The Extant Works of Aretæus, The Cappadocian.* The Sydenham Soc, London.

Aran FA (1843). *Practical Manual of the Diseases of the Heart and Great Vessels.* Translation by Harris WA. Barrington and Haswell, Philadelphia.

Arcieri JP (1945). *The Circulation of the Blood and Andreas Cesalpino of Arezzo.* SF Vanni, New York.

Bell J (1802). *The Anatomy of the Human Body,* 2nd ed. Strahan, London.

Bertin RJ (1833). *Treatise on the Diseases of the Heart and Great Vessels.* Translation by Chauncy CW. Carey, Lea and Blanchard, Philadelphia.

Bing RF (1999). *Cardiology. The Evolution of the Science and the Art.* Rutgers University Press, New Brunswick, New Jersey.

Bramwell B (1884). *Diseases of the Heart and Thoracic Aorta.* Appleton, New York.

Broadbent WH, Broadbent JFH (1898). *Heart Disease: With Special Reference to Prognosis and Treatment.* Wood, New York.

Corvisart JN* (1812). *An Essay on the Organic Diseases and Lesions of the Heart and Great Vessels.* Translation by Gates J. Bradford & Read, Boston.

Cournand A (1964). Air and blood. In Fishman AP, Richards DW, eds. *Circulation of the Blood: Men and Ideas.* Oxford University Press, New York.

East T (1958). The Story of Heart Disease. Lecture 4. *Failure of the Circulation and Its Treatment.* Dawson and Sons, London, pp. 127–145.

Fishman AP, Richards DW (1964). *Circulation of the Blood: Men and Ideas.* Oxford University Press, New York, New York.

Flint A (1870). *Diseases of the Heart*, 2nd ed. HC Lea, Philadelphia.

Fothergill JM (1879). *The Heart and Its Diseases,* 2nd ed. Lindsay & Blakiston, Philadelphia.

Furley DJ, Wilkie JS (1984). *Galen. On Respiration and the Arteries.* Princeton University Press, Princeton, NJ.

Harris CRS (1973). *The Heart and Vascular System in Ancient Greek Medicine.* University Press, Oxford.

Harvey W (1957) *Movement of the Heart and Blood in Animals.* Translation by Franklin KJ.

Horace. *The Complete Odes and Epodes.* Translation by Shepherd WG. Penguin, London, 1983.

Jarcho S (1980). *The Concept of Heart Failure. From Avicenna to Albertini.* Harvard University Press, Cambridge, Massachusetts.

Jones WHS (1923–1931). *Hippocrates.* William Heinemann, London.

Kuhn TS (1970). *The Structure of Scientific Revolutions*, 2nd ed. The University of Chicago Press, Chicago.

Lathan PM (1845). *Lectures on Subjects Connected with Clinical Medicine Comprising Diseases of the Heart.* Longman, Brown, Green and Longmans, London.

Littré E (1839–1861). *Oeuvres Complètes d'Hippocrate.* JB Baillière, Paris.

MacKenzie J (1918). *Diseases of the Heart*, 3rd ed. Oxford University Press, London.

MacKenzie J* (1908). *Diseases of the Heart,* Oxford University Press, London.

Major RH (1945). *Classic Descriptions of Disease*, 3rd ed. CC Thomas, Springfield, IL.

Major RH (1954). *A History of Medicine.* CC Thomas, Springfield, IL.

Mettler CC* (1947). *History of Medicine.* Blakiston Philadelphia.

Morgagni JB*. *The Seats and Causes of Diseases Investigated by Anatomy, in Five Books.* Translation by Alexander B. Millar and Cadell, London, 1769.

NHLBI Report of the Task Force on Research in Heart Failure (1994). US Department of Health and Human Services, Bethesda, Maryland.

Osler W* (1892). *The Principles and Practice of Medicine.* Appleton, New York

Osler W* (1921). *The Evolution of Modern Medicine.* Yale University Press, New Haven, CT.

Paul C (1884). *Diseases of the Heart.* Wood, New York.

Paul JR (1930). *The Epidemiology of Rheumatic Fever.* The Metropolitan Life Insurance Co., New York.

Schroetter L (1876). Diseases of the heart substance. In Ziemssen H, ed. *Practice of Medicine,* Vol. VI. *Diseases of the Circulatory System.* Wood, New York.

Sénac J-B (1749). *Traité de la Structure du Coeur, de son Action et de ses Maladies.* Vincent, Paris.

Singer C* (1988). *The Fasciculus Medicinae of Johannes de Ketham.* Classics of Medicine, Birmingham, AL.

Snellen HA (1984). *History of Cardiology.* Donker, Rotterdam.

Spann JF Jr, Buccino RA, Sonnenblick EH, Braunwald E (1967). Contractile state of cardiac muscle obtained from cats with experimentally produced ventricular hypertrophy and heart failure. *Circ Res* 21:341–354

Spencer WG (1938). *Celsus. De Medicina,* Vol. I. Heinemann, London.

Starling EH (1918). *The Linacre Lecture on the Law of the Heart.* Longmans, Green & Co, London.

Traube L (1856). *Über den Zusammenhang von Herz und Nieren Krankheiten.* A Hischwald, Berlin.

Traube L (1878). *Gesammelte Beiträge zur Pathologie und Physiologie.* Berlin 3:167–169.

Vaquez H (1924). *Diseases of the Heart.* Translation by Laidlaw GF. WB Saunders, Philadelphia.

Virchow R* (1860). *Cellular Pathology.* Translation by Chance F. Churchill, London.

Wiggers CJ (1928). The Pressure Pulses in the Cardiovascular System. Longmans, Green & Co, London.

Wiggers CJ (1949). Physiology in health and disease. In *Dynamics of Valvular Lesions,* 5th ed. Lea & Febiger, Philadelphia, pp 786–801.

Wilson MG (1940). *Rheumatic Fever.* The Commonwealth Fund, New York.

Wright WC (1952). *Lancisi's Aneurysms.* MacMillan, New York.

*Reprints published by the Classics in Medicine Library.

REFERENCES

Bright R (1836). Cases and observations illustrative of renal disease accompanied with secretion of albuminous urine. *Guy's Hosp Rep* 1:339–379.

Burch GE, Ray CT, Cronvich JA (1952). Certain mechanical properties of the human cardiac pump in normal and diseased states. The George Fahr Lecture. *Circulation* 5:504–512.

Burton AC (1957). The importance of the shape and size of the heart. *Am J Physiol* 54:801–810.

Cohn AE (1927). Heart disease from the point of view of the public health. *Am Heart J* 2:275–301 and 386–407.

Coombs CF (1927). The aetiology of cardiac disease. *Bristol Med Chir J* 43:1.

Garg R, Packer M, Pitt B, Yusuf S (1993). Heart failure in the 1990s: evolution of a major public health problem in cardiovascular medicine. *J Am Coll Cardiol* 22:3A–5A.

Grossman W, Jones D, McLaurin LP (1975). Wall stress and patterns of hypertrophy in the human left ventricle. *J Clin Invest* 56:56–64.

Gull WW, Sutton HG (1872). On the pathology of the morbid state commonly called "Bright's disease with contracted kidney" ("arterio-capillary fibrosis"). *Med-Chir Tr (Lond)* 55:273–329.

Hamilton A (1997). Academic distinctions. How competition blighted Europe's universities. *Times Literary Suppl.* No. 4915:9–10.

Hennen J, Krumholz HM, Radford MJ (1995). Twenty most frequent DRG groups among Medicare inpatients age 65 or older in Connecticut hospitals, fiscal years 1991, 1992, and 1993. *Conn Med* 59:11–15.

Ho KKL, Anderson KM, Kannel WB, Grossman W, Levy D (1993a). Survival after the onset of congestive heart failure in Framingham heart study subjects. *Circulation* 88:107–115.

Ho KKL, Pinsky JL, Kannel WB, Levy D (1993b). The epidemiology of congestive heart failure: the Framingham Study. *J Am Coll Cardiol* 22:6A–13A.

Hood WP Jr, Rackley CE, Rolett EL (1968). Wall stress in the normal and hypertrophied human left ventricle. *Am J Cardiol* 22:5550–5558.

Jarcho S (1980). *The Concept of Heart Failure. From Avicenna to Albertini.* Harvard University Press, Cambridge, Massachusetts.

Johnson G (1868). I. On certain points in the anatomy and pathology of Bright's disease of the kidney. II. On the influence of the minute blood vessels upon the circulation. *Med-Chir Tr (Lond)* 51:57–78.

Katz AM (1988). Molecular biology in cardiology, a paradigmatic shift. *J Mol Cell Cardiol* 20:355–366.

Katz AM (1997). Evolving concepts of heart failure: cooling furnace, malfunctioning pump, enlarging muscle. Part I. Heart failure as a disorder of the cardiac pump. *J Cardiac Failure* 3:319–334.

Katz AM (1998). Evolving concepts of heart failure: cooling furnace, malfunctioning pump, enlarging muscle. Part II. Hypertrophy and dilatation of the failing heart. *J Cardiac Failure* 4:67–81.

Katz AM, Katz LA (1991). What is a paradigm and when does it shift? *J Mol Cell Cardiol* 23:403–408.

Katz AM, Katz PB (1962). Diseases of the heart in the works of Hippocrates. *Br Heart J* 24:257–264.

Katz AM, Katz PB (1995). Emergence of scientific explanations of nature in ancient Greece: the only scientific discovery? *Circulation* 92:637–645.

MacMahon B, McKeown T, Record RG (1953). The incidence and life expectancy of children with congenital heart disease. *Br Heart J* 15:121.

Mahomed FA (1881). Chronic Bright's disease without albuminuria. *Guy's Hosp Rep,* 3rd ser, 24:363.

Mancia G (1997). Scipione Riva-Rocci. *Clin Cardiol* 20:503–504.

Riva-Rocci S (1896). Un nuovo sfigmomanometro. *Gazz Med Torino* 50-51:1001–1007.

Riva-Rocci S (1897). La tecnica sfigmomanometra. *Gazz Med Torino* 9-10:161–172.

Sandler H, Dodge HT (1963). Left ventricular tension and stress in man. *Circ Res* 13:91–104.

2

Organ Physiology: The Failing Heart as a Weakened Pump

The heart, like any pump, imparts the energy needed to "lift" fluid from a low pressure system (the veins) to one at higher pressure (the arteries). Impairment of the cardiac pump, therefore, can have one or both of two consequences. One the one hand, there can be inadequate forward flow of blood from the heart into the aorta and pulmonary artery; on the other hand, there can be inadequate emptying of the venous reservoirs, which causes blood to back up behind the heart. A simple analogy is to compare the failing heart to a pump that is forcing water out of a flooded basement through a garden hose (Fig. 2-1); when the pump fails, less water emerges from the hose and flooding of the basement increases.

In reality, however, the consequences of heart failure are far more complex than shown in the simple analogy in Fig. 2-1. In the first place, the heart is not one pump, but is two pumps arranged in series: the right and left ventricles. Furthermore, as pointed out by Harvey, blood flows in a circle. This means that if less blood is pumped out of one ventricle, then less returns to the other, and that blood backing up behind either ventricle increases the load on the other. Another complication arises because the interventricular septum is shared by both ventricles, so that failure of one ventricle can modify the function of the other by ventricular interaction. An important feature of the failing cardiac pump is that impaired emptying of either ventricle reduces its capacity to fill. The reason is that reduced ejection during systole increases the residual volume at the beginning of diastole, which impedes filling during the next beat. Conversely, reduced filling during diastole means that the ventricle contains less blood that can be ejected in the following systole. Stated simply, a heart that ejects poorly during systole cannot fill normally during diastole, and a heart that fills poorly during diastole cannot eject normally during systole.

Changes in the peripheral and pulmonary circulations also complicate the hemodynamics of heart failure. The reason is that the vascular system is far more than a network of rigid tubes; instead, both arterial resistance and venous capacitance respond vigorously to changes in blood pressure and cardiac output. When the cardiac pump fails, decreased forward flow of blood into the arterial system and increased venous pressure activate a powerful hemodynamic defense reaction. This neurohumoral response, which is discussed at length in Chapter 4, is very important and very complex in heart failure; its influence is so great that the hemodynamic defense reaction generally dominates the clinical picture in these patients. In terms of the paradigm of *organ physiology* (see Table 1-2), the hemodynamic defense reaction modifies both circulatory hemodynamics and cardiac pump function. In response to a decrease in cardiac output, for example, this neurohumoral response increases both ejection and the capacity of the heart to fill, accelerates heart rate, constricts

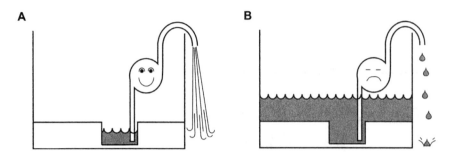

FIG. 2-1. "Leaky basement" analogy. The heart can be viewed as a pump that removes water from a leaky basement. The manifestations of the pump failure can be inadequate emptying of the basement, which then floods ("backward failure"), inadequate flow into a hose ahead of the pump ("forward failure"), or both.

both arteries and veins, and, by promoting salt and water retention by the kidney, increases blood volume. At the level of *cellular biochemistry*, these reflexes increase myocardial contractility, accelerate relaxation, speed the sinoatrial (SA) node pacemaker, modify the energetics of working cardiac myocytes, and alter the properties of the ion channels that control membrane potential (see Chapter 3). These neurohumoral responses also modify the signal transduction systems that control *cell growth*, the final paradigm listed in Table 1-2. The result is a hypertrophic response that changes the molecular structure and architecture of the failing heart. By shortening myocardial cell survival, maladaptive features of this growth response have a major impact on prognosis. Heart failure, therefore, triggers a dazzling array of responses, both compensatory (adaptive) and deleterious (maladaptive), that influence organ physiology, cell biochemistry, and growth.

This chapter focuses on the immediate hemodynamic consequences of a damaged cardiac pump, emphasizing the interplay between the failing heart and the circulation whose needs it cannot fulfill. Some of the simpler short-term reflex adjustments to reduced emptying of the great veins and reduced ejection of blood under pressure into the aorta and pulmonary artery are also described. These immediate hemodynamic consequences of depressed cardiac function are discussed in terms of classic concepts of organ physiology, such as ventricular function curves (Starling's Law of the Heart), end-systolic and end-diastolic pressure-volume relationships, pressure-volume loops, and the interplay between venous return and stroke volume (Guyton diagrams). The concepts of backward and forward failure are reviewed, as are the often ambiguous concepts of systolic and diastolic dysfunction. The description of the physiologic basis for the major hemodynamic manifestations of heart failure ends with an examination of the relationship between these pathophysiologic abnormalities and the signs and symptoms caused by *right* and *left* heart failure.

CLASSIFICATIONS OF HEART FAILURE

Several classifications of heart failure are commonly used in clinical practice. These are largely descriptive, although some imply the operation of underlying pathophysiologic mechanisms. The link between causal mechanisms and many of these classifications is quite complex, which can generate considerable confusion. The following paragraphs describe several classifications that are based on abnormalities in the heart's function as a pump.

Backward and Forward Failure

As already noted, the hemodynamic abnormalities in patients with heart failure are conceptually simple because, like any pump, the heart has only two ways to fail: inadequate emptying of the venous reservoirs (often called *backward failure*) and reduced ejection of blood under pressure into the aorta and pulmonary artery (*forward failure*). The terms "backward" and "forward" failure, however, are oversimplifications that must be used with caution in describing the hemodynamic responses to a failing cardiac pump. The "purest" causes of backward failure of the left heart include mitral stenosis, in which narrowing of the mitral valve orifice impedes venous return into a normal left ventricle, and hypertrophic cardiomyopathy, in which left ventricular cavity obliteration caused by inappropriate concentric hypertrophy reduces diastolic filling. Forward failure of the left ventricle can occur when a mechanical obstruction inhibits ejection, as in aortic stenosis; when myocardial damage or weakness reduces systolic shortening, as occurs with myocarditis; or when the ventricle becomes scarred after a large myocardial infarction. Similar mechanisms can impair right ventricular ejection, although left ventricular dysfunction is by far the most common cause of heart failure. As already noted, backward and forward failure invariably coexist. Moreover, reflex adjustments, such as arteriolar vasoconstriction and fluid retention, generally modify these hemodynamic patterns, as do many drugs commonly used to treat heart failure, notably diuretics and vasodilators. For these reasons, backward and forward failure are useful mainly as concepts that help in the understanding of the immediate hemodynamic consequences of specific pathophysiologic processes in a failing heart.

It is common for forward failure to be equated with depressed myocardial contractility (decreased inotropy), and backward failure with impaired relaxation (decreased lusitropy). However, the link between altered hemodynamics and these abnormalities of muscle biochemistry and biophysics is so tenuous as almost to lack meaning. This is because the manifestations of forward and backward failure can be influenced as much by interactions between the heart and the peripheral circulation as by the extent to which myocardial contractility and relaxation are impaired. Increased afterload, a consequence of the peripheral vasoconstriction that accompanies the hemodynamic defense reaction, reduces cardiac output and so worsens forward failure. Conversely, increased preload, as occurs when salt and water retention by the kidney (also a consequence of the hemodynamic defense reaction) increases intravascular volume, can be more important than impaired diastolic filling in causing the increased venous pressure that is the hallmark of backward failure.

The different patterns of hypertrophy seen in failing hearts also influence the manifestations of forward and backward failure. Concentric hypertrophy of the pressure-overloaded left ventricle, while aiding ejection, reduces left ventricular cavity volume, which impairs filling and so increases the severity of backward failure. Conversely, progressive left ventricular dilatation (remodeling), commonly seen in patients with a dilated cardiomyopathy or after a large myocardial infarction, puts the failing heart at a mechanical disadvantage by increasing systolic wall tension (according to the Law of Laplace) and so worsens forward failure. For these reasons, the severity of either forward or backward failure, defined as reduced cardiac output and increased venous pressure, respectively, generally provides little information as to whether the primary abnormality in muscle function is impaired relaxation or depressed contractility.

Therapy is also a major determinant of the extent of forward and backward failure in the patient with heart failure. Vasodilator drugs, which reduce the impedance to ejection by a failing left ventricle, increase stroke volume and so alleviate symptoms of forward failure (low cardiac output) without directly affecting inotropy. Even more dramatic are the effects of diuretics, which by depleting vascular volume alleviate backward failure (elevated venous pressure) without altering the lusitropic state of the heart. Diuretics also reduce preload, so that, according to Starling's Law of the Heart, they can worsen forward failure. For these reasons, the severity of the manifestations of forward and backward failure provides little information about either etiology or the biochemical state of the myocardium in patients with heart failure.

Systolic and Diastolic Dysfunction

A more useful classification than that based on the concepts of forward and backward failure is the distinction between systolic and diastolic dysfunction, which in general terms refer to impaired ability of the heart to eject (systolic dysfunction) and to fill (diastolic dysfunction). These terms have different pathophysiologic meanings in acute and chronic heart failure.

In acute heart failure, systolic and diastolic dysfunction reflect different biochemical abnormalities in the myocardium. Acute systolic dysfunction impairs ejection in patients with viral myocarditis, or with toxic and metabolic abnormalities such as alcohol intoxication and anemia. Acute diastolic dysfunction impairs filling when the heart becomes ischemic, as occurs during coronary spasm or balloon angioplasty, when coronary flow is suddenly interrupted. In these settings, acute systolic and diastolic dysfunction are due to abnormalities in the biochemical processes responsible for cardiac contraction and relaxation, respectively (Chapter 3). In chronic heart failure, however, the terms systolic and diastolic dysfunction are most appropriately defined in terms of abnormal ventricular architecture (cavity size, shape, and wall thickness) (Table 2-1).

Chronic systolic dysfunction of the left ventricle, which from an architectural standpoint describes a dilated, thin-walled heart (eccentric hypertrophy), is usually caused by diseases that damage or weaken the myocardium. Systolic dysfunction can be either diffuse (global) or regional (see Table 2-1); diffuse systolic dysfunction is seen in conditions such as idiopathic dilated cardiomyopathy or myocarditis, which weaken contraction in all regions of the ventricle, whereas regional impairment of systolic function is usually seen after a myocardial infarction. Chronic diastolic dysfunction, which describes a noncompliant, thick-walled ventricle with normal, or even reduced cavity size (concentric

---

TABLE 2-1. *Systolic and diastolic dysfunction[a]*

Systolic dysfunction
  Impaired ejection (forward failure), depressed inotropy (contractility)
    Global: dilated cardiomyopathies, viral or toxic myocarditis
    Regional: myocardial infarction
Diastolic dysfunction
  Impaired filling (backward failure), depressed lusitropy (relaxation)
    Hypertrophic cardiomyopathy, hypertensive heart disease

---

[a]Systolic dysfunction refers to a pathophysiologic abnormality in which ejection is reduced in a dilated ventricle. This is seen when inotropy (contractility) is depressed, or when the ventricle dilates as the result of global or regional damage to its walls. In diastolic dysfunction, the primary hemodynamic abnormality is impaired filling, as occurs in a thick-walled ventricle or where the major biochemical defect is a lusitropic (relaxation) abnormality. Systolic and diastolic dysfunction are often associated with forward and backward failure, respectively; however, these hemodynamic syndromes are also influenced by changes in the circulation as well as ventricular architecture (concentric and eccentric hypertrophy).

hypertrophy), is commonly seen in patients with left ventricular hypertrophy secondary to aortic stenosis or long-standing, inadequately treated systemic hypertension. These patterns appear in patients with heritable forms of heart disease: diastolic dysfunction in the familial hypertrophic cardiomyopathies and systolic dysfunction in a growing number of inherited syndromes characterized by the late appearance of dilated cardiomyopathy. As discussed in later chapters, even in the more common forms of heart failure, these different patterns of abnormal ventricular architecture result from different growth responses in an overloaded or diseased heart.

Systolic dysfunction, the impaired ability of a dilated ventricle to eject its contents, is readily quantified by measuring ejection fraction (EF), the ratio between the decreased stroke volume (SV), and the increased end-diastolic volume (EDV):

$$EF = \frac{SV}{EDV} \qquad \text{Equation 2.1}$$

It is important to recognize that ejection fraction is not an accurate measurement of contractile function. This is because this ratio is reduced in the patient with a dilated ventricle, even when stroke volume is normal or nearly normal, simply because EDV, the denominator in Equation 2.1, is increased. Furthermore, ejection fraction can be normal, or even increased in patients with diastolic dysfunction, where hypertrophy reduces cavity volume, the denominator in Equation 2.1. As stroke volume, the numerator in Equation 2.1, can be depressed to a similar extent in patients with systolic and diastolic dysfunction, the distinction between these two types of heart failure depends mainly on whether ventricular cavity size is increased or decreased. Ventricular diastolic pressure can also be elevated to a similar extent in systolic and diastolic dysfunction, so that these two types of heart failure cannot be distinguished on the basis of hemodynamic measurements. Instead, this distinction is made on the basis of ventricular architecture.

It is an oversimplification to equate chronic systolic and diastolic dysfunction with forward and backward failure respectively, or the former with abnormal contractility and the latter with impaired relaxation. As already noted, a ventricle that does not empty normally cannot fill normally, and vice versa. Furthermore, diuretic therapy, by depleting vascular volume, readily converts backward failure to forward failure without directly affecting ventricular function. For these reasons, chronic systolic and diastolic dysfunction cannot be distinguished from one another on the basis of measurements of such hemodynamic variables as filling pressures and cardiac output. Instead, this distinction requires that the architecture of the failing ventricle be determined, for example, by echocardiography.

Right and Left Heart Failure

The distinction between right and left heart failure is especially useful in patients with congenital and valvular heart disease, in whom a narrowed or leaky valve, or an intracardiac shunt, can affect predominantly the right or left side of the heart. In developed countries, where the major etiologies of heart failure are coronary and hypertensive heart disease, left heart failure is especially common (Table 2-2). The clinical picture in patients with a dilated cardiomyopathy is also generally dominated by the symptoms of left heart failure. Right heart failure, which is much less common, occurs most often in congenital heart disease and cor pulmonale; the latter can be caused by chronic lung disease, multiple pulmonary emboli, or primary pulmonary hypertension. Right heart failure can come to dominate the clinical picture in some patients with left heart failure; this occurs when chronically elevated left atrial and pulmonary venous pressures lead to vasocon-

TABLE 2-2. *Common causes of heart failure in the industrialized world[a]*

Etiology	Right/left heart failure	Systolic/diastolic dysfunction	Global/regional wall motion abnormality
Ischemic heart disease			
Myocardial infarction	Left	Systolic	Regional
Ischemic cardiomyopathy	Left	Systolic	Generally regional
Dilated cardiomyopathy/myocarditis	Left	Systolic	Global
Hypertensive	Left	Diastolic	Global
Hypertrophic cardiomyopathy	Left	Diastolic	Often regional
Valvular/congenital	Depends on structures affected		Global
Cor pulmonale	Right	Both	Global
Tachycardia-induced	Left	Diastolic	Global
Pericardial effusion tamponade	Right	Diastolic	Global

[a]This overview of common causes of heart failure is much oversimplified. "Ischemic cardiomyopathy" includes to a functional disorder often called "hibernation," whereas the dilated cardiomyopathies can be caused by a variety of infectious, toxic, metabolic, and a growing number of familial disorders. The hypertrophic cardiomyopathies include patients with several different genetic defects, whereas a variety of structural abnormalities are causal in valvular and congenital heart disease. Tachycardia-induced cardiomyopathy, which contributes to atrial dilatation in patients with chronic atrial fibrillation, is an uncommon cause of ventricular failure. Pericardial effusions generally result from such noncardiac conditions as autoimmune diseases and metastatic malignancies.

striction and proliferative changes in the pulmonary arterioles, which increase pulmonary artery pressure (pulmonary hypertension). The increased pulmonary arterial resistance in these patients, by reducing pulmonary blood flow, "protects" against pulmonary congestion, albeit at the cost of replacing the clinical picture of left heart failure with that of right heart failure. This sequence of events is elegantly described by Paul Wood in one of the outstanding clinical papers of the 20th century (Wood, 1954).

ALTERED INOTROPIC AND LUSITROPIC PROPERTIES

Myocardial contractility (inotropy) and relaxation (lusitropy) are impaired in most patients with heart failure. The molecular mechanisms responsible for these abnormalities are discussed in Chapter 3; at this point, their consequences are reviewed in terms of their impact upon the ability of the heart to eject and to fill.

Historically, more attention has been paid to reduced ejection than to impaired filling. It is interesting to speculate as to why earlier investigators focused more on systole than diastole. In part, this probably reflects the fact that ejection of blood under pressure during systole is a more dramatic event than filling of the heart during diastole. Another explanation for the emphasis on systolic function is that myocardial contractility is readily estimated clinically using pressure data, most often the rate of pressure increase (+dP/dt), which have been available since the introduction of cardiac catheterization in the 1940s. Measurements of diastolic function based on the rate of pressure decrease (-dP/dt), however, are much more difficult to interpret. For this reason, little attention was paid to lusitropy until the late 1970s, when advances in echocardiography and nuclear cardiology provided the high quality measurements of wall motion needed to quantify the rate and extent of ventricular filling in humans.

Even in modern times, heart failure is commonly viewed mainly as a disorder of ejection. Even though this is correct in many patients, notably those who suffer from chronic ischemic heart disease and dilated cardiomyopathies, the primary abnormality in the grow-ing number of elderly patients with heart failure is impaired ventricular filling. Table 2-2, which lists the major causes of heart failure in the United States, provides an overview of the etiology of this syndrome in developed countries. (For further information about this important clinical syndrome, refer to standard cardiology and internal medicine textbooks.)

Impaired ejection and filling in a failing heart are often equated with inotropic and lusitropic abnormalities, respectively. Although ejection is often impaired as the result of defects in the molecular processes responsible for myocardial contraction, and slow, in-complete filling can be caused by abnormalities in the molecular mechanisms that relax heart muscle, the correlation between cellular and pump function is quite complex. The reason is that systemic hemodynamics and ventricular architecture (cavity size, shape, and wall thickness), in addition to inotropic and lusitropic properties, determine filling and ejection by a failing heart.

Heart Failure and Starling's Law of the Heart

Discovery of the relationship between end-diastolic volume and ventricular function at the beginning of the 20th century led early investigators to postulate that abnormal length-dependent changes in cardiac performance play a major role in the pathophysiol-ogy of heart failure. This interesting chapter in the history of heart failure research has its origins in the middle of the 19th century, when the length-tension relationship was de-scribed for skeletal muscle (Fig. 2-2). Otto Frank's demonstration in the 1890s that this relationship also applied to the frog heart led to Starling's classic studies of the isolated canine heart, which showed that changes in end-diastolic volume were a major determi-nant of the work of the heart (Fig. 2-3). As noted in Chapter 1, rapid acceptance of the

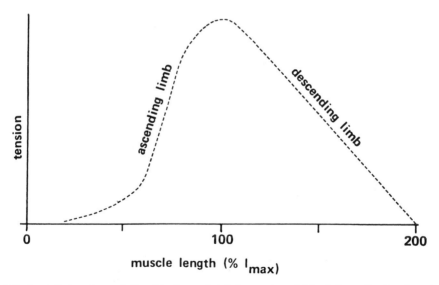

FIG. 2-2. Length-tension relationship in a skeletal muscle, which defines the tension devel-oped during isometric tetanic contractions that begin at different rest lengths. Muscle tension is expressed as percent of I_{max}, which is defined as the rest length at which developed tension is maximal. Curves of this sort are generally scanned from left to right, so that the *ascending* limb is to the left, and the *descending* limb, where tension decreases with increasing length, is to the right. [From Katz, 1992.]

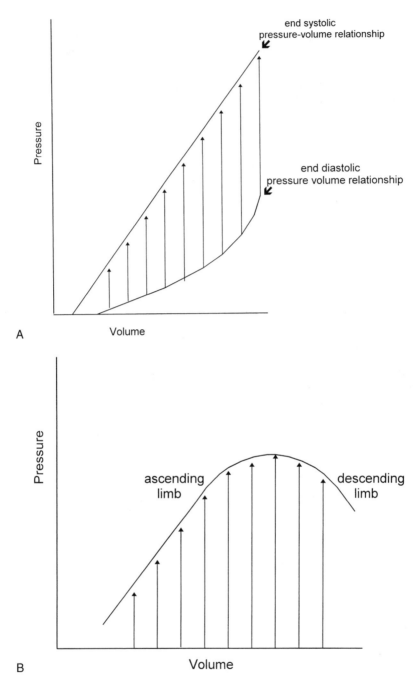

FIG. 2-3. The Frank–Starling relationship (Starling's Law of the Heart). **A:** The pressure developed in a series of isometric contractions that start from different end-diastolic volumes (*vertical arrows*) increases with increasing end-diastolic volume. **B:** Plot of the vertical arrows shown in A, showing ascending and descending limbs of the Starling curve. The decline in developed pressure at very high end-diastolic pressures (the descending limb) is not seen at physiologic end-diastolic pressures.

importance of Starling's Law of the Heart led to a paradigm shift in efforts to understand heart failure, from the role of the architecture of the failing heart to abnormalities in the physiologic response to changing end-diastolic volume.

Starling's curves, like the length-tension relationship in skeletal muscle (see Fig. 2-2), often showed a "descending limb" where, at high end-diastolic volumes, increasing ventricular filling reduces cardiac output. In his 1914 paper describing the role of end-diastolic volume in regulating the heart beat, Starling wrote:

> Fatigue of the heart may go on to heart failure. This occurs when the dilatation, which is the mechanical result of unchanging inflow and failing outflow...proceeds to such an extent that the tension of the muscle fibres becomes increasingly inadequate in producing rise of intracardiac pressure. The mechanical disadvantage, at which in the dilated spherical heart the skein of muscle fibres must act, finally smashes up the system and the circulation comes to an end. (Patterson et al., 1914)

Although Starling may have been thinking of acute left heart failure (pulmonary edema) and not chronic congestive heart failure when he wrote this paragraph, a number of later writers came to view the weakness of the failing heart as due, at least in part, to the operation of the failing ventricle on the descending limb of the Starling Curve (Fig. 2-4) (McMichael, 1950; Wiggers, 1952; Guyton, 1961). Currently, though, it is known that this is not a valid explanation for chronic heart failure. In the first place, it is unlikely that diastolic pressure in the intact ventricle ever becomes sufficiently high to force the heart onto the descending limb (Spiro and Sonnenblick, 1962; Elzinga, 1992). Furthermore, the heart cannot achieve at a steady state on the descending limb, where increased filling decreases ejection because, as I noted more than 30 years ago (Katz, 1965):

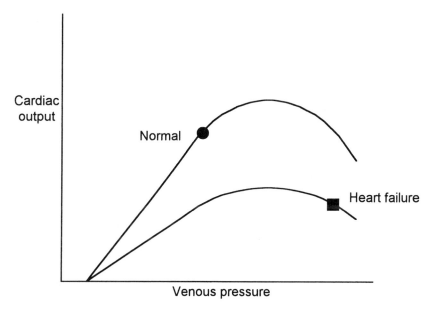

FIG. 2-4. Hypothetical Starling Curves from normal and failing hearts in which the normal heart operates on the ascending limb of the curve (●) and the failing heart is on the descending limb of a depressed curve (■). [Adapted from McMichael (1950).]

The geometry of the heart imposes certain functional requirements upon the physiology of its muscular walls. The most important is that contractile force *must* increase with increasing ventricular volume; failure to meet this requirement (operation of the heart on the descending limb of the Starling Curve) sets the stage for the establishment of a vicious cycle that, in the absence of length-independent increases in contractile force or rapid adjustments of the peripheral circulation, will lead to progressive cardiac dilatation and death of the organism.

It is well known that ventricular dilation in patients with eccentric hypertrophy is not caused by overstretching of cardiac myocytes; in fact, sarcomere length remains normal in the failing heart. Instead, as discussed later in this text, failing hearts dilate as the result of a maladaptive growth response in which cell elongation, uncoiling of the spiral musculature of the heart's walls, and possibly fiber slippage cause "remodeling" of damaged or chronically overloaded hearts. Of interest, the fallacy that the failing heart operates on the descending limb of the Starling Curve, which as recently as the 1980s was believed by a majority of medical students at a prominent United States medical school, was selected to illustrate "a pervasive and powerful misconception" in medical education (Feltovich et al., 1989).

There remains some controversy as to whether the ascending limb of the Frank–Starling relationship operates at all in the failing heart; that is, whether increased venous return increases the ability of the heart to eject. Although one group recently reported that failing hearts are unable to use this mechanism (Schwinger et al., 1994), contrary views have been published (Holubarsch et al, 1996; Weil et al., 1998). In view of the essential role of length-dependent changes in cardiac performance in allowing the heart to equalize stroke volume and venous return (see earlier discussion), it seems unlikely, probably impossible, for this hemodynamic adjustment to be lost completely in these patients.

Impaired Ejection: Depressed Myocardial Contractility in the Failing Heart

In the 1950s, when biochemistry and biophysics—the fifth paradigm listed in Table 1-2—was incorporated into the mainstream of cardiovascular research, it became clear that factors other than end-diastolic fiber length play a major role in regulating the performance of the heart. Demonstration that neurotransmitters like norepinephrine and drugs like digitalis increase the force of contraction at any given end-diastolic fiber length, while anemia and anoxia weaken the heart in a manner that does not depend on end-diastolic volume, shifted the emphasis in studies of heart failure to the inotropic state of the myocardium, which came to be called *myocardial contractility*. Efforts to measure myocardial contractility in patients with valvular and other forms of structural heart disease were stimulated by the realization that the contractile state of the myocardium (Mackenzie's "reserve force," see Chapter 1) plays an important role in determining the heart's ability to pump in the face of a hemodynamic overload. Following the advent of open heart surgery, the state of the myocardium was found to have an important influence on the outcome after surgical repair of structural abnormalities of the heart. For example, when mitral valve replacement is delayed too long in a patient with mitral insufficiency, the risk of operative mortality is greatly increased by deterioration of the myocardium. The need to identify the optimal time to operate, that is, before the overloaded myocardium has deteriorated to the point that patients cannot recover after a mechanically perfect operation, highlighted the need to quantify this myocardial factor. Efforts to use clinical determinations of myocardial contractility in this context, however, have proven to be a difficult challenge.

A *change* in myocardial contractility is readily demonstrated as a shift in the Starling Curve (Fig. 2-5), which simply documents a change in the amount of work done at any given end-diastolic fiber length. However, quantification of the *absolute level* of contractility is, for all practical purposes, impossible. This is because myocardial contractility is the expression of *all* of the many biochemical and biophysical factors that influence the number and turnover rate of the interactions between the contractile proteins, as well as the transmission of shortening and tension developed by the sarcomeres to the ends of the individual muscle fibers in the complex three-dimensional structure of the heart (Katz, 1992). Even if these factors could be easily evaluated in an isolated strand of cardiac muscle, which is not the case, evaluation of myocardial contractility in the intact heart is even more difficult. The interplay between the heart and the circulation makes it necessary to distinguish the hemodynamic effects of altered myocardial contractility from those caused by changes in preload and afterload. In the patient with heart failure, for example, it is not always obvious whether worsening congestion (backward failure) is due to increased venous return, such as occurs when fluid retention by the kidney augments blood volume, or whether the congestion has worsened because progressive impairment of myocardial contractility has impaired ejection. Similarly, cardiac output can be reduced when peripheral arteriolar vasoconstriction increases impedance to ejection, as well as by depressed myocardial contractility. These considerations highlight the importance of understanding both the interplay between length-dependent changes in contractile performance (Starling's Law

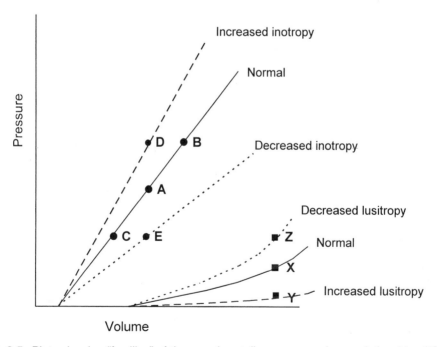

FIG. 2-5. Plots showing "families" of three end-systolic pressure-volume relationships ("Starling Curves," above), and three end-diastolic pressure volume relationships (filling curves, below). The Starling Curve *CAB* can be increased (curve containing point *D*) or decreased (curve containing point *E*) by interventions that modify inotropy, whereas the filling curve containing point *X* can be shifted to curves containing points *Y* and *Z* by changes in lusitropy as shown on the figure.

of the Heart), myocardial contractility, and changes in preload and afterload. All have important effects on hemodynamics in patients with heart failure.

The interplay between Starling's law and changing contractility in regulating the work of the heart is shown in Fig. 2-5, in which points *A*, *B*, and *C* lie along a control Starling Curve. Because myocardial contractility is, by definition, the ability of the cardiac muscle to do work *at constant end-diastolic fiber length*, a Starling Curve obtained under control conditions, such as *CAB*, defines baseline contractility. At this, or any level of contractility, increased end-diastolic volume, by the operation of Starling's law, increases the ability of the heart to perform work (*A→B*), whereas work decreases when end-diastolic volume decreases (*A→C*). A change in myocardial contractility, which by definition alters the ability of the heart to do work at any given end-diastolic volume, allows any intervention that alters the inotropic state of the heart to generate a new Starling Curve. This means that, as shown by the top three curves in Fig. 2-5, the heart can operate on any of a "family of Starling Curves," each of which represents a different inotropic state (Sarnoff, 1955). A positive inotropic intervention, which by definition increases work capacity at any given end-diastolic volume (or fiber length), shifts the heart to a new, higher Starling Curve (*A→D*), while a negative inotropic intervention, by causing a downward shift in the Starling Curve (*A→E*), reduces the work of the heart at any given end-diastolic volume.

Starling Curves, such as those shown in Fig. 2-5, can be recorded in laboratory animals, where they provide useful measurements of changing myocardial contractility. This approach, however, is difficult clinically. Although infusion and removal of blood volume in patients with heart failure could be used to generate a family of Starling Curves, the altered circulatory dynamics also evoke neurohumoral responses that modify contractility (Chapter 4). From a practical standpoint, the hazards of these interventions preclude this approach to measuring contractility in these sick patients.

Clinical Estimation of Myocardial Contractility

A solution to the challenge described in the preceding paragraph was suggested in the early 1960s, when the biophysical principles described in frog sartorius muscle by A. V. Hill in the 1930s were applied to heart muscle in a new area of research called "cardiac mechanics" (for review, see Braunwald et al., 1976; Katz, 1992). Central to this approach are plots of the *force-velocity relationship*, which in skeletal muscle are readily obtained from measurements of the load-dependence of developed tension and shortening velocity during brief tetanic contractions. In the 1960s and 1970s, many viewed the maximal velocity of unloaded shortening (V_{max}, the intercept of the force-velocity curve at zero force) as a definitive measurement of contractility, while P_o, the maximal tension developed when the ends of the muscle are fixed so that shortening cannot take place (isometric tension, the other intercept of the force-velocity curve), was believed to reflect the length-dependent properties of the heart; that is, Starling's law. Unfortunately, several properties of cardiac muscle, for example, its complex architecture, the slow onset of active state, and inability to generate a tetanic contraction, make it impossible to achieve the precision of Hill's determinations in amphibian skeletal muscle (Abbott and Mommaerts, 1959). Despite these limitations, this approach was used in heart muscle (Sonnenblick, 1964) and helped make it possible to confirm the long-held view that myocardial contractility is depressed in the failing heart (Spann et al., 1967). A more detailed discussion of both the force-velocity relationship and this loss of contractile function is deferred to Chapter 3, where the biochemical basis for the depressed contractility seen in failing heart muscle is considered.

Impaired Filling: Relaxation Abnormalities in the Failing Heart

It is only over the past 10 to 15 years that the importance of abnormal filling has come to be recognized in many of these patients (Grossman and Lorell, 1988). This delay, as discussed earlier, was due in part to the widely held view that the major problem in heart failure was simply reduced ejection. In addition, the pressure measurements initially used to quantify the heart's lusitropic properties, while providing some useful indices, lack the precision of the newer indices based on determinations of ventricular volume (Smith et al., 1986). Quantification of the relaxation abnormalities in heart failure therefore remained difficult and clinically impractical until technologic advances in echocardiography and nuclear cardiology provided safe and accurate means by which to document slowed, incomplete filling in the failing heart. These noninvasive methods allow estimates of the rate and extent of filling, which provide excellent clinical indices of lusitropic function.

Many different mechanisms can cause lusitropic abnormalities in patients with heart failure; these range from the mechanical obstruction caused by a stenotic mitral valve to molecular changes that reduce the density of calcium pump molecules in the sarcoplasmic reticulum membrane. Because so many different pathophysiologic mechanisms interact to cause structural and functional disorders that impair filling, efforts to classify and define the mechanistic basis for clinical relaxation abnormalities (including the one that follows) are far from perfect.

This text considers four different pathologic mechanisms that depress lusitropy in the failing heart (Table 2-3). These are *structural abnormalities*, such as the mechanical obstruction to ventricular filling caused by mitral stenosis, pericardial effusion, and concentric hypertrophy; *physiological abnormalities*, such as excess blood remaining in the ventricle after a weak systole and reduced filling time caused by tachycardia; *nonmyocyte abnormalities*, notably the impaired filling caused by connective tissue proliferation within (fibrosis) or at the surface (constrictive pericarditis) of the heart; and *myocyte abnormalities*. The latter can result from a number of different molecular abnormalities, which are discussed in Chapter 3. The pathologic mechanisms listed in Table 2-3, unfortunately, do not correspond to the different hemodynamic manifestations of impaired diastolic function described herein.

A simple way to view changes in the lusitropic properties of the ventricle is depicted in the lower part of Fig. 2-5, which shows a "family" of filling curves analogous to the

---

TABLE 2-3. *Causes of impaired filling by the failing heart*

1. Structural abnormalities
    Valvular disorders, e.g., mitral stenosis
    Pericardial effusion
    Architectural abnormalities, e.g., concentric hypertrophy
2. Physiologic abnormalities
    Increased end-systolic (residual) volume
    Abbreviation of systole (tachycardia)
3. Nonmyocyte abnormalities
    Increased connective tissue, fibrosis
    Constrictive pericarditis
4. Cardiac myocyte abnormalities
    Decreased rate of calcium uptake by the sarcoplasmic reticulum
    Decreased extent of calcium uptake by the sarcoplasmic reticulum
    Increased calcium affinity of the contractile proteins

Starling curves discussed earlier. Here, the curve containing the point "X" is the control, the curve containing point "Y" shows increased lusitropy, and the curve containing point "Z" shows the effects of a negative lusitropic change that impairs filling and so increases diastolic pressure. When examined from a hemodynamic standpoint, diastolic function can be impaired in at least four different ways (Fig. 2-6): a decrease in the rate of pressure fall during isovolumic relaxation (-dP/dt), slowed filling during early diastole, reduced filling throughout diastole, and a volume-dependent increase in diastolic pressure seen as the heart fills late in diastole. The latter can be viewed either as a decrease in compliance (dV/dP, the slope of the curve relating the change in volume for each increment of pressure), or an increase in stiffness (dP/dV, the slope of the curve relating the change in pressure for each increment of volume); these are shown schematically in Fig. 2-7.

Diastolic function can be impaired by changes in the biochemical systems that relax the heart, notably reduced calcium uptake into the sarcoplasmic reticulum, a lower calcium affinity of the pump, and an increase in the calcium affinity of troponin C. Both concentric and eccentric hypertrophy also impair ventricular filling. The impaired filling caused by concentric hypertrophy is readily understood as a consequence of the small cavity volume

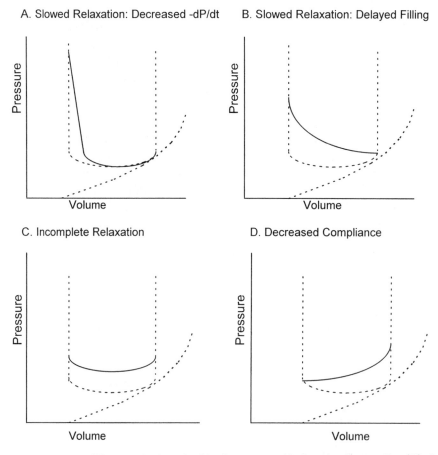

FIG. 2-6. Ventricular filling can be impaired by four types of lusitropic abnormality: **(A)** slowed relaxation with decreased rate of pressure fall (-dP/dt) during isovolumic relaxation; **(B)** slowed relaxation with delayed filling during early diastole; **(C)** incomplete relaxation with impaired filling throughout diastole; **(D)** decreased compliance (increased stiffness).

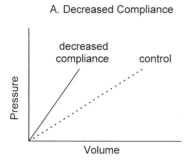
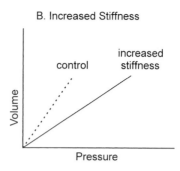

FIG. 2-7. Diagrammatic representations of decreased compliance **(A)** and increased stiffness **(B).** The difference is simply in the way that the variables are plotted.

(Fig. 2-8A), which by decreasing compliance (compare Fig. 2-8A with Fig. 2-7), impedes venous return. The less obvious causes of the reduced filling seen in the eccentrically hypertrophied heart include the higher end-diastolic pressure and volume that occur when end-systolic volume is increased by reduced ejection, the greater wall tension in a dilated ventricle, which according to the Law of Laplace increases as the cavity becomes larger, and fibrosis that occurs following myocardial cell death (Chapter 8).

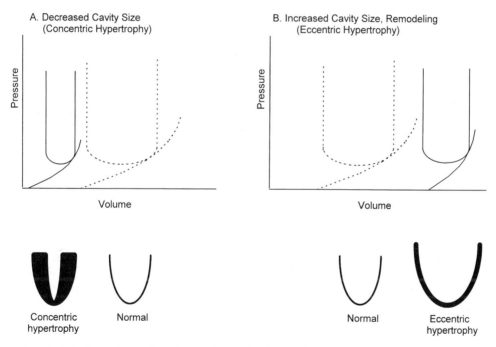

FIG. 2-8. Effects of different patterns of hypertrophy on diastolic function. Normal curves are shown as dotted lines. **A:** Concentric hypertrophy reduces both ventricular volume and compliance. **B:** Eccentric hypertrophy, which increases ventricular volume, is also generally accompanied by a decrease in compliance. Sketches of the architecture of these ventricles are provided in the text; note that the intercept of the diastolic pressure-volume curve at zero pressure is equal to the volume of the relaxed, opened ventricle, which is proportional to the cross-sectional areas shown in these sketches.

Biochemical mechanisms that impair relaxation in the failing heart can be classified as abnormalities that slow relaxation rate (see Fig. 2-6A and B), those in which relaxation is incomplete (see Fig. 2-6C), and those that decrease compliance (see Fig. 2-6D). The physiologic consequences of these three relaxation abnormalities are most prominent at different times during diastole (Table 2-4). Slowed relaxation can reduce the rate of pressure decrease (-dP/dt) during isovolumic relaxation, and the rate of rapid filling during early diastole, or both. Incomplete relaxation increases the steady-state level of diastolic tension, while at the same time decreasing the extent of filling. Loss of compliance causes a steep increase in diastolic pressure as the ventricle fills.

It is difficult to assign specific biochemical mechanisms to these different patterns of impaired lusitropy. Potential causes of slowed relaxation include reduced density of calcium pump ATPase molecules in the sarcoplasmic reticulum membrane, decreased calcium sensitivity of this calcium transport system, and increased calcium-affinity of the troponin complex. Incomplete relaxation can result from persistence of rigor bonds linking the thick and thin filaments when calcium is not removed from troponin; the latter can be caused by a decreased calcium-sensitivity of the sarcoplasmic reticulum calcium pump and an increased calcium affinity of troponin C. Compliance can be decreased by fibrosis and cytoskeletal abnormalities, as well as such dynamic mechanisms as a decrease in the calcium sensitivity of the sarcoplasmic reticulum calcium pump and formation of rigor bonds between the thick and thin filaments of the sarcomere. Calcium overloading of the cytosol, which can be caused by excessive calcium influx or incomplete calcium removal across the plasma membrane, can exacerbate all of these abnormalities.

The classification of the lusitropic abnormalities in the failing heart shown in Table 2-4 and Fig. 2-6 is both oversimplified and incomplete. In the first place, more than one of these different hemodynamic patterns of diastolic dysfunction is generally found; furthermore, as shown in Table 2-4, the biochemical mechanisms that cause these hemodynamic abnormalities overlap significantly. For example, abnormalities of the sarcoplasmic reticulum that impair calcium uptake can both slow relaxation (see Fig. 2-6A and B) and cause relaxation to be incomplete (see Fig. 2-6C). Furthermore, several biochemical abnormalities can slow calcium dissociation from the cardiac contractile proteins, which is essential for the heart to relax. These include a reduced density of calcium pump molecules in the sarcoplasmic reticulum membrane, isoform shifts and heritable abnormalities of the proteins of the thin filament that increase the calcium affinity of troponin C, energy-starvation that impairs calcium removal from the cytosol by lowering the free energy of adenosine triphosphate (ATP) hydrolysis, allosteric effects of a decrease in ATP concentration that slows the

TABLE 2-4. *Biochemical mechanisms that can impair filling in the failing heart*

Hemodynamic abnormality	Biochemical causes
Slowed relaxation	
Decreased rate of pressure fall (-dP/dt)	Slowed turnover rate of SR Ca pump
Decreased filling rate in *early* diastole	Increased Ca affinity of troponin
Incomplete relaxation	
Increased pressure and impaired filling	Increased collagen (fibrosis)
throughout diastole	Incomplete Ca removal from troponin
	Decreased Ca affinity of SR Ca pump
	Rigor bonds linking thick and thin filaments
	Calcium overloading of the cytosol
Decreased compliance	
Increased pressure and impaired filling *at end*	Increased collagen (fibrosis) and cytoskeletal
of diastole	abnormalities
	Persistent bonds linking thick and thin filaments

Na/Ca exchanger and both the sarcoplasmic reticulum and plasma membrane calcium pumps, and calcium overload. The multiplicity and complexity of the causes of impaired relaxation in the failing heart, which are discussed further in Chapter 3, make it virtually impossible to relate the lusitropic abnormalities commonly seen in these patients to specific biochemical mechanisms.

INTERPLAY BETWEEN THE FAILING HEART AND THE CIRCULATION

To this point, the discussion has focused on the failing heart, highlighting the reduced ejection and impaired filling seen in most of these patients. At this point, the focus is turned to the effects of abnormal pump function on the circulation, focusing first on the immediate hemodynamic consequences of reduced forward flow out of, and impaired venous return into, a damaged ventricle. Chapter 4 completes this aspect of the discussion by detailing the hemodynamic defense reaction that helps the body compensate for the resulting hemodynamic abnormalities.

Heart failure not only involves contractile (inotropic) and relaxation (lusitropic) abnormalities in the myocardium but also altered interactions between the heart and the circulation. The immediate consequences of impaired pump performance are not difficult to predict: reduced forward flow out of the heart decreases filling of the arterial system, while reduced venous return causes blood to back up in the veins behind the failing ventricle (see Fig. 2-1). The clinical manifestations in heart failure, however, are caused not only by the impaired cardiac pump but also by changes that occur throughout the circulation, which is much more than a passive victim in this syndrome.

The interactions between the heart and circulation can be visualized in several ways. Most useful in describing this interplay are pressure-volume loops and Guyton diagrams, which plot the relationships between venous return, cardiac output, and ventricular filling pressure. Pressure-volume loops define the interactions between ventricular filling and venous pressure, and between ejection and arterial pressure; as each loop is inscribed during a single beat, it provides no information regarding the effects of changes in heart rate. Curves that relate venous return and cardiac output to ventricular filling pressure (Guyton diagrams) highlight the interplay between the lusitropic properties of the heart and venous return, and between inotropic properties and cardiac output, but provide little direct information about arterial pressures. Yet each provides a unique view of the interaction between a failing heart and the circulation whose needs it cannot satisfy.

In the current era of physiologic therapy, an appreciation of the interactions between the heart and the circulation is needed to optimize the care of the cardiac patient. A clear understanding of the impact of the failing heart on the peripheral circulation and the way in which altered hemodynamics modify cardiac loading are essential in predicting the clinical consequences of therapeutic strategies that alter arteriolar resistance, blood volume, and cardiac performance. The following discussion first reviews these interactions on a beat to beat basis, using the pressure-volume loop as a guide to understanding, and then in terms of the interplay between central venous pressure, venous return, and cardiac output. To facilitate understanding of these relationships, a few simple concepts and definitions are reviewed.

Factors That Determine Work and Energy Expenditure by the Heart

The ejection of a volume of blood under pressure represents a form of mechanical work, as is readily seen in the product of pressure (dynes/cm^2) times volume (cm^3), which has the correct units for work (dynes cm). This mechanical work, called *stroke work*, is the work performed during each beat, and is readily calculated as the product of the volume of blood ejected during each beat (stroke volume, or SV) and the pressure (P) at which the blood is ejected:

$$\text{Stroke work} = P \times SV \qquad \text{Equation 2.2}$$

Because arterial pressure changes throughout ejection, stroke work is more accurately the integral PdV, where P is the pressure at which each increment (dV) of the stroke volume is ejected. This refinement, however, is cumbersome and adds little to a practical understanding of heart failure, and so is almost never used clinically.

Stroke volume is equal to end-diastolic volume (EDV) minus end-systolic volume (ESV), the "residual" volume remaining in the ventricle at the end of systole. This allows the equation for stroke work to be expanded:

$$\text{Stroke work} = P \times (EDV - ESV) \qquad \text{Equation 2.3}$$

Equation 2.3 indicates that three variables determine stroke work: EDV, ESV, and ejection pressure. The importance of this equation lies in the fact that each of these determinants of stroke work has different energetic implications.

The *Law of Laplace* defines the relationship between the geometry of the heart, the pressure within its cavity, and wall tension. Even though the complex shape of the human heart makes precise calculations virtually impossible, wall tension can be seen to be directly proportional to cavity pressure and cavity size, and inversely proportional to wall thickness:

$$\text{Wall tension} \propto \frac{\text{Pressure} \times \text{Radius}}{\text{Wall Thickness}} \qquad \text{Equation 2.4}$$

The importance of the Law of Laplace lies in the fact that wall tension is a major determinant of both cardiac energy expenditure and efficiency; a higher wall tension increases the first and decreases the second.

The *external work* of the heart is generally expressed as *minute work*, the work performed per minute. Minute work, which in physical terms is a *power*, is simply stroke work (SV × P, see Equation 2.2) multiplied by heart rate (HR):

$$\text{Minute work} = HR \times SV \times P \qquad \text{Equation 2.5}$$

Cardiac output (CO) is the product of HR × SV, so that:

$$\text{Minute work} = CO \times P. \qquad \text{Equation 2.6}$$

Because stroke volume = EDV - ESV, there are actually four determinants of minute work:

$$\text{Minute work} = P \times HR \times (EDV - ESV) \qquad \text{Equation 2.7}$$

Two types of work must be considered (Table 2-5) in evaluating the energetics of cardiac contraction. The first is the *external work* done to eject blood under pressure into the great vessels; this is the "useful" work of the heart. More than three fourths of the energy expended by the heart, however, is normally degraded into heat (see Table 2-5). Some of this energy is expended in such chemical processes as metabolism and ion transport (see Katz, 1992). A major contribution to the inefficiency of cardiac contraction is the *internal work* that is performed in stretching elastic and viscous elements in the walls of the contracting heart because most of this energy is degraded to heat when the heart relaxes.

TABLE 2-5. *Major forms of left ventricular work*

External (useful) work: (15%–25% of total work); energy used to pump blood
  Pressure-volume work: (approximately 95% of external work). Energy imparted to "lift" blood from the pulmonary veins to the aorta.
  Kinetic work: (approximately 5% of external work). Energy imparted to move the column of blood through the aortic valve as it leaves the ventricle; subsequently converted to pressure-volume work as blood flow slows in the aorta.
Internal (wasted) work: (75%–85% of total work); degraded to heat during diastole
  Work done to stretch elasticities and to rearrange myofibrillar structure during tension development

This table does not consider the large amount of energy expended by the biochemical reactions involved in such processes as oxidative phosphorylation, excitation-contraction coupling, and relaxation.

A portion of this internal work can help the heart to eject because the energy stored in these elasticities contributes to the decrease in ventricular volume during ejection. The fact that ejection allows internal work to be converted to useful work explains some of the beneficial energetic effects of unloading the failing heart with vasodilators.

The product BP × HR, called the *double product*, provides a useful clinical index of left ventricular energy consumption. The reason is that these two variables contribute both to external (useful) work and to the internal work that stretches elasticities in the walls of the heart. Stroke volume, while an important determinant of external work, has much less impact on internal work because shortening of these elasticities during ejection converts some of the stored potential energy into useful work.

Internal work is directly proportional to wall tension, so that the progressive dilatation (remodeling) generally seen in failing hearts reduces efficiency. According to the laws of geometry, less wall shortening is needed to eject a given volume of blood from a large ventricle than from a small ventricle. It therefore follows that less sarcomere shortening is needed to eject a given stroke volume in a dilated heart (see Katz, 1992); for this reason, dilatation of the failing heart (see Chapter 1) reduces efficiency. High wall tension also reduces efficiency by increasing the stretch on the elasticities and viscosities in the walls of the heart; as a result, elevation of wall tension in decompensated heart failure increases internal work and so worsens the state of energy starvation discussed in Chapter 3. These considerations define an important goal in managing the patient with heart failure: to minimize cardiac energy expenditure by minimizing wall tension. Tachycardia also increases internal work simply by increasing the number of times tension must be developed in the walls of the ventricle. Drugs that slow heart rate, like those that reduce wall tension, can therefore be expected to improve cardiac energetics in patients with heart failure.

The fact that the energy requirements of the heart are determined not only by the external (useful) work but also by how this work is performed is of central importance in the management of heart failure. As discussed earlier, this reflects the importance of internal work (see Table 2-5). The most efficient way to increase cardiac work is to decrease ESV, which can be done either by increasing contractility or reducing arterial impedance (afterload). Increasing sarcomere shortening during ejection not only reduces wall tension and internal work, according to the Law of Laplace, but also allows more of the energy stored in the stretched elasticities in the walls of the heart to be converted to useful work, rather than being degraded to heat during diastole.

The four determinants of minute work in Equation 2.7 have different effects on energy demands. A decrease in ESV, which increases stroke volume, is energetically the most advantageous means by which to increase the work of a failing heart because, according to the Law of Laplace (Equation 2.4), wall tension—and thus internal work—is less in the smaller heart. More expensive are increases in P, HR, and EDV. These considerations provide an important rationale for afterload reduction in the treatment of heart failure: the ability of vasodilators to unload the heart not only facilitates ejection and increases cardiac output, but by reducing ESV, these drugs reduce myocardial energy demands. However, as discussed later in this text, vasodilator therapy in heart failure often worsens long-term prognosis because too great or too rapid a decrease in blood pressure can evoke a maladaptive neurohumoral response.

Afterload, the pressure at which the aortic valve opens to allow the heart to eject, is determined by both peripheral resistance and aortic impedance. Resistance and impedance, while related, are not identical to one other; in fact, they are determined by different regions of the arterial system. Resistance, the main determinant of mean arterial pressure and the rate at which blood flows out of the arteries to perfuse the peripheral tissues, is regulated mainly by the diameter of small arterioles, which are often called resistance vessels. Aortic impedance, which determines the increase in pressure for a given increment of blood volume in the aorta, is influenced largely by the elasticities of the aorta and other large arteries. Loss of this elasticity, which occurs during normal aging and is accelerated by arteriosclerotic changes in the large arteries, increases impedance. The result is that ejection of a given stroke volume causes a greater increase in aortic systolic pressure even though mean aortic pressure remains unchanged because aortic diastolic pressure is decreased. The elevated aortic pressure increases afterload, which, as discussed earlier, is a major determinant of myocardial energy expenditure, while the reduced aortic diastolic pressure, which is a major determinant of nutrient coronary flow, exacerbates the state of energy starvation commonly encountered in the failing heart (Chapter 3).

Effects of Heart Failure on Pressure-Volume Loops

A useful way to examine the interactions between the heart and circulation is to construct a pressure-volume loop, which plots the changes in ventricular pressure and volume that occur during a single cardiac cycle (Fig. 2-9). Inscription of the pressure-volume loop begins at end-diastole and is inscribed in a counterclockwise direction, passing through four phases. The first, *isovolumic contraction*, begins at the end of diastole when tension develops in the walls of the left ventricle. The increasing intraventricular pressure closes the mitral valve so that until ventricular pressure exceeds that in the aorta and the aortic valve opens, blood can neither enter nor leave the ventricle. Because pressure increases at constant volume during this phase of the cardiac cycle, isovolumic contraction causes an upward deflection of the loop. The second phase, that of *ejection*, begins after the aortic valve opens and blood flows into the aorta. The reduction in ventricular volume during ejection causes the pressure-volume loop to turn to the left. Aortic pressure first increases because ejection is initially rapid, and then decreases when slowing of ejection allows blood to run out of the aorta into the periphery more rapidly than it enters from the ventricle. Systole ends at a point along the end-systolic pressure-volume relationship, which as described later can be viewed as a "Starling curve" that defines the inotropic state of the ventricle. The third phase, *isovolumic relaxation*, begins after the aortic valve closes and ends after the decrease in left ventricular pressure allows the mitral valve to open. The final phase, that of *filling*, begins when the mitral valve opens and blood flows from the atrium into the relaxed ventricle. Left ventricular pressure and volume then increase gradually to end at a point along the end-diastolic pressure-volume relationship that is determined by the lusitropic properties of the relaxed ventricle. The blood that enters the ventricle from the left atrium generates the preload for the next contraction. Atrial systole, which provides a final "kick" that completes ventricular filling at the end of diastole, cannot be seen on these loops.

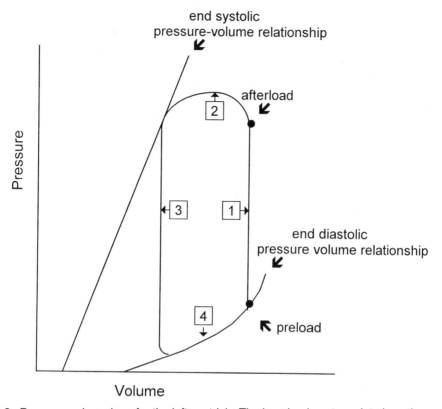

FIG. 2-9. Pressure-volume loop for the left ventricle. The loop begins at a point along the end-diastolic pressure-volume relationship that is determined by venous return (preload). After pressure is developed during the phase of isovolumic contraction (*1*), ejection (*2*) begins when ventricular pressure exceeds that in the aorta (i.e., the heart meets its afterload) and the aortic valve opens. The increase and subsequent decrease in aortic pressure during this phase reflect the fact that ejection is more rapid than runoff from the aorta during early ejection, whereas the opposite is true later in systole. Ejection ends at a point along the end-systolic pressure-volume relationship, which is determined by the inotropic properties of the ventricle, after which the aortic valve closes and pressure decreases during the phase of isovolumic relaxation (*3*). Filling (*4*) begins after left ventricular pressure decreases below that in the left atrium, which allows the mitral valve to open. Filling follows the end-diastolic pressure volume relationship, which is determined by the lusitropic properties of the ventricle. The points along the end-diastolic and end-systolic pressure volume relationships at which systole begins and ends are determined by preload and afterload, respectively.

Each pressure-volume loop is constrained by two pressure-volume relationships, each of which reflects one of the two key properties of the heart (see Fig. 2-9). These are the *end-diastolic pressure-volume relationship*, which reflects the lusitropic properties of the relaxed heart, and the *end-systolic pressure-volume relationship*, which is determined by the inotropic state of the contracting ventricle (myocardial contractility). The interactions between the heart and circulation at end-diastole and at end-systole are best understood by considering the end-diastolic and end-systolic points that lie on each of these relationships. The end-diastolic point, which is located along the end-diastolic pressure-volume relationship, is determined by the venous return that fills the ventricle at the end of diastole (preload) and by the lusitropic properties of the ventricle. The end-systolic point, which is located along the end-systolic pressure-volume relationship, is determined by aortic diastolic pressure (afterload) and the inotropic state. When the heart "meets" its afterload (the aortic diastolic pressure) at the end of isovolumic contraction, the aortic valve opens. Although aortic pressure first increases and then decreases during ejection, wall tension decreases throughout this phase of the cardiac cycle because of progressive reduction of cavity volume and thickening of the walls of the heart (see Equation 2.4). For this reason, afterload, as viewed by a cardiac myocyte, decreases steadily during ejection.

The two pressure-volume relationships shown in Fig. 2-9 represent limits that enclose all possible pressure-volume loops at all possible levels of inotropy and lusitropy. Although changing preload and afterload shift intraventricular pressure and volume along these two relationships, these limits cannot be exceeded. Only a change in either the inotropic and lusitropic state of the ventricle can alter these limits. In this way, the properties of the ventricle determine the two pressure-volume relationships, while the positions of the end-diastolic and end-systolic points along these lines are determined by the circulatory hemodynamics (preload and afterload, respectively).

Decreased Inotropy

A sudden decrease in contractility, as occurs clinically when a region of the left ventricle loses its blood supply following coronary occlusion (acute myocardial infarction), shifts the end-systolic pressure-volume relationship (the Starling Curve) to the right and downward (Fig. 2-10). In the pressure-volume loop generated by the first beat after such a decrease of contractility, afterload has not changed (see Fig. 2-10); however, because the heart has become weaker, ejection is reduced ("forward failure"). Subsequent adjustments to the circulation modify these pressure-volume loops; these include a rapid increase in preload, caused when reduced ejection increases end-systolic volume, and changes in the peripheral circulation caused by the neurohumoral responses (see Chapter 4).

Decreased Inotropy

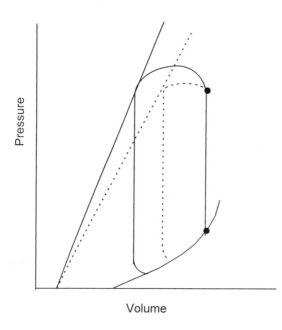

FIG. 2-10. Effects of decreased inotropy on the pressure-volume relationship. (The normal curve is shown as a *solid line.*) The downward shift in the end-systolic pressure-volume relationship (*dotted line*, which represents a shift to a lower Starling Curve) reduces ejection, even though preload and afterload (*circles*) have not changed.

Decreased Inotropy Followed by a Rise in End-Diastolic Pressure and Volume

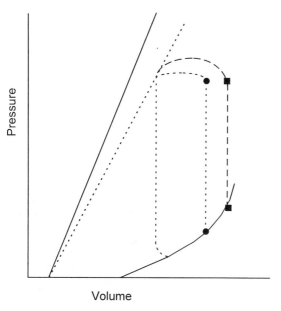

FIG. 2-11. Effects of increased end-diastolic volume (dashed line), caused by the reduced ejection that follows the decrease in inotropy shown in Fig. 2-10 (dotted line). Although afterload has not changed in this example (compare upper square and circle), the increased preload (lower square) increases stroke volume.

The reduced ejection in the cycle shown in Fig. 2-10 increases end-systolic (residual) volume, as shown in Fig. 2-11. If, for simplicity, it is assumed that venous return remains unchanged, addition of this constant venous return to the increased end-systolic volume at the end of the cycle chown in Fig. 2-10 increases end-diastolic volume. This moves the end-diastolic point upward and to the right along the end-diastolic pressure-volume relationship. As shown in Fig. 2-11, this increases stroke volume, albeit at the expense of an increase in filling pressure ("backward failure"). This response is one manifestation of Starling's Law of the Heart. In real life, this compensation becomes even more complex because the increased end-diastolic pressure reduces venous return, as discussed later when the effects of a decrease in contractility on the Guyton diagrams are described.

Decreased Lusitropy

A sudden loss of lusitropy, for example, an increase in diastolic compliance, shifts the end-diastolic pressure-volume relationship to the left and upward, which increases the pressure needed to achieve a given increment in diastolic volume (Fig. 2-12). This situation can occur during an transient coronary occlusion, as occurs when a thrombus forms on a ruptured atherosclerotic plaque, or when an interventional cardiologist inflates an angioplasty balloon in a diseased coronary artery. If, as in the preceding example, the first beat after such an abrupt decrease in diastolic compliance is examined, the increased resistance to filling elevates end-diastolic pressure while at the same time decreasing end-diastolic volume (see Fig. 2-12). The result is a leftward shift of the pressure-volume loop in which, even

Decreased Lusitropy

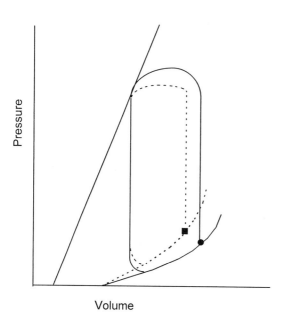

FIG. 2-12. Effects of decreased lusitropy on the pressure-volume relationship. (The normal curve is shown as a *solid line.*) The upward shift in the end-diastolic pressure-volume relationship (*dotted line*), which represents a loss of compliance, increases end-diastolic pressure, decreases end-diastolic volume, and at the constant afterload shown in this figure, reduces ejection.

though diastolic pressures are increased, ventricular volume has decreased. As long as inotropic properties (i.e., the end-systolic pressure-volume relationship) remain unchanged, stroke volume is decreased.

The decreased stroke volume depicted in Fig. 2-12 increases residual (end-systolic) volume, as shown in Fig. 2-13, and causes the ventricle to dilate. As a result, the stiff heart op-

Decreased Lusitropy Followed by
a Rise in End-Diastolic Pressure and Volume

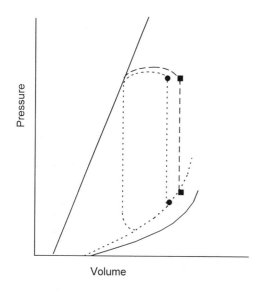

FIG. 2-13. Compensation for decreased lusitropy shown in Fig. 2-12 (dotted line) when end-systolic volume is increased by reduced ejection (*dashed line*). Although afterload has not changed in this example (compare upper circle and square), the increased preload (lower circle and square) leads to an increase in stroke volume, but at the price of a further increase in diastolic pressure.

erates at increased diastolic pressure and volume, which, according to Starling's Law of the Heart, helps this situation by increasing stroke volume. As discussed in Chapter 4, these simple hemodynamic adjustments are modified by the neurohumoral responses to the decrease in cardiac performance.

Combination of Decreased Inotropy and Lusitropy

Both ejection and filling are commonly impaired in heart failure. This "compresses" the pressure volume loop, as shown in Fig. 2-14, which depicts the effects of a decrease in both inotropy and lusitropy where neither preload nor afterload has changed. The smaller area within the pressure-volume loop, which reflects the reduced work of the failing heart, is expressed in this example mainly by a decrease in stroke volume.

Circulatory adjustments initiated by the decrease in stroke volume modify this pressure-volume loop. These include increases in end-diastolic pressure and volume, caused by the reduced ejection, which tends to restore stroke volume, albeit at the expense of a further increase in end-diastolic pressure that worsens the signs and symptoms of backward failure (Fig. 2-15). Another major adjustment is provided by the hemodynamic defense reaction discussed in Chapter 4, which by increasing contractility, shifts the end-systolic pressure-volume relationship upward and to the right, which allows the heart to eject more blood at a given end-diastolic volume (Fig. 2-16).

Decreased Inotropy and Lusitropy

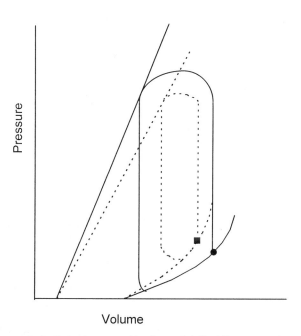

FIG. 2-14. A decrease in both inotropy and lusitropy (*dotted line*; normal curves are shown as *solid lines*), as commonly occurs in the failing heart. These abnormalities severely reduce stroke volume even though end-diastolic pressure has increased (compare circle and square). In this, as in the preceding examples, afterload has been assumed to remain constant; in real life, a variety of compensatory mechanisms modify the pressure-volume loops in these figures.

Decreased Inotropy and Lusitropy Followed by
a Rise in End-Diastolic Pressure and Volume

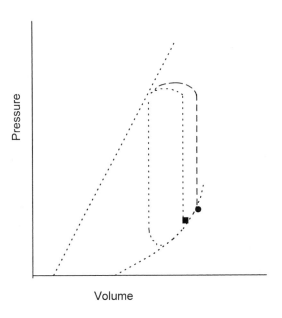

Volume

FIG. 2-15. Compensation for a decrease in both inotropy and lusitropy (*dotted lines*; for simplicity, the control curves are omitted in this figure) by increased end-diastolic pressure and volume. The increased preload (*circle*) has increased stroke volume (*dashed line*), even though afterload has not changed.

Decreased Inotropy and Lusitropy Followed by
an Increase in Contractility

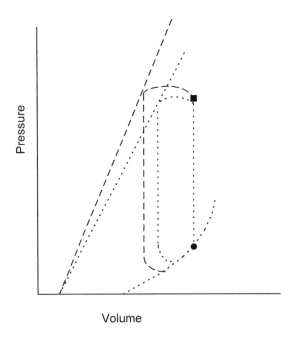

Volume

FIG. 2-16. Compensation for a decrease in both inotropy and lusitropy (*dotted lines*; for simplicity, the control curves are omitted in this figure) by an increase in contractility. The latter, which shifts the end-systolic pressure-volume relationship upward and to the left (*dashed line*), increases stroke volume, even though preload (*circle*) and afterload (*square*) are unchanged.

INTERPLAY BETWEEN VENOUS RETURN AND CARDIAC OUTPUT

The interplay between venous return and cardiac output, which must be equal to one another at any steady state, is depicted in Fig 2-17. This figure, which shows how blood flow into and out of the right ventricle depends on right atrial pressure, is often referred to as a Guyton diagram, named for Arthur Guyton, who made many contributions to physiology over the past 4 decades. Fig. 2-17 shows the opposite influences of changing right atrial pressure on cardiac output and venous return. An increase in right atrial pressure increases cardiac output and decreases venous return, whereas a decrease in this pressure decreases cardiac output and increases venous return. Similar curves showing a similar relationship can be drawn for the left heart.

The effects of atrial pressure on cardiac output reflect the increased ability of the heart to do work at a higher filling pressure—this is, of course, simply another way to plot Starling's Law of the Heart. The other curve, which shows that increasing right atrial pressure reduces venous return, is readily understood because the right atrium is "downstream" from the systemic veins that return blood to the right atrium. Increased right atrial pressure impedes the return of blood from the veins to the heart, so that the slope of this curve is opposite to that relating right atrial pressure to cardiac output.

The intercept of the curve relating right atria pressure to venous return falls to zero as right atrial pressure increases; the pressure at which blood flow ceases (both venous return and cardiac output become zero) is the *mean circulatory filling pressure*. This is the pressure that would be found in all parts of the circulation if the heart were to stop and pressures throughout the vascular system came to equilibrium. In reaching this equilibrium, of course, arterial pressures would decrease and venous pressures would increase.

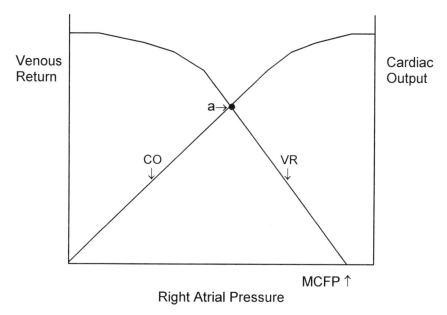

FIG. 2-17. Curves showing the dependence of venous return and cardiac output on right atrial pressure ("Guyton diagrams"). At steady state, there is a unique value for both dependent variables (*point a*). Mean circulatory filling pressure (MCFP), the arrow along the abscissa at the left, is the right atrial pressure seen when the circulation is stopped and all pressures throughout the vascular system come to equilibrium.

The mean circulatory filling pressure is closer to the low pressure in the veins than the higher pressures in the arteries because there is much more blood in the venous circulation. Mean circulatory filling pressure, which is about 7 mmHg in anesthetized dogs, is shown by the small arrow at the lower right in Fig. 2-17.

In the intact circulation, a steady state is reached where blood flow from the veins into the heart equals that from the heart into the arteries. This steady state is represented by the unique point where the curves relating right atrial pressure to venous return and cardiac output intersect (see Fig. 2-17). This intersection defines the right atrial pressure at which venous return and cardiac output are equal. Any deviation from this steady state will initiate adjustments that bring the circulation to a new steady state, where blood flow into and out of the heart again becomes equal.

The two curves in Fig. 2-17 show the effects of the circulation on the heart, where increasing venous return brings about a corresponding increase in cardiac output through the operation of Starling's Law of the Heart, and the effects of the heart on the circulation, where an increase in cardiac output lowers the pressure behind the heart (atrial pressure) and so facilitates venous return. Changes in the steady state described above, where venous return and cardiac output are equal, can be brought about by a variety of interventions, for example, by fluid retention and depressed contractility. The intersection between the two curves shown in Fig. 2-17, therefore, can shift in response to changes in the peripheral circulation (e.g., fluid overload), the heart (e.g., decreased contractility), or both.

In the failing heart, where a decrease in contractility causes atrial pressure to increase (see Fig. 2-11), venous return is reduced. These effects are seen in the Guyton diagrams depicted in Fig. 2-18, in which cardiac output is decreased by a fall in contractility. The

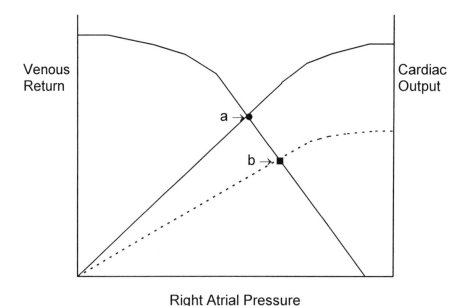

FIG. 2-18. Effect of a decrease in inotropy (*dotted line*) on the curves shown in Fig. 2-17, where point a is the initial steady state of venous return and cardiac output. At the new steady state, shown as point b, cardiac output and venous return are reduced, while right atrial pressure is elevated.

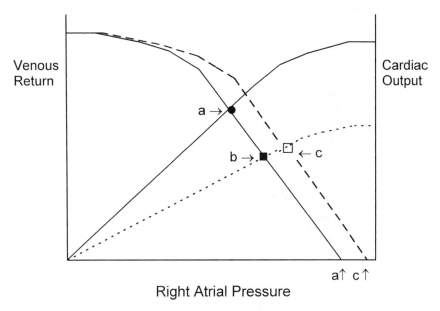

FIG. 2-19. Compensation for the decrease in contractility depicted in Fig. 2-18 by an increase in circulating blood volume (*dashed line*). The increase in mean circulatory filling pressure (from the control upward arrow a to the new arrow c) has shifted the relationship between venous return and right atrial pressure upward and to the right. The steady state, which in Fig. 2-18 shifted from the filled circle labeled "a" to the filled square labeled "b," is shifted to the open square labeled "c." This increases venous return and cardiac output (the latter along the depressed Starling Curve), but at the cost of a further increase in diastolic pressure.

resulting increase in right atrial pressure brings the circulation to a new steady state by reducing venous return.

One feature of the neurohumoral response to the decrease in cardiac output depicted in Fig. 2-18 is fluid retention by the kidneys (see Chapter 4). The result is an increase in blood volume that, as shown in Fig. 2-19, causes a rightward shift in the curve relating venous return to right atrial pressure. If the circulation is stopped, the extra blood volume would increase mean circulatory filling pressure. The compensation brought about by fluid retention increases cardiac output, but at the expense of a further increase in venous pressure. This example illustrates a general rule, which is that the compensatory responses to impaired cardiac function are "two-edged swords" in that they cut both ways, both alleviating and worsening the patient's condition. Because this rule also applies to virtually every form of therapy, an understanding of pathophysiology is essential in managing these patients.

SIGNS AND SYMPTOMS OF HEART FAILURE

In concluding this chapter on the hemodynamics of heart failure, to explain several clinical features of this syndrome the discussion returns to the concepts of forward and backward failure. Although the terms lack precision in describing pathophysiology, these concepts are valuable both for understanding the causes of the disability in these patients and as a guide to treatment.

The consequences of increased venous pressure (backward failure) are readily understood because transmission of this pressure upstream behind a failing ventricle raises capillary pressure, which increases the hydrostatic forces that cause fluid to be transudated across the capillary endothelium into the tissues. The result is edema in the lungs of patients with left heart failure, and in the soft tissues and body cavities in right heart failure. Gravity operates in both to favor fluid accumulation in dependent regions—the lower portions of the lungs in left heart failure and the lower extremities in right heart failure. In forward failure, which must involve both ventricles, the major symptom is fatigue; this symptom is not a direct consequence of the low cardiac output but instead is due mainly to a molecular disorder involving the skeletal muscles.

Backward Failure of the Left Ventricle

The shortness of breath (dyspnea) generally reported by patients with left heart failure is due in large part to the increased work required to ventilate the congested lungs, which like a water-logged sponge, become stiff and inelastic (Mancini et al., 1992). Whereas the normal work of breathing is barely perceived, elevated pulmonary venous pressure, by filling the lungs with water, increases respiratory effort to such a point that it cannot be ignored. The resulting difficulty in breathing, called *dyspnea,* is exacerbated by weakness of the respiratory muscles (Mancini et al., 1995; Poole-Wilson and Ferrari, 1996). Arterial hypoxia, caused by ventilation-perfusion mismatch and impaired oxygen exchange in the edematous pulmonary interstitium (Wasserman et al., 1997), probably plays only a minor role in causing cardiac dyspnea (Sullivan et al., 1988, Poole-Wilson and Ferrari, 1996). The extent to which left atrial pressure is elevated is not a good predictor of the severity of dyspnea in chronic left heart failure (Wilson et al., 1995) because reactive pulmonary vasoconstriction and obliteration of small pulmonary arteries in many of these patients protects the lungs from overfilling. This response exchanges one problem (pulmonary congestion) for another (pulmonary hypertension).

The fluid transudated through the pulmonary capillaries in left heart failure appears first in the interstitium, where it can be carried into the systemic veins via the lymphatics. This interstitial edema occurs mainly in the lower lobes of the lung because of the effects of gravity, which explains the common appearance of rales and Kerley B lines at the lung bases. The former are crackling sounds, described by Hippocrates as like the "seething of vinegar," whereas the latter are thin horizontal lines seen at the lung bases in the chest radiograph. Another radiologic feature of left heart failure is "cephalization" of the pulmonary venous shadows, which occurs when increased pulmonary venous pressure expands the veins supplying the upper lobes of the lungs; this reduces the normal difference in diameter between these vessels and the pulmonary veins supplying the lower lobes, which are normally engorged by the effects of gravity on the pressure distribution in these thin-walled vessels.

Dyspnea, which as noted in Chapter 1 is the major symptom of left heart failure, generally becomes more severe when the patient lies down (orthopnea). This occurs because elevation of the legs increases venous return to the right heart, which by increasing blood flow into the lungs and lung stiffness, exacerbates the symptom of dyspnea. Paroxysmal nocturnal dyspnea, another symptom described in Chapter 1, occurs when fluid is resorbed from the tissues in dependent parts of the body (mainly the legs) when these patients lie in bed. The slow expansion of blood volume increases mean circulatory filling pressure (see Fig. 2-19), which causes an increase in left ventricular diastolic and pulmonary capillary pressures. This generally occurs during the night, causing these patients to awaken suddenly with dyspnea.

As backward failure of the left heart becomes more severe, the amount of fluid transudated into the pulmonary interstitium begins to exceed the ability of the lymphatics to carry this out of the lungs. The result is fluid accumulation in the air spaces, which interferes with gas exchange. Because oxygen is much less water soluble than carbon dioxide, the major abnormality is arterial hypoxia.

Before the availability of powerful diuretics, end-stage left heart failure led eventually to pulmonary edema, in which the patient literally drowns in fluid that fills the lungs. Some protection against this catastrophe can be provided by pulmonary arterial vasoconstriction and a vascular growth response that obliterates the pulmonary arterioles. By reducing blood flow into the pulmonary capillaries, these responses can blunt some of the consequences of backward failure of the left heart (Wood, 1954). This does not, however, solve the problem; instead, by causing pulmonary artery pressure to increase (pulmonary hypertension), these responses convert left heart failure to right heart failure.

Backward Failure of the Right Ventricle

Backward failure of the right heart, as occurs in severe pulmonary hypertension, causes fluid to be transudated into the soft tissues and body cavities. When severe, this results in dropsy, a key feature of the horrible suffering described by Corvisart (see Chapter 1). This misery can generally be avoided by modern diuretics, which blunt the inappropriate fluid retention by the kidneys in these patients. By replacing backward failure with forward failure, these drugs have changed the major clinical manifestations of this syndrome. As a result, fatigue, rather than fluid retention, is generally the primary cause of disability in these patients. It is for this reason that the term *congestive heart failure* (*CHF*) is being replaced by the more general term *heart failure*.

Careful examination of the jugular veins provides an accurate measure of right atrial pressure and thus the severity of backward failure of the right heart. This is unlike left heart failure, in which considerable skill supplemented by expensive, invasive tests are often needed to quantify the extent to which left atrial pressure is elevated. Analysis of the waveform of the jugular venous pressure also provides valuable information regarding the state of the tricuspid valve and the stiffness of the right ventricle (for further details, refer to standard textbooks of medicine, cardiology, and physical diagnosis).

Forward Failure

As noted throughout this text, elimination of one problem in heart failure generally worsens other problems. The ability of diuretics to alleviate the signs and symptoms of backward failure is a clear example of this rule. By reducing preload, diuresis leads to a decrease in cardiac output that worsens forward failure. In end-stage heart failure, in which the heart has little reserve and can become preload dependent, diuresis can lower cardiac output to such an extent as to cause renal and hepatic failure. Yet from practical and humane considerations, death in the coma caused by renal and hepatic failure can be preferable to the agonizing death of an alert patient who drowns slowly with undertreated fluid retention. Such deaths, vividly described in 18th and 19th century texts, are rarely seen today.

The ability of diuretics to alleviate backward failure has caused fatigue to emerge as one of the most common and troublesome symptoms in heart failure. Once attributed to reduced perfusion of the skeletal muscles, it is now apparent that fatigue is not a *direct* consequence of low cardiac output. Instead, the major cause of this symptom is a skeletal muscle myopathy that, while initiated by forward failure, is due to structural and molecular changes in these muscles (Perreault et al., 1993; Wilson, 1995, 1996; Schaufelberger et al., 1995; Poole-Wilson and Ferrari, 1996). Skeletal muscle abnormalities include atrophy, rapid appearance of acidosis during exercise, accelerated phosphocreatine consumption, loss of mitochondria and oxidative enzymes, changes in fiber type, and alterations in myosin isoforms (Massie et al., 1987; Simonini et al., 1996a, 1996b). This myopathy, in some ways, resembles disuse atrophy (Hambrecht et al., 1995; Simonini et al., 1996a) and is accompanied by biochemical changes similar to those that cause fatigue (Fitts, 1994). The causes of these molecular abnormalities, which have many similarities to those seen in the failing heart, remain poorly understood. Among the potential causes of this myopathy are the actions of inflammatory cytokines (see Chapter 5). The severity of the skeletal muscle myopathy of heart failure correlates poorly with the severity of left ventricular dysfunction. Although ejection fraction is a good predictor of survival, it provides surprisingly little information about exercise intolerance or the extent of clinical disability (Benge et al., 1980; Franciosa et al., 1981; Lipkin and Poole-Wilson, 1986; Volterrani et al., 1994).

From a practical standpoint, evidence that the symptoms associated with the skeletal myopathy of heart failure can be alleviated when these patients are encouraged to exercise (Coats et al, 1990; McKelvie et al., 1995; Belardinelli et al., 1995; Hambrecht et al., 1997) is changing yet another dogma regarding this syndrome: that rest is a keystone of therapy. The symptomatic benefit of moderate exercise in these patients explains a "training effect," well known from clinical trials, in which effort tolerance increases markedly during a series of exercise tests even though there had been no change in therapy. These benefits of exercise contradict the once universal view that heart failure should be treated with prolonged rest (see Chapter 1), an approach that even led to the recommendation that these patients should spend up to a year at complete bed rest (Burch et al., 1963). Today's recognition that the disability caused by heart failure can be alleviated by carefully planned exercise program represents yet another major advance in the management of this condition (see Chapter 10).

SUMMARY

Although the hemodynamic abnormalities described in this chapter are responsible for most of the clinical features seen in the patient with heart failure, it is clear that this syndrome is much more than an abnormality of pump function. It is not apparent that changes in ventricular architecture (Fig. 2-20) play a major role in determining both pathophysiology and prognosis. As discussed in subsequent chapters, the body's efforts to compensate for a weakened pump, along with a maladaptive growth response in the failing heart, play a critical role in determining prognosis. In the patient with heart failure, both eventually cause more problems than they solve. The progressive, long-term deterioration of the failing heart, therefore, is more important but less evident than the obvious hemodynamic abnormalities described in this chapter.

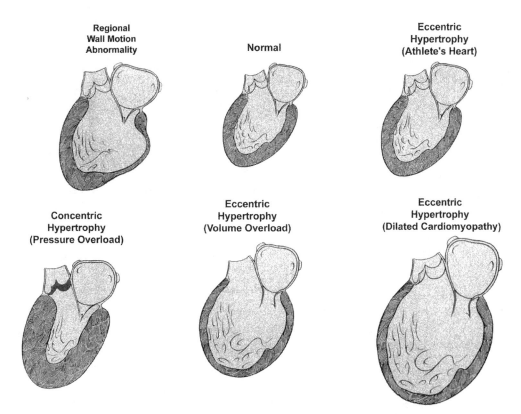

Regional Wall Motion Abnormality

Normal

Eccentric Hypertrophy (Athlete's Heart)

Concentric Hypertrophy (Pressure Overload)

Eccentric Hypertrophy (Volume Overload)

Eccentric Hypertrophy (Dilated Cardiomyopathy)

FIG. 2-20. Five examples of the many architectural patterns of cardiac hypertrophy; a normal left ventricle is depicted at the center of the top row. The eccentric hypertrophy seen in the "athlete's heart" (*top, right*) is a physiologic hypertrophy that differs from the pathologic eccentric hypertrophy (systolic dysfunction) seen in dilated cardiomyopathies (*bottom, right*) and following a chronic volume overload such as occurs in aortic insufficiency (*bottom, center*). The latter differ from one another in that ejection is impaired to a greater extent in dilated cardiomyopathy. A regional wall motion abnormality (*top, left*), commonly seen as the result of myocardial infarction, causes the noninfarcted regions of the ventricle to undergo eccentric hypertrophy. All are different from the concentric hypertrophy caused by chronic pressure overload (diastolic dysfunction), as occurs in chronic hypertension and aortic stenosis (*bottom, left*). Whereas physiologic eccentric hypertrophy (the athlete's heart) does not appear to shorten survival, all forms of pathologic eccentric hypertrophy lead to the progressive dilatation called "remodeling." Deterioration is generally more rapid in dilated cardiomyopathy and the eccentric hypertrophy caused by a regional wall motion abnormality than in chronic volume overload. Progressive dilatation (remodeling) of a concentrically hypertrophied heart is uncommon, but diastolic dysfunction, like systolic dysfunction, leads to deterioration of the overloaded myocardium.

REFERENCES

Abbott BC, Mommaerts WFHM (1959). Study of inotropic mechanisms in papillary muscle preparation. *J Gen Physiol* 42:533–551.

Belardinelli R, Georgiou D, Scocco, D, Barstow TJ, Purcaro A (1995). Low intensity exercise training in patients with chronic heart failure. *J Am Coll Cardiol* 26:975–982.

Benge W, Litchfield RL, Marcus ML (1980). Exercise capacity in patients with severe heart failure. *Circulation* 61:955–959.

Braunwald E, Ross J Jr, Sonnenblick EH (1976). *Mechanisms of Contraction of the Normal and Failing Heart.* Little Brown, Boston.

Burch GE, Walsh JJ, Black WC (1983). Value of prolonged bed rest in management of cardiomegaly. *JAMA* 183:81.

Coats AJS, Adamopoulos S, Meyer TE, Conway J, Sleight P (1990). Effects of physical training in chronic heart failure. *Lancet* 335:63–66.

Elzinga G (1992). Starling's Law and the rise and fall of the descending limb. *News Physiol Sci* 7:134–137.

Feltovich PJ, Spiro RJ, Coulson RL (1989). The nature of conceptual understanding in biomedicine: the deep structure of complex ideas and the development of misconceptions. In Evans DA, Patel VL, eds. *Cognitive Science in Medicine*. The MIT Press, Cambridge, MA, pp 113–165.

Fitts RH (1994). Cellular mechanisms of muscle fatigue. *Physiol Rev* 74:49–94.

Franciosa JA, Park M, Levine TB (1981). Lack of correlation between exercise capacity and indexes of resting left ventricular performance in heart failure. *Am J Cardiol* 47:33–39.

Grossman W, Lorell BH (1988). *Diastolic Relaxation of the Heart* Martinus Nijhoff, Boston.

Guyton A (1961). Cardiac failure. In *Textbook of Medical Physiology*. WB Saunders, Philadelphia.

Hambrecht R, Niebauer J, Fiehn E, Kälberer B, Offner B, Hauer K, Riede U, Schlierf G, Kübler W, Schuler G (1995). Physical training in patients with stable chronic heart failure: effects on cardiorespiratory fitness and ultrastructural abnormalities of leg muscles. *J Am Coll Cardiol* 25:1239–1249.

Hambrecht R, Fiehn E, Yu J, Niebauer J, Weigl C, Hilbrich L, Adams V, Riede U, Schuler G (1997). Effects of endurance training on mitochondrial ultrastructure and fiber type distribution in skeletal muscle in patients with stable chronic heart failure. *J Am Coll Cardiol* 29:1067–1073.

Holubarsch C, Ruf T, Goldstein D, Ashton RC, Nickl W, Pieske B, Pioch K, Lüdemann J, Weisner S, Hasenfuss G, Posival H, Just H, Burkhoff D (1996). Existence of the Frank-Starling mechanism in the failing human heart. Investigations on the organ, tissue and sarcomere levels. *Circulation* 94:683–689.

Katz AM (1965). The descending limb of the Starling curve and the failing heart. *Circulation* 32:871–875.

Katz AM (1992). *Physiology of the Heart*, 2nd ed. Raven, New York.

Lipkin DP, Poole-Wilson PA (1986). Symptoms limiting exercise capacity in chronic heart failure. *BMJ* 292:653–655.

Mancini DM, LaManca J, Henson D (1992). The relation of respiratory muscle function to dyspnea in patient with heart failure. *Heart Failure* 8:183–189.

Mancini DM, Henson D, La Manca J, Donchez L, Levine S (1995). Benefit of selective respiratory muscle training on exercise capacity in patients with chronic heart failure. *Circulation* 91:320–329.

Massie B, Conway M, Yonge R, Frostick S, Ledingham J, Sleight P, Radda G, Rajagopalan B (1987). Skeletal muscle metabolism in patients with congestive heart failure; relation to clinical severity and blood flow. *Circulation* 76:1009–1019.

McKelvie RS, Teo KK, McCartney N, Humen D, Montague T, Yusef S (1995). Effects of exercise training in patients with congestive heart failure: a critical review. *J Am Coll Cardiol* 25:789–796.

McMichael J (1950). *Pharmacology of the Failing Heart*. Blackwell, London.

Patterson SW, Piper H, Starling EH (1914). The regulation of the heart beat. *J Physiol (London)* 48:465–513.

Perreault CL, Gonzalez-Serratos H, Litwin SE, Sun X, Franzini-Armstrong C, Morgan JP (1993). Alterations in contractility and intracellular Ca^{2+} transients in isolated bundles of skeletal muscle fibers from rats with chronic heart failure. *Circ Res* 73:405–412.

Poole-Wilson P, Ferrari R (1996). Role of skeletal muscle in the syndrome of chronic heart failure. *J Mol Cell Cardiol* 28:2275–2285.

Sarnoff SJ (1955). Myocardial contractility as described by ventricular function curves. *Physiol Rev* 35:107–122.

Schaufelberger M, Eriksson BO, Grimby G, Held P, Swedberg K (1995). Skeletal muscle composition and capillarization in patients with chronic heart failure: relation to exercise capacity and central hemodynamics. *J Cardiac Failure* 1:267–272

Schwinger RHG, Böhm M, Koch A, Schmidt U, Morano I, Eissner H-J, Überfuhr P, Reichart B, Erdmann E (1994). The failing human heart is unable to use the Frank-Starling mechanism. *Circulation* 74:959–969.

Simonini A, Long CS, Dudley GA, Yue P, McElhinny J, Massie BM (1996a). Heart failure in rats causes changes in skeletal muscle morphology and gene expression that are not explained by reduced activity. *Circ Res* 79:128–136.

Simonini A, Massie BM, Long CS, Qi M, Samarel AM (1996b). Alterations in skeletal muscle gene expression in the rat with chronic congestive heart failure. *J Mol Cell Cardiol* 28:1683–1691.

Smith VE, Weisfeldt ML, Katz AM (1986). Relaxation and diastolic properties of the heart. In Fozzard H, Haber E, Katz A, Jennings R, Morgan HE, eds. *The Heart and Cardiovascular System*. Raven, New York, pp 803–818.

Sonnenblick EH (1964). Force-velocity relations in mammalian heart muscle. *Am J Physiol* 202:931–939.

Spann JF Jr, Buccino RA, Sonnenblick EH, Braunwald E (1967). Contractile state of cardiac muscle obtained from cats with experimentally produced ventricular hypertrophy and heart failure. *Circ Res* 21:341–351.

Spiro D, Sonnenblick EH (1962). Comparison of the ultrastructural basis of the contractile process in heart and skeletal muscle. *Circ Res* 14:II-14–II-36.

Sullivan M, Higgenbotham M, Cobb F (1988). Increased exercise ventilation in patients with chronic heart failure: intact ventilatory control despite hemodynamic and pulmonary abnormalities. *Circulation* 77:552–559.

Volterrani M, Clark AJ, Ludman PF, Swan JW, Adamopoulos S, Piepoli M, Coats AJS (1994). Predictors of exercise capacity in chronic heart failure. *Eur Heart J* 15:801–809.

Wasserman K, Zhang Y-Y, Gitt A, Belardinelli R, Koike A, Lubarsky L, Agostini PG (1997). Lung function and gas exchange in chronic heart failure. *Circulation* 96:2221–2227.

Weil J, Eschenhagen T, Hirt S, Magnussen O, Mittmann C, Remmers U, Scholz H (1998). Preserved Frank-Starling mechanism in end stage heart failure. *Cardiovasc Res* 37:541–548.

Wiggers CJ (1952). *Circulatory Dynamics*. Grune & Stratton, New York.

Wilson JR (1995). Exercise intolerance in heart failure. Importance of skeletal muscle. *Circulation* 91:559–661.

Wilson JR (1996). Evaluation of skeletal muscle fatigue in patients with heart failure. *J Mol Cell Cardiol* 28: 2287–2292.

Wilson JR, Rayos G, Yeoh TK, Gothard P, Bak K (1995). Dissociation between exertional symptoms and circulatory function in patients with heart failure. *Circulation* 92:47–53.

Wood P (1954). An appreciation of mitral stenosis. *BMJ* 1:1051–1063, 1113–1124.

3

Cell Biochemistry: Abnormal Excitation-Contraction Coupling, Contraction, and Relaxation; Arrhythmias; Energy Starvation

But when the parenchyma of the heart has been harmed by various diseases, its motion also is necessarily much altered; for if the parenchyma of the heart is burdened with too much fat, labours under inflammation, abscess, ulcer or wound, so that it cannot vibrate or contract without great trouble or difficulty, it soon gives up its motions; whence the movement of blood also to the same degree becomes weak and languid.

Lower R (1669), trans. East (1958)

The basic question "Is failure of chronically overloaded hearts the result of abnormalities within the myocardial fiber?" remains unanswered. . . . Is myocardial failure due to weakness of the myofibril itself; if so, what functions are altered?

Katz AM (1964)

In the 1960s, shortly after myocardial contractility had been recognized as a major determinant of the heart's ability to perform work, the focus in heart failure research shifted from the hemodynamic abnormalities reviewed in Chapter 2 to the heart itself. Growing appreciation of the complex interplay between the heart and circulation, discussed at length in Chapter 2, redirected studies of this syndrome to isolated cardiac muscle, cardiac muscle homogenates, and components purified from the myocardium. Although this reductionistic approach drew attention away from the patient, it became possible, for the first time, to confirm directly the suggestion made by Lower almost three centuries earlier that the failing heart contracted with "great trouble [and] difficulty." This, in turn, led to a search for the causes of an increasing number of cellular and molecular abnormalities that weaken the failing heart, an effort that dominated thinking in this field until the early 1990s.

Although it has become clear that many biochemical abnormalities can be found in the cells of the failing heart, their clinical significance, and especially the value of efforts to correct the observed defects in the systems that control myocardial contraction and relaxation, have recently been called into question (see Chapter 9). The following discussion reviews abnormalities in excitation-contraction coupling, contraction, and relaxation that contribute to the impaired contraction of the failing heart. These considerations provide the background for a brief discussion of the mechanisms that cause arrhythmias in these patients. A state of energy starvation that probably plays an important role causing these abnormalities, as well as the progressive deterioration of the failing heart, is also discussed. Although this chapter highlights the biochemistry of failing cardiac myocytes, it is apparent that the impaired pump performance of the failing heart is due not only to these biochemical abnormalities, which are not found in all models of heart failure (Anand et al., 1998), but also to myocardial cell death and fibrosis (see Chapters 5 through 8), which contribute to the architectural changes discussed in Chapter 2. This chapter, therefore, deals with only one aspect of the mechanisms that reduce ejection and filling in the failing heart.

BIOCHEMICAL CAUSES OF IMPAIRED EJECTION AND FILLING OF THE FAILING HEART

Cardiac contraction and relaxation are abnormal in virtually every patient with heart failure. These abnormalities are generally attributed to changes in a number of cellular processes, including the metabolic pathways that oxidize fats and carbohydrates to generate high-energy phosphates, the ion pumps and ion channels that control excitation-contraction coupling, contraction and relaxation, and the contractile proteins whose interactions are directly responsible for the heart's pumping. These abnormalities in cell function can be either primary, wherein a disease process involves the myocardium itself, or they can be secondary to changes initiated by chronic overloading of previously normal heart muscle.

Two general types of biochemical abnormality impair excitation-contraction coupling, depress myocardial contractility, and slow relaxation in the failing heart (Table 3-1). The first includes abnormalities in the proteins, membranes, and other structures responsible for these processes, for example, isoform shifts that replace the high ATPase myosin heavy chain isoform with an isoform that has a lower rate of energy turnover, and alterations in membrane architecture that decrease in the density of calcium pump ATPase molecules in the sarcoplasmic reticulum. The second type of abnormality is caused by a state of energy starvation that, by somewhat arcane mechanisms, inhibits the interactions of the contractile proteins and slows virtually all of the processes involved in excitation-contraction coupling, contraction and relaxation. These abnormalities are described after brief review of the biochemical mechanisms responsible for systole and diastole in the normal heart.

TABLE 3-1. *Biochemical mechanisms that depress cellular function in the failing heart*

I. Abnormalities in the proteins, membrane and other structures responsible for excitation-contraction coupling, contraction, and relaxation
II. Energy starvation

OVERVIEW OF CONTRACTION AND RELAXATION IN THE NORMAL HEART

Cardiac contraction, which is brought about by energy-dependent interactions between the heart's contractile proteins, is "turned on" when calcium enters the cytosol through open calcium channels. Contraction is "turned off" and the heart relaxes when this activator is actively transported out of the cytosol. An old debate, whether energy is required for contraction and relaxation, has been settled: energy is needed for *both*. However, the way in which this energy is used is quite different during these two phases of the cardiac cycle.

The process that activates contraction is referred to as *excitation-contraction coupling* because it couples the signal generated by action potential at the cell surface (excitation) to the delivery of calcium into the cytosol that initiates contraction. *Contraction* occurs when the contractile proteins transduce chemical energy released by ATP hydrolysis into the mechanical work that allows cardiac myocytes to shorten and develop tension, and so to propel blood under pressure from the systemic veins into the pulmonary artery, and from the pulmonary veins into the aorta. *Relaxation*, which depends on calcium removal from the cytosol, is not simply a reversal of the steps in excitation-contraction coupling; instead, different structures are responsible for excitation-contraction coupling and relaxation.

The calcium fluxes responsible for excitation-contraction coupling, contraction and relaxation, can be viewed as two "calcium cycles," in which this activator moves back and forth between different "pools" (for review, see Katz, 1992). In the *extracellular cycle*, calcium moves between the extracellular space and the cytosol, while the *intracellular cycle* involves calcium fluxes between the sarcoplasmic reticulum, the cytosol, and calcium-binding proteins located in the myofilaments (Fig. 3-1). The sarcoplasmic reticulum provides most of the calcium that activates contraction in adult mammalian cardiac myocytes; in these cells, the major role of the extracellular calcium cycle is to "trigger" calcium release from these intracellular stores. This situation is quite different in the embryonic heart and smooth muscle. These more primitive cells lack a well-developed sarcoplasmic reticulum and so depend mainly on the extracellular calcium cycle.

In both cycles, calcium enters the cytosol by passive, "downhill" fluxes through calcium-selective ion channels. In the extracellular cycle, these are the *L-type calcium channels* found in the plasma membrane; a different family of channels, the *calcium release channels* located in the membranes of the sarcoplasmic reticulum, admit a much larger amount of calcium into the cytosol via the intracellular cycle. Calcium that enters the cytosol via the plasma membrane calcium channels serves as a "trigger" that opens intracellular calcium release channels in the sarcoplasmic reticulum.

The calcium transport out of the cytosol that relaxes the heart is an active, "uphill" process that is effected by ion pumps and ion exchangers in both the plasma membrane and sarcoplasmic reticulum. Ion pumps are membrane proteins that use energy derived from ATP hydrolysis to transport calcium out of the cytosol against an electrochemical gradient, while ion exchangers use the energy of the sodium gradient for the uphill movement of calcium (and other substances) into the extracellular space. The sodium gradient is maintained by the ATP-dependent sodium pump (Na-K ATPase). As already noted, energy is used in both contraction and relaxation, although it is used by different systems, and in different ways.

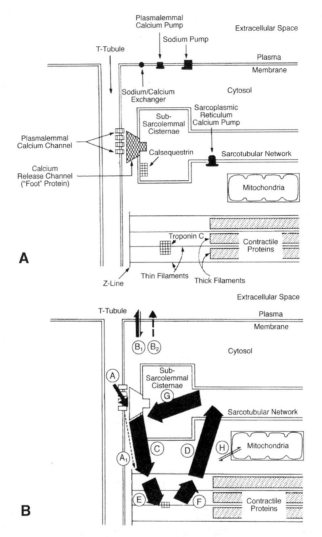

FIG. 3-1. Schematic diagram showing **(A)** key structures and **(B)** major calcium fluxes involved in cardiac excitation-contraction coupling. The thickness of the arrows indicates the magnitude of the calcium fluxes, and their directions describe the "energetics" of the calcium fluxes: downward arrows describe passive calcium fluxes and upward arrows describe energy-dependent calcium transport.

Calcium enters the cell from the extracellular fluid via plasma membrane calcium channels. Arrow A: while most of this calcium triggers calcium release from the sarcoplasmic reticulum, a small portion directly activates the contractile proteins (*arrow A_1*). Calcium transport back into the extracellular fluid involves two plasma membrane systems: sodium/calcium exchange (*arrow B_1*), and the plasma membrane calcium pump (*arrow B_2*). The sarcoplasmic reticulum membrane regulates two calcium fluxes: calcium release from the subsarcolemmal cisternae (*arrow C*), and active calcium uptake by the calcium pump located in the sarcotubular network (*arrow D*). Calcium diffuses within the sarcoplasmic reticulum in a third calcium flux (*arrow G*), returning to the subsarcolemmal cisternae where it is stored in complex with calsequestrin and other calcium-binding proteins. The contractile proteins are regulated by calcium binding to (*arrow E*) and dissociation from (*arrow F*) the high affinity calcium-binding sites of troponin C. Movements of calcium into and out of mitochondria (*arrow H*) buffer cytosolic calcium concentration. [From Katz (1992).]

Myocyte Structure

More than half of the volume of working myocardial cells is made up of the contractile proteins, which are organized in a manner that gives rise to a characteristic repeating pattern of light and dark striations (Fig. 3-2). The more darkly staining A-bands contain the thick filaments, whereas the lightly staining half I-bands at either side of the A-band contain only thin filaments. Each I-band is bisected by a narrow, darkly staining, Z-line that delimits the sarcomere, which is the fundamental morphologic unit of striated muscle. Each sarcomere, which is defined as the region between two Z-lines, consists of a central A-band plus the two adjacent half I-bands. The A-bands of the contracted heart contain not only thick filaments, but also the ends of thin filaments that penetrate from the Z-lines at either end of the sarcomere. At physiologic sarcomere lengths, the thin filaments of the resting heart extend almost to the center of the A-band, so that when the muscle shortens, the thin filaments from each half of the sarcomere cross into the opposite half ("double overlap").

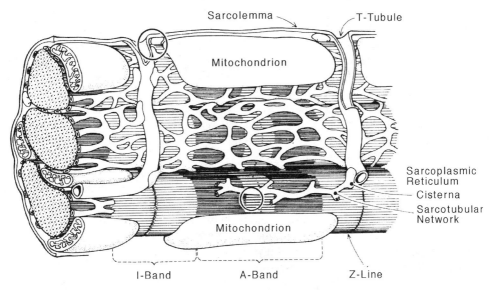

FIG. 3-2: Ultrastructure of the working myocardial cell. Contractile proteins are arranged in a regular array of thick and thin filaments (seen in cross section at the left). The A-band represents the region of the sarcomere occupied by the thick filaments into which thin filaments extend from either side. The I-band is the region of the sarcomere occupied only by thin filaments; these extend toward the center of the sarcomere from the Z-lines, which bisect each I-band. The sarcomere, the functional unit of the contractile apparatus, is defined as the region between adjacent Z-lines and so contains two half I-bands and one A-band. The sarcoplasmic reticulum, an intracellular membrane system that surrounds the contractile proteins, consists of the sarcotubular network at the center of the sarcomere and the subsarcolemmal cisternae that abut on the t-tubules and the sarcolemma. The transverse tubular system (t-tubule) is lined by a membrane that is continuous with the sarcolemma, so that the lumen of the t-tubules carries the extracellular space toward the center of the myocardial cell. The arrangement allows the action potential to be propagated into the center of the cell. Mitochondria are shown in the central sarcomere and in cross section at the left. [Copyright 1975, Massachusetts Medical Society. All rights reserved. From Katz, *New Eng J Med* 1975;293–1184.]

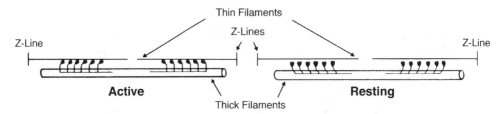

FIG. 3-3. Changes in the positions of the myosin cross-bridges during systole. In resting muscle (*right*) the cross-bridges project at almost right angles to the longitudinal axis of the thick filament. In active muscle (*left*) the cross-bridges interact with actin in the thin filaments, which are pulled toward the center of the sarcomere by a "rowing" motion caused by a shift in cross-bridge orientation. [From Katz (1992).]

The A-bands are composed largely of myosin, which is arranged so that the active sites of these molecules project from the thick filament as the cross-bridges. The thick filaments contain several additional supporting proteins, including titin, nebulette, and myosin-binding protein C (Small et al., 1992; Moncman and Wang, 1995; Helmes et al., 1996; Trombitás and Granzier, 1997; Linke et al., 1997; Koston et al., 1998). Titin and nebulette are oriented along the long axis of the filament, whereas myosin-binding protein C links adjacent thick filaments to each other. The thin filaments are double-stranded structures whose backbone is made up of two strands of polymerized actin to which are attached the regulatory proteins: tropomyosin and the three components of the troponin complex. Troponin C, one of the latter, binds calcium and so plays a central role in excitation-contraction coupling. The other proteins of the thin filament, along with myosin in the thick filament, participate in cooperative interactions that regulate both the development and intensity of the contractile process.

Sarcomere shortening in the contracting heart occurs when the thin filaments are pulled toward the center of the A-band by a rowing motion of the myosin cross-bridges (Fig. 3-3). The latter, as already noted, represent the heads of myosin molecules that project from the thick filaments. The interactions between the myosin cross-bridges of the thick filament and actin in the thin filaments are powered by energy released from hydrolysis of the terminal high-energy phosphate of ATP; this occurs when actin activates catalytic sites in the myosin cross-bridges.

THE PLASMA MEMBRANE AND SARCOPLASMIC RETICULUM

Excitation-contraction coupling and relaxation use the two different calcium cycles shown in Fig. 3-1. Each cycle is regulated by its own set of membrane structures. The extracellular calcium cycle is controlled by the plasma membrane, which separates the cytosol from the extracellular space; this membrane is divided structurally into the sarcolemma, which surrounds the body of the cell, and the transverse tubular (t-tubular) system that penetrates the cell interior (see Fig. 3-2). The lumens of the t-tubules open freely to the extracellular space, which allows these plasma membrane extensions to propagate the action potential into the cell interior, thereby providing for rapid activation of the central regions of the myocardial cell.

The intracellular calcium cycle is regulated by the sarcoplasmic reticulum, an intracellular membrane system that contains the large supply of calcium needed for rapid activation

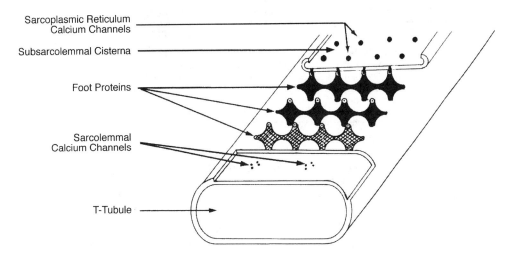

Sarcoplasmic Reticulum Calcium Channels

Subsarcolemmal Cisterna

Foot Proteins

Sarcolemmal Calcium Channels

T-Tubule

FIG. 3-4. Schematic diagram of a dyad, a composite structure made up of the membranes of the t-tubule (below) and the subsarcolemmal cisternae of the sarcoplasmic reticulum (above). The t-tubules, which are invaginations of the sarcolemma, are lined by extensions of the plasma membrane. Excitation-contraction coupling in the heart occurs when a small amount of calcium enters the space between these membranes through calcium channels in the plasma membrane. When this calcium is "sprayed" on the calcium release channels (foot proteins) of the sarcoplasmic reticulum, the latter open. As shown in this sketch, there are about half as many plasma membrane calcium channels as sarcoplasmic reticulum calcium release channels in the dyad. [From Katz (1992).]

of cardiac contraction. Because this membrane system is analogous to the endoplasmic reticulum of nonmotile cells, it is sometimes referred as the *sarcoendoplasmic reticulum.* Proteins associated with these membranes take up, store, and release activator calcium. The sarcoplasmic reticulum in the adult mammalian heart is divided into two regions (see Fig. 3-2). One is the *subsarcolemmal cisternae*, which are dilated extensions of the sarcoplasmic reticulum that abut the t-tubules and sarcolemma to form structure called dyads. The cisternae contain both calcium-binding proteins, which store this activator, and calcium release channels, through which calcium is delivered into the cytosol at the onset of systole. The second region is the more extensive *sarcotubular network*, which surrounds the contractile proteins in the center of the sarcomere. This network contains a dense array of calcium pump ATPase proteins that use the energy obtained from ATP hydrolysis to relax the heart by transporting calcium out of the cytosol into the sarcoplasmic reticulum.

A critical link in excitation-contraction coupling is provided by the dyads, which are composite structures made up of membranes of the sarcolemma (and its extensions, the t-tubules) and the subsarcolemmal cisternae of the sarcoplasmic reticulum (Fig. 3-4). These structures bring portions of these two membranes into close proximity, which allows calcium entry through plasma membrane calcium channels to spray onto the calcium release channels of the sarcoplasmic reticulum, causing these channels to open. The resulting calcium flux provides most of the activator calcium for excitation-contraction coupling.

THE CONTRACTILE (MYOFIBRILLAR) PROTEINS

Six proteins found in the myofilaments are responsible for the contractile process and its control (Table 3-2). These are myosin, actin, tropomyosin, and the three components

TABLE 3-2. *Contractile proteins of the heart*

Protein	Location	Salient properties
Myosin	Thick filament	Hydrolyzes adenosine triphosphate (ATP); interacts with actin
Actin	Thin filament	Activates myosin ATPase; interacts with myosin
Tropomyosin	Thin filament	Modulates actin-myosin interaction
Troponin C	Thin filament	Binds calcium
Troponin I	Thin filament	Inhibits actin-myosin interactions
Troponin T	Thin filament	Binds troponin complex to tropomyosin

of troponin; as noted earlier, additional proteins provide structural support to the myofilament lattice. Myosin and actin suffice to convert the chemical energy of ATP into the mechanical work that pumps blood out of the heart's cavities. Physiologic control of the force-generating reactions between actin and myosin is provided by allosteric interactions within the thin filament that involve tropomyosin, troponins C, I, and T.

Mutations in many of these proteins, as discussed in Chapter 8, are responsible for a number of familial cardiomyopathies. In addition, overload causes a reversion to the fetal pattern of gene expression that is accompanied by isoform shifts involving many of these proteins.

Myosin

Myosin is an elongated, dimeric molecule that contains a filamentous "tail" and a globular "head" (Fig. 3-5). In living muscle, myosin is aggregated in the thick filament so that the myosin heads, which contain both the ATPase and actin-binding sites, project as the cross-bridges (Fig. 3-6). Shortening and tension development occur when the cross-bridges, which in resting muscle are perpendicular to the long axis of the thick filament,

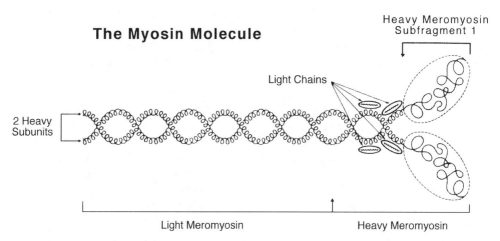

FIG. 3-5. Myosin is an elongated molecule consisting of two heavy subunits and four light subunits. The "tail" of the molecule (*left*) is a coiled coil (two α-helical chains wound around each other) that extends into the paired globular "head" of the molecule (*right*). Enzymatic cleavage at the point indicated by the lower arrow produces heavy and light meromyosins, while enzymatic cleavage of heavy meromyosin at the point indicated by the upper arrow yields heavy meromyosin subfragment 1. [From Katz (1992).]

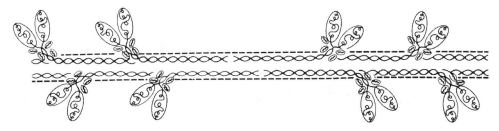

FIG. 3-6. Organization of individual myosin molecules in the thick filament. The "backbone" of the thick filament, delineated by dashed lines, is made up of the tails of the individual myosin molecules, which have opposite polarities in the two halves of the sarcomere (right and left). The bare area in the center of the thick filament is a region devoid of cross-bridges, which can be seen to arise from the "tail-to-tail" organization of myosin molecules unique to the center of the thick filament. The cross-bridges represent the "heads" of the individual myosin molecules, which project from the long axis of the thick filament. [From Katz (1992).]

bind to the thin filaments and, using energy derived from ATP hydrolysis, shift toward the center of the sarcomere (see Fig. 3-3).

The mechanical energy generated by the "rowing" motion of the myosin cross-bridges can be used to develop pressure or to eject blood, the extent of either being determined by the manner in which the muscle is loaded. If afterload is very high, as when aortic pressure is elevated or the heart is dilated (see Chapter 2), sarcomere shortening is limited by the high wall tension, so that stroke volume is reduced. At a low afterload, the energy released by the contractile proteins is used for sarcomere shortening, rather than tension development, which increases stroke volume. As noted in Chapter 2, shortening allows the energy stored in the stretched elasticities of the ventricular walls to be converted to mechanical work, rather than being degraded to heat, which is largely responsible for the relatively low-energy cost of ejection and some of the benefits of afterload reduction in heart failure.

The intrinsic rate at which myosin hydrolyses ATP is of considerable importance because it determines both muscle shortening velocity and myocardial contractility (Alpert et al., 1991). This property is determined by the cardiac myosin heavy chains, which include both high and low ATPase isoforms (Swynghedauw et al., 1986; Schwartz et al., 1990, 1993). The higher ATPase myosin heavy chain, called α, determines a rapid muscle shortening velocity and high myocardial contractility, whereas the lower ATPase myosin heavy chain, called β, is associated with a weaker, slower contraction. The latter, however, yields a more efficient contraction when the heart ejects against a heavy afterload (Awan and Goldspink, 1972). The role of the cardiac myosin light chains, which are located near hinge regions of the molecule, is less clear. These small proteins are members of the family of E-F hand proteins, which, in some muscle types, contain the calcium-binding sites that control contraction. In vascular smooth muscle, phosphorylation of some myosin light chains by a calcium, calmodulin–activated protein kinase causes vasoconstriction, whereas in the heart, these proteins probably serve as substrates for phosphorylation reactions that regulate the intensity of the contractile process. As discussed later, isoform changes involving both the heavy and light chains play a role in heart failure.

Actin

Actin is a smaller globular protein that forms a double-stranded macromolecular helix that makes up the backbone of the thin filament (Fig. 3-7). As already noted, the interac-

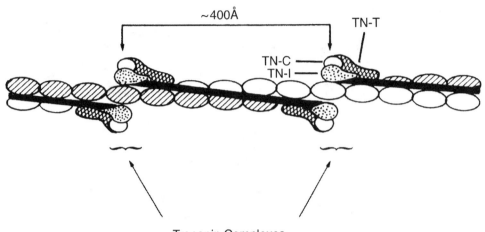

Troponin Complexes

FIG. 3-7. Structure of the thin filament. Tropomyosin (heavy lines) lies in the grooves between the two strands of actin filaments (*shaded* and *unshaded ovals*). Troponin complexes, containing troponins C, I, and T, are distributed at 400Å intervals. [From Katz (1992).]

tion of actin with the myosin cross-bridges allows the chemical energy released by ATP hydrolysis to power the physicochemical changes responsible for the contractile process. Actin, like myosin, is found in several isoforms that can change when the heart is overloaded or fails.

Tropomyosin

Tropomyosin, an elongated molecule made up of two helical peptide chains, lies in each of the two longitudinal grooves between the two strands of actin in the thin filament (see Fig. 3-7). The major function of tropomyosin, along with the troponin complex, is to regulate the interactions between actin and myosin.

The Troponin Complex

The troponin complex is made up of three discrete proteins. *Troponin I*, in concert with tropomyosin, reversibly inhibits the interactions between actin and myosin, *troponin T* binds the troponin complex to tropomyosin, and *troponin C* contains the high-affinity calcium-binding sites that bind to the calcium released into the cytosol in the final step of excitation-contraction coupling. These proteins interact with one another, and with actin and myosin, to regulate contraction in the living heart.

Troponin C is a member of a family of calcium-binding proteins called "E-F hand proteins" because their calcium-binding sites resemble a hand in which the cation is bound by negatively charged oxygen atoms located between two α-helices (E and F). The latter resemble the extended thumb and forefinger of a right hand (for review, see Katz, 1996a). Other E-F hand proteins include calmodulin and the myosin light chains. Cardiac troponin C contains the key calcium-binding site that recognizes the appearance of calcium in the cytosol as the signal that initiates systole.

Troponin I, which binds the troponin complex to actin in the thin filament, regulates the interactions between actin and the myosin cross-bridges. Calcium-binding to troponin C initiates conformational changes in the proteins of the thin filament that loosen the

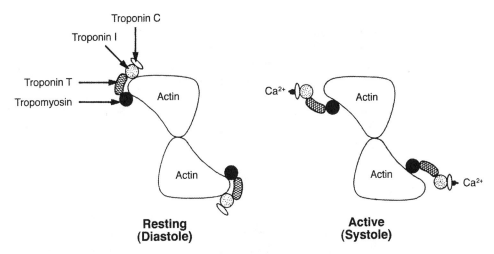

FIG. 3-8. Cross section of a thin filament in the resting (*left*) and active (*right*) states. At rest, the troponin complex holds the tropomyosin molecules toward the periphery of the groove between adjacent actin strands so as to prevent actin from interacting with the myosin cross-bridges. In active muscle, calcium binding to troponin C weakens the bond linking troponin I to actin, causing a structural rearrangement of the regulatory proteins that shifts the tropomyosin deeper into the groove between the strands of actin. This rearrangement exposes active sites on actin for interaction with the myosin cross-bridges. [From Katz 1992.]

bond linking troponin I to actin. The result is a shift in the position of the elongated tropomyosin molecules in the grooves between actin chains (Fig. 3-8). By exposing binding sites on actin that interact with the myosin cross-bridges, this conformational change plays a central role in excitation-contraction coupling. Cardiac troponin I can be phosphorylated by cyclic AMP-dependent protein kinase in a reaction that, by reducing the calcium-sensitivity of troponin C, participates in the lusitropic response to β-adrenergic stimulation.

Troponin T, which binds the troponin complex to tropomyosin, participates in the allosteric reactions that activate and inactivate the contractile process. Isoform switches involving the more than 30 isoforms of this protein can modify the calcium sensitivity of tension development.

INTERACTIONS BETWEEN
THE CONTRACTILE PROTEINS

Cooperative interactions among the contractile proteins allow subtle changes in one protein to have marked effects on both the intensity of the contractile process and its response to changes in cytosolic composition. The most important physiologic regulator of these interactions is, of course, the calcium released by excitation-contraction coupling. Other variables that regulate their interactions include allosteric effects of ATP and changing muscle length. Another example is the response to a change in pH. Protons compete with calcium for binding sites on many proteins, so that the acidosis that occurs in the energy-starved heart blunts the response to a given increase in cytosolic calcium, thereby reducing myocardial contractility (Jacobus et al., 1982). There is growing evidence that interactions with structural proteins, like titin and myosin-binding protein C, also modify mechanical performance.

Control of cardiac performance by changing end-diastolic volume (the Frank-Starling relationship) is due mainly to sarcomere length-dependent changes in the calcium sensitivity of the contractile proteins (Hibberd and Jewell, 1982) and, to a lesser extent, length-dependent changes in calcium release from the sarcoplasmic reticulum (Fabiato et al, 1975). Myocardial contractility, the other physiologically important determinant of the interactions among the heart's contractile proteins, is regulated largely by changes in the level of cytosolic calcium achieved during excitation-contraction coupling. Isoform shifts involving these proteins in the failing heart influence both myocardial contractility and the calcium sensitivity of the contractile response.

EXCITATION-CONTRACTION COUPLING AND RELAXATION

Excitation-contraction coupling, as already noted, describes the processes that link plasma membrane depolarization to the release of calcium into the cytosol, where it can bind to troponin C. Relaxation is an energy-dependent process in which calcium is actively transported out of the cytosol by structures that are entirely different than those that activate the heart. Relaxation, therefore, is not simply a reversal of the steps involved in excitation-contraction coupling. The major structures that participate in excitation, excitation-contraction coupling, and relaxation are depicted schematically in Fig. 3-1 and listed in Table 3-3.

TABLE 3-3. *Structure-function relationships in working cardiac myocytes*

Structure	Role In E-C coupling	Role in relaxation
Plasma membrane		
Sarcolemma		
Sodium channel	Depolarization	
Calcium channel (dihydropyridine receptor)	Action potential plateau, calcium-triggered calcium release	
Potassium channels	Repolarization	
Calcium pump (PMCA)		Calcium removal
Sodium/calcium exchanger	Calcium entry	Calcium removal
Sodium pump		Establish sodium gradient
Transverse tubule		
Sodium channel	Action potential propagation	
Calcium channel (dihydropyridine receptor)	Calcium-triggered calcium release	
Sarcoplasmic reticulum		
Subsarcolemmal cisternae		
Calcium release channel (ryanodine receptor)	Calcium release	
Sarcotubular network		
Calcium pump (SERCA)		Calcium removal
Phospholamban		Sensitizes SERCA to Ca
Myofilaments		
Myosin	Energy transducer (ATPase site)	
Actin	Activates and binds myosin	
Troponin C	Calcium receptor	
Tropomyosin, Troponins I and T	Allosteric regulation	

Voltage-Gated Ion Channels

Plasma membrane ion channels play a key role in excitation, and so initiate excitation-contraction coupling. Sodium and calcium channels, whose opening and closing are controlled by changes in membrane voltage, are responsible for the generation and propagation of the action potentials that depolarize the myocardium. A detailed discussion of cardiac electrophysiology is beyond the scope of this discussion. The second function, initiation of excitation-contraction coupling, is highly relevant to this discussion of the molecular abnormalities in the failing heart; a brief description follows.

Depolarization of the working myocytes of the atria and ventricles begins when sodium ions cross the hydrophobic barrier in the center of the membrane bilayer. These physiologic ion currents are generated by the opening of voltage-gated ion channels, a family of membrane proteins that provide for the highly regulated control of membrane potential (for review, see Catterall, 1988, 1992; Hille, 1992; Jan and Jan, 1992; Katz, 1993, 1998; Clapham and Ackerman, 1997). In the working myocytes of the atria and ventricles, and the rapidly conducting cells of the His-Purkinje system, the flux of sodium ions into the cell carries the major inward (depolarizing) currents. In nodal cells, where action potentials are smaller and more slowly rising, depolarization depends mainly on the inward movement of calcium ions. Resting potential in all of these cell types is restored by outward (repolarizing) currents that are generated when potassium moves out of the cell through a diverse group of potassium channels.

Plasma membrane ion channels can contain as many as five subunits, called α_1, α_2, β, γ, and δ. Most important are the large tetrameric α- and α_1-protein subunits that, in most voltage-gated ion channels, surround the ion-selective pore. The other channel subunits are smaller proteins that serve mainly to regulate ion channel function; for example, some mediate the effects of cyclic AMP-dependent protein kinases, which generally promote channel opening (Ruth et al., 1988; Nunoki et al., 1989).

The large α-subunits of sodium and calcium channels contain four domains (Fig. 3-9), which are connected covalently in a tetrameric structure by relatively short linking segments (Fig. 3-10). Each domain in most ion channels contains six α-helical transmembrane segments, designated S_1 to S_6. The S_5 and S_6 segments of the four domains, along with the connecting peptide chains, surround the channel pore (see Fig. 3-9). The S_4 transmembrane segments contain positively charged arginine and lysine residues that represent the "voltage sensor," a charged region that responds to membrane depolarization by opening the channel. Most potassium channels are also tetrameric structures made up of domains such as shown in Fig. 3-9; however, unlike the sodium and calcium channels, the four domains are not linked covalently. Some classes of potassium channels are assembled from smaller proteins that contain only two transmembrane segments that are analogous to the S_5 and S_6 membrane-spanning helices and the intervening peptides that make up the pore region.

The four domains of the α subunits of most plasma membrane ion channels are organized in the phospholipid bilayer so that in the open state of the channel, the S_5 and S_6 segments, along with the intervening peptide chains, line a water-filled pore. A "selectivity filter," determined by the amino acid sequence of this pore region, restricts passage to a given ion species. Channel inactivation occurs when intracellular peptide chains of the α-subunit, called "inactivation particles," occlude the inner mouth of the channel pore. In sodium channels, the inactivation particles are made up of the cytoplasmic peptide chain, called the III-IV linker (see Fig. 3-10), which connects the S_6 transmembrane

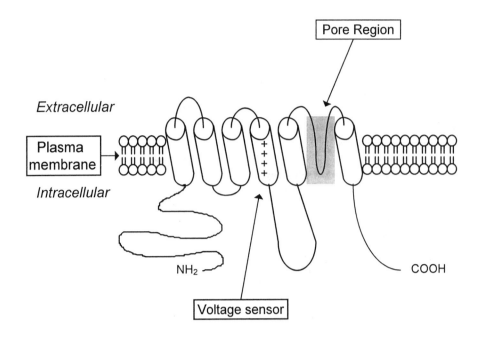

ION CHANNEL DOMAIN

FIG. 3-9. Schematic representation of an ion channel domain. The major domains in sodium and calcium channels, and in the *Shaker* class of potassium channels, contain six transmembrane α helices. Four of these domains are covalently linked to make up the major subunits of the sodium and calcium channels; in the case of the *Shaker* potassium channels, which also contain four of these domains, the domains are not covalently linked. The positively charged S_4 transmembrane segment in each domain represent the voltage sensor that responds to membrane depolarization by opening the channel. The "pore region" of the ion channels (*shaded*) is made up of the S_5 and S_6 transmembrane segments and the intervening loop that "dips" into the membrane bilayer.

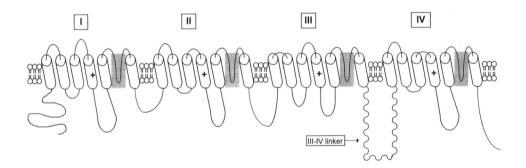

ION CHANNEL SUBUNIT

FIG. 3-10. Schematic representation of the major subunit of a tetrameric voltage-gated channel. The channel is a covalently linked tetramer made up of four of the domains as shown in Figure 3-9, which are numbered I to IV. The transmembrane segments S_5 and S_6 of the four domains, along with the intervening peptide chains, are assembled so as to surround the pore through which ions cross the lipid barrier in the core of the membrane bilayer (*shaded*). The gating mechanism that opens (activates) the channel is provided by the four charged S_4 transmembrane segments, whereas the channel inactivates (shifts to its closed, inactive state) when the peptide chain that connects the III and IV domains (the III-IV linker or inactivation particle) binds to the inner surface of the channel so as to occlude the pore.

segment of domain III to the S_1 segment of domain IV (Stühmer et al., 1989; Hartmann et al., 1994; Bennett et al., 1995; Kellenberger et al, 1996). Channel inactivation can be viewed as a ball moving at the end of a chain, where the inactivation particle (the "ball") responds to membrane repolarization by swinging into the inner mouth of the pore to close the channel. In some potassium channels, a similar mechanism uses other intracellular peptide chains to plug, and so inactivate, the channel (Isacoff et al., 1991; Jan and Jan, 1994; Antz et al., 1997).

The coordinated openings and closing of the heart's ion channels generate the ionic currents that control membrane potential. Conformational changes in L-type calcium channels also regulate excitation-contraction coupling, although the exact mechanisms for this coupling differ in skeletal and cardiac muscle.

Plasma Membrane Calcium Channels

The most important plasma membrane calcium channels in the heart are the L-type calcium channels, which bind the familiar classes of calcium channel blockers (*dihydropyridines* such as nifedipine, *phenylalkylamines* such as verapamil, and *benzothiazepines* such as diltiazem). These channels are sometimes called *dihydropyridine receptors* because of their high affinity for binding to this class of calcium channel blockers. Other types of plasma membrane calcium channels have been described and are referred to as T, N, P, Q, and R (for review, see Tsien and Tsien, 1990; Zhang et al., 1993; Katz, 1996a). In the heart, the L-type calcium channels serve a dual function: (1) they contribute inward, depolarizing currents that help maintain the plateau of the action potential, and (2) by opening intracellular calcium release channels in the sarcoplasmic reticulum, they play a central role in excitation-contraction coupling.

The functional link between depolarization of the plasma membrane (the action potential) and the opening of intracellular calcium release channels in skeletal muscle sarcoplasmic reticulum is effected by a mechanical coupling in which plasma membrane depolarization removes a "plug" that, in the resting muscle, occludes the intracellular calcium release channel. The plug itself is a portion of an L-type plasma membrane calcium channel that moves in response to changes in the electrical potential across the plasma membrane. A different L-type plasma membrane calcium channel isoform couples a change in membrane potential to calcium release from the cardiac sarcoplasmic reticulum. The cardiac calcium channel couples membrane depolarization to calcium release from the cardiac sarcoplasmic reticulum by causing a localized increase in cytosolic calcium concentration, called a "calcium spark" (Cheng et al., 1993). This area of high calcium concentration, which in effect "sprays" calcium onto the adjacent intracellular calcium release channels in the sarcoplasmic reticulum, causes a much greater calcium release from the latter in a process often referred to as "calcium-induced calcium release" (Fabiato, 1983; Wier et al, 1994).

Intracellular Calcium Release Channels

The intracellular calcium release channels in the sarcoplasmic reticulum (Fig. 3-11), which differ considerably from those of the plasma membrane, are members of a family that includes at least two classes of related proteins (for review, see Fleischer et al., 1989; Henzi et al., 1992; Berridge, 1993). These are the *ryanodine receptors*, so named because they bind to this plant alkaloid, and the *InsP₃ receptors,* which bind to and are activated by inositol trisphosphate ($InsP_3$). The ryanodine receptors are located in the dyads across

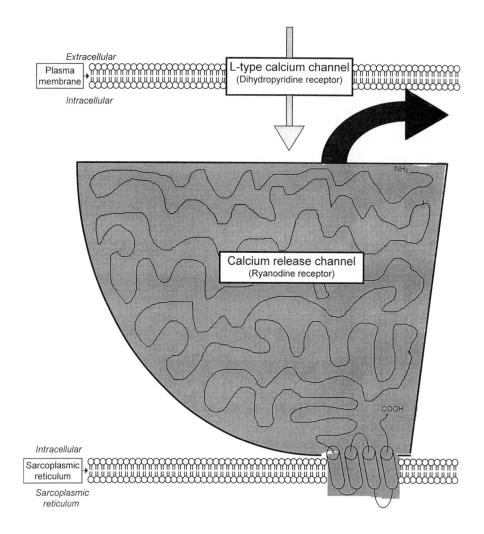

Molecular structure of the dyad

FIG. 3-11. Molecular structure of the dyad showing a subunit of a tetrameric calcium release channel (ryanodine receptor) in the membrane of the subsarcolemmal cisterna (*below*), which contains four membrane-spanning regions and a very large asymmetrical cytoplasmic domain. The latter is positioned adjacent to an L-type calcium channel (dihydropyridine receptor) in the t-tubular membrane (*above*). Depolarization of the plasma membrane allows calcium to enter the intracellular space through the L-type calcium channels, which when "sprayed" onto the calcium release channel, initiates a conformational change that opens the latter.

from the L-type plasma membrane calcium channels (see Figs. 3-4 and 3-11), an arrangement that is key to the calcium-induced calcium release discussed earlier. Less is known about the role of the InsP₃ receptors, which carry much smaller calcium currents. While of primary importance in smooth muscle excitation-contraction coupling, in the heart they carry too little calcium to have effects on mechanical function other than to regulate diastolic tension. As discussed in Chapter 7, InsP₃-gated calcium channels probably play •13• an important role in mediating signals involved in cell growth and proliferation.

The ryanodine receptors, by releasing large amounts of calcium from the sarcoplasmic reticulum, mediate the final step in excitation-contraction coupling. These channels are tetrameric structures, in which each subunit includes four α-helical transmembrane segments and a huge cytosolic domain (see Fig. 3-11). This structure differs markedly from that of the voltage-gated plasma membrane calcium channels described earlier.

Calcium Pump ATPases

The calcium pump ATPases are members of a family of closely related proteins, called P-type ion pumps, which are found in both the plasma membrane and sarcoplasmic reticulum. These ion pumps contain ten membrane-spanning α-helices and a large "head" region that projects into the cytosol (Fig. 3-12). All use a similar reaction mechanism to couple the hydrolysis of the high-energy phosphate bond of ATP to the uphill transport of calcium out of the cytosol (for review, see Carafoli, 1991; Lytton and MacLennan, 1991). In the heart, the plasma membrane calcium pump (PMCA) is larger than that of the sarcoplasmic reticulum, which is generally abbreviated *SERCA* for *sarcoendoplasmic reticulum ATPase*. Both calcium pumps are activated by an increase in cytosolic calcium.

Calcium pumping by SERCA is stimulated when a cyclic AMP-dependent protein kinase (PK-A, see Chapter 7) phosphorylates a regulatory protein called *phospholamban*. The latter is a small membrane protein, distinct from the much larger SERCA, that reg-

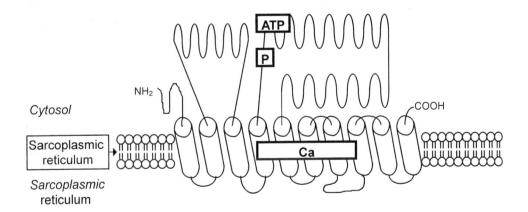

SARCOPLASMIC RETICULUM CALCIUM PUMP ATPase

FIG. 3-12. Depiction of the sarcoplasmic reticulum calcium pump ATPase. This P-type ion pump contains ten membrane-spanning segments and two large cytoplasmic loops. The ATP binding and phosphorylation sites are found on the larger cytoplasmic loop, and amino acids in several of the membrane-spanning loops participate in calcium binding and transfer across the bilayer.

ulates the calcium sensitivity of the calcium pump. In its dephospho form, phospholamban inhibits SERCA, so that phosphorylation of phospholamban, which reverses this inhibition, accelerates calcium uptake from the cytosol. This response accelerates relaxation, and by retaining calcium within the cell, increases contractility (for review, see Tada and Katz, 1982; Kim et al., 1990). The PMCA, on the other hand, is stimulated by calcium; this occurs when calcium forms a complex with an E-F hand protein called *calmodulin*, which binds to an inhibitory site located on the intracellular C-terminal peptide chain of the calcium pump molecule (Carafoli, 1991). The calmodulin-binding peptide, which is absent in the homologous SERCA, is analogous to phospholamban in that both stimulate calcium transport out of the cytosol. However, their physiologic roles differ. Cyclic AMP–activated phosphorylation of phospholamban accelerates cardiac relaxation and shortens mechanical systole during β-adrenergic stimulation, whereas the calcium-calmodulin-activated phosphorylation of the plasma membrane calcium pump promotes calcium efflux from the cell under conditions of calcium overload. Phospholamban in the sarcoplasmic reticulum membrane can also be phosphorylated by a calcium-calmodulin–dependent protein kinase, thereby providing the cardiac myocyte with an additional mechanism to rid the cytosol of excess calcium.

The Sodium/Calcium Exchanger

Sodium/calcium exchange plays a major role in the active transport of calcium out of the cytosol into the extracellular space. The sodium/calcium exchanger, which is a large membrane protein that contains 12 α-helical transmembrane segments (Nicoll et al., 1990; Levitsky et al., 1994), differs markedly from that of the calcium pump ATPases (Fig. 3-13). The mechanisms of action of the exchangers and the ATPases also differ markedly. In contrast to SERCA and PMCA, which directly couple ATP hydrolysis to osmotic work, the sodium/calcium exchanger uses the osmotic energy of the sodium gradient across the plasma membrane for this active transport. The ultimate energy source for the active calcium transport out of the cell by the sodium/calcium exchanger is ATP hydrolyzed by the Na-K ATPase (sodium pump), which establishes this sodium gradient.

The sodium/calcium exchanger generates a small repolarizing current when calcium, which carries two positive charges, leaves the cell in exchange for three monovalent

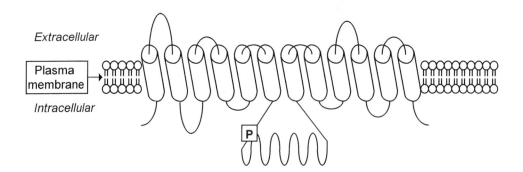

SODIUM/CALCIUM EXCHANGER

FIG. 3-13. Structure of the sodium-calcium exchanger. This membrane protein contains 12 membrane-spanning peptides and contains a large intracellular loop that can be regulated by phosphorylation.

sodium ions; as a result, calcium efflux via the exchanger causes positive charge to enter the cell. The currents generated by the sodium/calcium exchanger are small, and probably contribute less than a few millivolts to membrane potential.

The Sodium Pump

The Na-K ATPase, like the calcium pump ATPases described earlier, is a P-type ion pump. This pump uses energy derived from ATP hydrolysis to exchange the small amount of sodium that enters the cell during each action potential for the small amount of potassium lost from the cytosol during repolarization (Horisberger et al., 1991). Because three sodium ions are exchanged for only two potassium ions moved in opposite directions during each turnover of the pump, the Na-K ATPase generates a small, repolarizing current; this is normally less than 10 mV. In addition to restoring the intracellular concentrations of sodium and potassium after each action potential, the sodium pump generates the sodium gradient across the plasma membrane that provides the osmotic energy used to couple the transport of a number of molecules, including calcium, by several exchange systems.

Calcium Storage Proteins Within the Sarcoplasmic Reticulum

Some of the calcium stored in the sarcoplasmic reticulum is in a free, ionized form, but much of this cation is associated with calcium-binding proteins within this intracellular membrane system (Lytton and MacLennan, 1991). Most important of the latter is *calsequestrin*, a 45,000-dalton protein that traps calcium within this membrane system. Other calcium-binding proteins found in smaller amounts include the 44,000-dalton protein *calreticulin* and a 170,000-dalton *histidine-rich calcium-binding protein*. These calcium-binding proteins are concentrated in the subsarcolemmal cisternae, where they maintain a calcium store that is readily released through the calcium release channels during excitation-contraction coupling.

ARRHYTHMOGENIC MECHANISMS AND SUDDEN DEATH IN HEART FAILURE

Sudden cardiac death has become a major cause of death in patients with heart failure; this change is due largely, if not entirely, to the ability of modern therapy to prevent the once common slow, lingering death described in Chapter 1. The clinical definition of "sudden death," however, is far from obvious because most deaths that occur when the heart stops are "sudden," even when they occur at the end of a long period of clinical deterioration. Better terms might be "unexpected sudden death" or "death from arrhythmia." In the context of the present description of the biochemical abnormalities in the failing heart, the following discussion reviews mechanisms that can cause the sudden, unexpected cardiac deaths that result from arrhythmias.

General Causes of Cardiac Arrhythmias

Several key features of arrhythmogenic mechanisms provide a basis for understanding the role of abnormal ion channel function. Extensive and systematic discussions of the arrhythmias can be found in standard textbooks of medicine, cardiology, and cardiovascular physiology.

Arrhythmias are often divided into two classes (Table 3-4): the *bradyarrhythmias*, in which the heart beats too slowly, and the *tachyarrhythmias*, in which ventricular rate is

TABLE 3-4. *Mechanisms responsible for cardiac*
arrhythmias in patients with heart failure

Bradyarrhythmias
   Depressed impulse formation (pacemaker slowing)
   Impaired impulse conduction
Tachyarrhythmias
   Accelerated pacemaker activity
   Triggered depolarizations: early and late
   Reentry caused by slow impulse conduction
      Inhomogeneities in action potential characteristics
      Inhomogeneities of resting potential
      Inhomogeneities of depolarization
      Inhomogeneities of repolarization and refractoriness

either too rapid to allow the heart to pump normally or else ventricular depolarization becomes so disorganized as to cause effective contractions to cease; the latter is ventricular fibrillation. Both of these arrhythmogenic mechanisms operate in heart failure; both can cause sudden death.

The mechanisms responsible for the bradyarrhythmias are not, as might be expected, the opposite of those that cause the tachyarryhthmias. This is because abnormalities in ion channel function that slow impulse conduction provide a substrate for *reentry*, in which excitation of the heart becomes disorganized. Disorganization of the spread of the wave of depolarization over the heart is among the most important causes of sudden death in patients with heart failure.

Bradyarrhythmias

Abnormally slow heart rate is generally of little consequence in a normal individual, unless heart rate decreases to less than 40 to 50 beats/min. Moderate bradycardias are easily tolerated because the circulation provides many mechanisms to maintain cardiac output and to shunt blood to such vital organs as the brain. The most important compensation for a decrease in heart rate is an increase in stroke volume (cardiac output equals heart rate times stroke volume). The increased stroke volume brought about when end-diastolic volume is increased by elevated filling pressure (the Starling mechanism) allows normal individuals to maintain a nearly normal cardiac output at slow heart rates. As discussed in Chapter 2, however, the ability of an increase in end-diastolic volume to increase stroke work is attenuated in heart failure, which means that when heart rate slows, these patients have difficulty in maintaining an already depressed cardiac output. A second mechanism that normally compensates for bradycardia is shunting of blood away from such organs as the viscera and skin to maintain blood flow to the brain. Although most persons would feel light-headed if their heart rate decreased to less than 40 to 50 beats/min (as in a vasovagal reaction), the disability would be only minor because constriction of nonessential vascular beds would maintain enough arterial pressure to perfuse the brain. The same heart rate in a patient with heart failure, however, often causes unconsciousness because these vasoconstrictor defenses are already activated by the hemodynamic defense reaction discussed in Chapter 4. A third problem lies in the heart itself. Whereas the normal heart has a considerable inotropic reserve, these inotropic reserves are exhausted in patients with heart failure. One dangerous consequence of a bradyarrhythmia in heart failure reflects the vulnerability of the failing heart to ischemia, a situation that can allow even a modest decrease in blood pressure, as occurs when heart rate slows, to reduce coronary flow and cause a lethal arrhythmia.

Bradyarrhythmias can be caused by slowing of the normal sinoatrial (SA) node pacemaker and by impaired impulse conduction (Table 3-4). Pacemaker slowing occurs when myocardial disease affects the (SA) node; more commonly this occurs as a side effect of drugs commonly used to treat heart failure, notably the cardiac glycosides and β-adrenergic blocking agents (Chapter 9). Depressed impulse conduction, which can slow normal propagation of impulses arising in the SA node, can be caused by a variety of diseases, drugs, and metabolic disorders. As discussed later, both energy starvation, which leads to resting membrane depolarization, and molecular changes in the voltage-gated ion channels slow conduction velocity in the failing heart.

Tachyarrhythmias

The most obvious cause of a tachyarrhythmia is accelerated pacemaker activity. Sinus tachycardia, in which the normal SA node pacemaker is accelerated by mediators of the hemodynamic defense reaction, represents a serious problem in patients with heart failure. This is because a major effect of increased heart rate is to impair filling by shortening diastole. In normal subjects, this rarely causes hemodynamic problems at heart rates of less than 140 to 160 beats/min because the normal heart relaxes rapidly. Furthermore, during exercise and other situations that are accompanied by sympathetic stimulation, phospholamban phosphorylation shortens systole by accelerating calcium uptake into the sarcoplasmic reticulum. In the failing heart, however, filling is usually impaired, even under basal conditions, and abbreviation of diastole by phospholamban phosphorylation is attenuated. As a result, the failing heart may not have sufficient time to fill, even during a modest tachycardia, an effect that reduces stroke volume and increases venous pressure.

The abnormal mechanisms listed in Table 3-4 include more important, and more deadly, causes of tachyarryhthmias. These mechanisms include triggered activity, often referred to as afterdepolarizations, which can lead to ventricular tachycardia and fibrillation (for review, see Wit and Rosen, 1991). This complex group of abnormalities is exacerbated by the calcium overloading commonly seen in the cells of a failing, energy-starved heart.

Inhomogeneities in the distribution of different ion channel isoforms can also disorganize the spread of the wave of depolarization over the heart. Such heterogeneities are very dangerous because the resulting electrical disorganization represents an important cause of sudden cardiac death. These molecular abnormalities can involve the channels that carry the inward currents that depolarize the heart; more commonly they result form nonuniform changes in the plastic potassium channels that are responsible for repolarization.

Disorganized repolarization, by disrupting the uniformity of recovery from the prior wave of depolarization, can allow areas of the heart that have recovered electrically to be activated by other regions that remain depolarized. The resulting ectopic activation not only causes single premature systoles, but in a failing heart that has other electrophysiologic abnormalities, it can also trigger a lethal arrhythmia.

Another group of mechanisms that cause tachyarryhthmias in the failing heart are abnormalities that slow conduction. Slowed impulse propagation is arrhythmogenic because it tends to disorganize the spread of the wave of depolarization, thereby setting the stage for reentry. Mechanisms that slow conduction include the decreased resting potential seen in the energy-starved heart. This occurs because sodium pump inhibition lowers intracellular potassium concentration, which by decreasing the potassium concentration gradient across the plasma membrane (K_i/K_o in the Nernst equation), reduces the potassium potential. Sodium channel inactivation, one of the major consequences of a decrease in resting potential, slows the inward, depolarizing, sodium currents by inactivating sodium channels, and so reduces conduction velocity. Another potential cause of slow conduction in the failing heart is increased resistance across the gap junctions in the intercalated disc (DeMello, 1996). The latter, which contain low-resistance channels made up of proteins called *connexins*, facilitate the ion movements that are essential to maintain a rapid conduction velocity. Acidosis and calcium overload, both of which are seen in failing hearts, tend to close the gap junction channels, so that, by increasing internal resistance, this change slows conduction. These, along with additional mechanisms that slow impulse conduction, often generate reentrant arrhythmias that cause sudden cardiac death in patients with heart failure.

A third class of abnormalities that leads to tachyarryhthmias is seen when inhomogeneities among action potentials in adjacent cells set the stage for reentry. In addition to differences in resting potential, localized variations in action potential duration can allow a cell that has recovered ahead of its neighbors to be depolarized by nearby cells whose action potentials are more long-lasting. Local variations in channel recovery time and refractoriness are arrhythmogenic because these heterogeneities create populations of cells that may not have recovered from the passage of an action potential; such cells respond to subsequent depolarization by generating a small, slowly increasing action potential that, because it is conducted slowly, sets the stage for a reentrant arrhythmia.

Architectural abnormalities in the hypertrophied ventricle represent a different, but very important cause for lethal tachyarryhthmias in patients with heart failure. Both thickening of the walls of a hypertrophied ventricle, which increases the length of the conducting pathways, and fibrosis, which slows and disorganizes conduction, increase the likelihood for reentry, and thus the appearance of lethal arrhythmias.

Molecular Changes Involving the Ion Channels of the Failing Heart

There is growing evidence that the molecular properties of the heart's voltage-gated ion channels are altered by chronic overload. Action potential prolongation, among the most prominent electrophysiologic abnormalities in hypertrophied myocardial cells (Tritthart et al., 1975; Aronson, 1980; Heller and Stauffer, 1981; Hemwall et al., 1984; ten Eick et al., 1992) can be caused by delayed inactivation of L-type calcium channels (Keung, 1989) and abnormalities involving the potassium channels that repolarize the heart (Beuckelmann et al., 1993; Tomaselli et al., 1994; Koumi et al., 1995). Among the most important of the latter are changes in the i_{to} potassium channels, which normally shorten action potential duration by opening briefly after initial depolarization (Näbauer et al., 1993; Rosen et al., 1998; Tomita et al., 1994; Bailly et al., 1997). The abnormal appearance of a hyperpolarization-activated inward current, i_f, which plays a key role in the SA node pacemaker, has also been found in failing ventricles (Cerbai et al., 1997; Hoppe et al., 1998). These and other molecular abnormalities can create regional variations in channel function and so cause electrical inhomogeneities that can kill patients with heart failure (Shipsey et al., 1997). Because this is a relatively young field, it is not yet possible to assess the role of these and other molecular abnormalities in generating lethal arrhythmias in heart failure.

MECHANISMS RESPONSIBLE FOR ABNORMAL EXCITATION-CONTRACTION COUPLING, CONTRACTION, AND RELAXATION IN THE FAILING HEART

Two entirely different mechanisms can inhibit the interactions between the cardiac contractile proteins and the calcium fluxes that regulate contraction and relaxation in the failing heart. The first is a state of energy starvation, discussed later, that is caused by an imbalance between increased energy demands and impaired energy production; the second is altered composition of the cardiac myocyte. Although both of these mechanisms have been studied for almost 40 years, neither their pathophysiology nor their clinical significance is fully understood.

A decrease in ATP level that deprives substrate-binding sites on the contractile proteins and ion pumps of their energy source, the simplest explanation by which energy-starvation can impair inotropy and lusitropy, is not the most important consequence of this lack of energy. Instead, the most important effects of energy starvation on contraction and relaxation are due to attenuation of the allosteric effects of ATP and to a reduction in the free energy released during ATP hydrolysis.

The second cause of the inotropic and lusitropic abnormalities in the failing heart are the molecular changes that accompany the hypertrophic response of a damaged or overloaded heart. This mitogenic response not only increases the mass of the failing heart but also changes the expression of genes that encode the proteins and membrane structures responsible for excitation-contraction coupling, contraction, and relaxation. Changes in the molecular composition of the hypertrophied heart involve many of the proteins of the contractile apparatus, the cytoskeleton, and the sarcoplasmic reticulum. Increased expression of a low ATPase isoform of the myosin heavy chain, for example, reduces myocardial contractility by slowing cross-bridge turnover, whereas decreased density of sarcoplasmic reticulum calcium pump ATPase molecules impairs relaxation by slowing calcium removal from the cytosol during diastole. Other maladaptive features of the hypertrophic response, which both weaken the failing heart and impair its ability to relax, include myocardial cell death and proliferation of fibrous tissue (see Chapters 5 through 8).

REVERSION TO THE FETAL PHENOTYPE

The following passage, a slightly modified Shakespeare's "seven ages of man" speech in *As You Like It*, reveals the bard's understanding of both the similarities and differences between infancy and old age:

> All the world's a stage, and all the men and women merely players. They have their exits and their entrances, and one man in his time plays many parts, his act being seven ages. At first the infant, mewling and puking in the nurse's arms. Then the whining schoolboy with his satchel and shining morning face, creeping like snail unwillingly to school. And then the lover, sighing like furnace, with a woeful ballad made to his mistress' eyebrow. Then a soldier, full of strange oaths and bearded like the pard, jealous in honor, sudden and quick in quarrel, seeking the bubble Reputation e'en in the cannon's mouth. And then the justice, in fair round belly with good capon lin'd, with eyes severe and beard of formal cut, full of wise saws and modern instances; and so he plays his part. The sixth age shifts into the lean and slipper'd pantaloon, with spectacles on nose and pouch on side; his youthful hose well sav'd, a world too wide for his shrunk shank, and his big manly voice, turning again toward childish treble, pipes and whistles in his sound. Last scene of all, that ends this strange eventful history, is second childishness and mere oblivion—sans teeth, sans eyes, sans taste, sans cardiac output, sans everything. (Apologies to Wm. Shakespeare.)

Shakespeare's description of the similarities between infancy and senescence, to which I have taken the liberty of adding a decrease in cardiac output, clearly shows his recognition that the second childhood is not like the first, but instead represents a progressive loss of function that tends toward oblivion. Shakespeare's view of old age also applies to the heart, where the molecular changes that accompany normal aging share many similarities with those seen in the fetal heart (for review, see Lakatta et al., 1997). Similar changes occur in the failing heart, where they tend to recreate the more primitive cardiac myocyte phenotype seen in fetal life. The result is that the failing heart, like the fetal heart, comes to depend on glycolytic energy production, becomes weakened, and depends more on the extracellular calcium cycle, which slows both excitation-contraction coupling and relaxation. Although the latter changes further impair the hemodynamic abnormalities in these patients, they offer some advantage to these patients in that they reduce the energy consumption of the failing heart.

MOLECULAR CHANGES IN THE OVERLOADED AND FAILING HEART

In 1962, Alpert and Gordon reported a reduction in the intrinsic rate of ATP hydrolysis (ATPase activity) of myofibrils isolated from failing hearts. This abnormality was immediately recognized as a potential explanation for the depressed myocardial contractility in these patients. Awan and Goldspink (1972) compared the energetics of skeletal muscles with different types of myosin and noted that, although shortening velocity was slower in muscles that had a low myosin ATPase activity, the efficiency of tension development was higher. These findings provide yet another example of the principle of "unexpected consequences" encountered throughout his text. In this case, changes in the contractile proteins that weaken the failing heart have beneficial energetic consequences.

Over the past 40 years, knowledge of the molecular changes responsible for the observations of Alpert and Gordon (1962) has been expanded considerably, although some aspects of the molecular changes associated with heart failure remain controversial. This is due in part to technical and other experimental problems, comparisons using both mRNA and protein levels (which do not always change in the same way), differences among heart failure models used in these studies, the age of the animals studied, and the time after an intervention that causes the heart to fail when the molecular studies are carried out. The availability of explanted human hearts, obtained at the time of heart transplantation, has added considerably to current knowledge of the molecular biology of clinical heart failure. However, because most tissue studied has come from end-stage heart failure, much remains to be learned about the progressive deterioration of the failing heart in humans. The following discussion provides an overview of the more important abnormalities seen in the failing heart, along with a discussion of the clinical significance of these changes. A personal interpretation of this difficult literature is provided in Table 3-5.

TABLE 3-5. *Contractile protein alterations in the failing heart*

Protein	Experimental heart failure	Human heart failure
Myosin heavy chain	Reversion to fetal phenotype	Reversion to fetal phenotype
Myosin light chains	Reversion to fetal phenotype	Reversion to fetal phenotype
Actin	Reversion to fetal phenotype	No change
Troponin I	Reversion to fetal phenotype	Reversion to fetal phenotype
Troponin T	Reversion to fetal phenotype	?Reversion to fetal phenotype
Troponin C	No change	No change
Tropomyosin	No change	No change

The Contractile Proteins

The isoform shifts seen in experimental models of heart failure often differ from those found in humans. Most important are the differences between the rat, which because this represents an inexpensive model, has been studied extensively, and larger animals. For this reason, the following discussion considers each of these separately.

Experimental Models

Isoform shifts involving most of the contractile proteins discussed earlier have been reported in experimental heart failure (for review, see Scheuer and Buttrick, 1985; Swynghedauw, 1986, 1989; Nadal-Ginard and Mahdavi, 1989; Bugaisky et al., 1992; Schiaffino and Reggiani, 1996; James and Robbins, 1997). The most extensively studied of these responses takes place in myosin, where a shift from the high ATPase α heavy chain to the slower β heavy chain reduces contractility. Changes are also seen in the myosin light chains, the smaller regulatory proteins discussed earlier. Another isoform shift occurs in actin, where pressure overload causes some of the cardiac α actin to be replaced by skeletal α actin, which is the gene product found in fetal heart. Studies using transgenic animals indicate that the actin isoform switch increases contractility (Hewett et al., 1994) and so has an effect opposite to that caused by the myosin heavy chain isoform shift.

There are many reports that the calcium-sensitivity of the contractile proteins is reduced in the failing heart. These changes cannot be attributed to isoform shifts involving troponin C, the calcium-binding protein of the thin filament. The latter, which is the least mutable of the myofibrillar proteins, appears not to be subject to the isoform shifts seen for the other myofibrillar proteins. Similarly, no changes were found when tropomyosin isoforms were examined in the failing heart (Morano et al., 1997). For this reason, isoform shifts involving troponin T, troponin I, the other regulatory proteins of the thin filament, appear to modify calcium-binding by troponin C by allosteric effect.

The molecular changes in hypertrophied hearts are not due simply to an overall stimulation of myocyte growth; instead, the altered protein isoforms appear at different times and in different places. In the initial response to overload, for example, appearance of the slow myosin and fetal actin isoforms follow different time courses (Izumo et al., 1987), and the abnormal isoforms of myosin and actin are initially found in different locations in the overloaded rat heart (Schiaffino et al., 1989). Different molecular changes are caused by pressure overload and volume overload (Calderone et al., 1995), which means that different signal pathways operate in different types of heart failure (see Chapters 6-8).

Heart Failure in Humans

The patterns of isoform replacement in the contractile proteins of the human heart are generally similar to those seen in laboratory animals. Once again, changes involving myosin have been studied most extensively. In the human atrium, where the normal myosin heavy chains are mostly the high ATPase isoform, chronic overload causes an isoform shift that replaces the fast atrial myosin heavy chains with the low ATPase isoform (Tsuchimochi et al., 1984; Bouvagnet et al., 1985; Mercadier et al, 1987). The normal human ventricle contains about 90% slow myosin heavy chain, which allows a less extensive, but similar, isoform shift to occur in clinical heart failure (Nakao et al., 1997). There is general agreement that myofibrillar function is depressed in the failing human heart, but the causal role of changes in myosin ATPase activity remains controversial (Nguyen et al., 1996).

Isoform shifts in the chronically overloaded human heart have also been found in the myosin light chains (Morano et al., 1997) and troponin I (Bodor et al., 1997). In contrast to the rat, where the fetal isoform of actin is upregulated in the failing heart, this feature of the reversion to the fetal phenotype appears not to occur in humans (Boehler et al., 1991). The status of troponin T remains unclear in that reversion to the fetal phenotype has been found by some (Anderson et al., 1991, 1995) but not all groups (Mesnard et al., 1995); this isoform shift probably varies among individual patients (Solaro et al., 1993). Altered phosphorylation of troponin I, a posttranslational modification that differs fundamentally from the isoform shifts caused by changes in gene expression, has been observed in the failing heart (Wolff et al., 1996; Bodor et al., 1997). As in the case of the animal models of heart failure discussed earlier, isoform shifts involving troponin C, the actual calcium-binding protein, do not appear to play a role in these functional changes.

The Sarcoplasmic Reticulum

Relaxation of the failing heart is impaired in experimental heart failure and end-stage heart failure in humans (Gwathmey et al., 1987; Smith and Zile, 1992; Perreault et al., 1993). In fact, delayed filling is probably one of the first hemodynamic abnormalities to appear in the pressure-overloaded human heart (Smith et al., 1986). The underlying causes of these lusitropic abnormalities, as noted in Chapter 2, are quite complex. There is general agreement that levels of all three of the major proteins that participate in calcium transport by the sarcoplasmic reticulum are reduced in the failing heart (Table 3-6); however, the proteins that store calcium within this membrane system appear to be unchanged (for review, see Arai et al., 1994; Lenhart et al., 1998). These changes appear not to be accompanied by isoform shifts like those described for the contractile proteins (Nagai et al., 1989; Komuro et al., 1990; De la Bastie et al., 1990), although a recent report describes a differential downregulation of the SERCA 2b isoform of the calcium pump ATPase (Anger et al., 1998). As was the case for the contractile proteins, not all reports have yielded the same results, discrepancies that are due in part to differences in the models used and the fact that mRNA and protein levels do not always change at the same time and in the same manner (Schwinger et al., 1995; Linck et al., 1996; Beuve et al., 1997).

The general pattern that emerges from studies of the sarcoplasmic reticulum in the failing heart, summarized in Table 3-6, indicates either a decrease or no change in the levels of the calcium pump ATPase, the calcium release channels, and the regulatory protein phospholamban. In experimental heart failure, there is lack of agreement in the published data, but as with clinical heart failure, levels of these transport proteins are generally

TABLE 3-6. *Sarcoplasmic reticulum alterations in the failing heart*

Protein	Change in human heart failure
Sarcoplasmic reticulum	
Calcium pump ATPase (SERCA)	Normal or decreased
Phospholamban	Normal or decreased
Calcium release channel (ryanodine receptor)	Normal or decreased
Calsequestrin	Normal
Calreticulin	Normal
Plasma membrane	
L-type calcium channels	?Increased channel opening
Sodium/calcium exchanger	Increased
Sodium pump	Reexpression of fetal isoforms

found either to be decreased or unchanged. A likely explanation for these discrepancies is that depressed levels of these sarcoplasmic reticulum proteins becomes more marked with the progressive deterioration of the failing heart (Feldman et al., 1993; Arai et al., 1996).

The reduced levels of the calcium pump ATPase generally observed in severe heart failure would decrease the rate of calcium uptake and so decrease both -dP/dt and filling rate (see Chapter 2). A decrease in the content of phospholamban, which in its dephospho form inhibits calcium transport into the sarcoplasmic reticulum, might be expected to accelerate calcium uptake into the sarcoplasmic reticulum, thereby accelerating relaxation. Lack of phospholamban in transgenic animals, by increasing the sequestration of calcium within internal stores, does have a positive inotropic effect (Luo et al., 1994). However, the observed downregulation of the calcium pump and phospholamban probably reflects a decreased content of sarcoplasmic reticulum, which would impair relaxation and, by reducing intracellular calcium stores, also depress contractility. The often observed decrease in the content of calcium release channels would also decrease contractility. This evidence that sarcoplasmic reticulum content decreases in severe heart failure fits the pattern of "reversion to the fetal phenotype" discussed earlier, because this internal membrane system is absent, or poorly developed, in primitive and embryonic hearts that depend mainly on the extracellular calcium cycle.

The Plasma Membrane

The protein composition of the plasma membrane appears to change less in the failing heart than that of either the myofilaments or sarcoplasmic reticulum. In the case of the voltage-gated calcium channels, published findings are conflicting (see Schröder et al., 1998, for a recent review of this literature). A recent report that the availability and open probability of the L-type plasma membrane calcium channels (dihydropyridine receptors) is increased in the failing human heart (Schröder et al., 1998) is congruent with evidence that expression of the sodium/calcium exchanger is increased in these hearts (Studer et al., 1994; Flesch et al., 1996; Reinecke et al., 1996). Taken together, these findings suggest that increased reliance of the extracellular calcium cycle in the failing heart might represent another manifestation of the reversion to a fetal pattern; in this case, that of excitation-contraction coupling. Support for this view is found in studies of the sodium pump, which have shown the reexpression of fetal isoforms in the hypertrophied heart (Charlemagne et al., 1986, 1994; Sweadner et al., 1994; Book et al., 1994). While many details remain to be filled in, increases in several plasma membrane activities in the failing heart are consistent with other data showing a reversion to the fetal pattern.

Proteins of the Cytoskeleton

Isoform shifts have been found in some of the cytoskeletal proteins in failing hearts of both laboratory animals and humans. Alterations have been reported in titin, α-actinin, myosin-binding protein C, microtubules, and fibronectin (Morano et al., 1994; Tsutsui et al., 1994; Farhadian et al., 1995; Kostin et al., 1998). Changes in the latter are found mainly in the coronary arteries (Farhadian et al., 1995), which is not surprising because nonmyocytes—which are capable of proliferation—participate in the growth response to overload. The response of nonmyocytes is discussed further in Chapter 6, when fibrosis of the failing heart is considered.

Summary

At least three lessons can be learned from the patterns of isoform shifts that occur in the failing heart. First, the mammalian heart, which is made up of terminally differentiated myocytes that have little or no capacity to divide (see Chapter 6), is a highly plastic organ that readily changes its composition in response to stress. Second, the details of the phenotypic change depend on the nature of the stress; for example, pressure overload and volume overload evoke different molecular responses (Calderone et al., 1995). Third, and from a practical standpoint the most important, the appearance of different phenotypic responses means that the heart is able to activate different signal transduction pathways to tailor its growth response to a specific stress (see Chapter 7). The latter interpretation is exciting in terms of efforts to treat the deadly clinical syndrome of heart failure, in which maladaptive growth appears to play a central role in the progressive deterioration of the failing heart. Some of the isoform shifts described in this section, for example, can be deleterious to the failing heart, whereas others may be beneficial. The existence of different mitogenic pathways provides opportunities for the development of selective growth inhibitors able to slow, and possibly reverse, the deterioration of these patients. These considerations raise the possibility of developing new means to optimize function and improve prognosis in this syndrome.

ENERGY STARVATION

High-energy phosphate levels have been found to be reduced in biopsy specimens taken from overloaded or failing animal hearts (Furchgott and Lee, 1961; Feinstein, 1962; Pool et al., 1967; Wexler et al., 1988; Sanbe et al., 1993; Neubauer et al., 1995; Liao et al., 1996) and failing human hearts (Peyton et al., 1982; Swain et al., 1982; Bashore et al., 1987; Hardy et al., 1991; Nascimben et al., 1996; Neubauer et al., 1997a). Phosphocreatine content is generally more depressed than that of ATP, largely because phosphocreatine buffers ATP concentration when the rate of energy use exceeds that of energy production. A more important role for phosphocreatine is its participation in a "shuttle" that transfers energy from the mitochondria, where high-energy phosphates are generated, to the cytosol, where they are consumed. A recent finding that, for the same degree of clinical symptoms, aortic insufficiency (volume overload) is accompanied by a much smaller decrease in myocardial high-energy phosphate levels than aortic stenosis (pressure overload) (Neubauer et al., 1997b), represents another example of the different phenotypes that appear in the failing heart (see Chapter 6).

The patterns of energy production in the failing heart, like those described above for excitation-contraction coupling, contraction, and relaxation, resemble those seen in the fetal heart, where there is less reliance on the efficient pathways of mitochondrial ATP production. The mitochondrial abnormalities in the failing heart are likely to be the result of damage to these intracellular organelles, rather than a "reversion to the fetal phenotype." Regardless of the pathogenic mechanisms involved, these changes reduce the availability of the high-energy phosphates needed to meet the increased work demands of an overloaded, failing myocardium.

Compartmentation of High-Energy Phosphates: "Glycolytic ATP"

There are two major problems in interpreting the significance of the depressed high-energy phosphate levels found in the failing heart. The first is that these compounds can be "compartmented" within the cell, owing largely to differences between concentrations within the cytosol and the mitochondria, which make up about one third of the volume of working myocardial cells. The second is a special role played by the ATP generated by glycolytic reactions. Even though there is no membrane barrier that can define an ultra-structural compartment for "glycolytic ATP," there is solid evidence that the ATP produced by these pathways is more readily used by ion pumps and other membrane structures than is the ATP generated by the mitochondria (Anderson and Morris, 1978; Bricknell et al., 1981; Weiss and Hiltbrand, 1985; Weiss and Lamp, 1987; Owen et al., 1990). This special role for the ATP generated by glycolytic enzymes explains reports that glycolytic inhibition is especially harmful in causing diastolic dysfunction in the failing heart (Apstein et al., 1976; 1983; Cunningham et al., 1990; Kagaya et al., 1995).

The Phosphocreatine Shuttle

The rate-limiting step in supplying high-energy phosphate to the contractile proteins and ion pumps is not, as might be expected, the delivery of ATP to these energy-consuming cytosolic structures. Instead, diffusion of ADP back to the mitochondria is rate-limiting because of the very low cytosolic ADP concentration, which is about 100-fold less than the ATP concentration (Illingworth et al., 1975; Rauch et al., 1994; Wallimann et al., 1992). To circumvent problems that could arise because of the extremely slow diffusion of these small amounts of ADP, creatine, which is present in the cytosol at much higher concentrations, rather than ADP serves as the high-energy phosphate receptor.

The phosphocreatine shuttle depends on reactions that are catalyzed by *creatine phosphokinase*, an enzyme that transfers high-energy phosphate in the cytosol from phosphocreatine to ADP according to the overall reaction:

$$\text{phosphocreatine} + \text{ADP} \leftrightarrow \text{ATP} + \text{creatine} \qquad \text{Equation 3.1}$$

Conversely, creatine provides the acceptor for the high-energy phosphates generated in the mitochondria when a similar reaction, catalyzed by mitochondrial creatine phosphokinase, regenerates phosphocreatine using the high-energy phosphate in ATP generated by oxidative phosphorylation. These reactions constitute the "phosphocreatine shuttle" (Jacobus, 1985; Kammermeier, 1987), so named because phosphocreatine transfers high-energy phosphates generated in the mitochondria to the contractile proteins and other energy-consuming systems in the cytosol. Slowing of the phosphocreatine shuttle, as discussed later, is probably a major cause of the state of energy starvation seen in the failing heart.

Reduced Oxygen Delivery

One of the most important abnormalities that impair high-energy phosphate production in the failing heart is reduced oxygen delivery to myocardial cells. Nutrient coronary flow is decreased by hypertrophy because of increased length of the arteries that penetrate the ventricular wall from their origins in the large epicardial coronary arteries. Diffusion of substrates, notably oxygen, is also impaired by increased intercapillary distance (Roberts and Wearn, 1941) and decreased density of transverse capillary profiles (Anversa et al., 1980). The resulting imbalance between energy production and consumption is especially marked in the relatively underperfused subendocardial regions of the thick-walled hypertrophied left ventricle (Hoffman, 1987), where a combination of high wall stress and reduced perfusion can lead to a state of energy starvation so severe as to cause myocyte necrosis. Although a recent study suggests that expansion of the capillary bed in the hypertrophied canine heart can maintain a virtually normal density and surface area of nutrient vessels (Bishop et al., 1996), there is abundant evidence that coronary flow reserve is reduced in the failing heart (Marcus et al., 1982; Wangler et al., 1982; Wicker et al., 1983).

Mitochondrial Changes

There is substantial evidence that mitochondrial energy production is impaired in the failing heart (Anderson et al., 1990; Sabbah et al., 1992; Sack et al., 1996; Allard et al., 1997; see Katz, 1996b for a review of the older literature) and that mitochondrial DNA is abnormal in the failing heart (Soumalainen et al., 1992; Obayashi et al., 1992; Remes et al., 1993). These abnormalities are due in part to the actions of free radicals, which damage the mitochondrial DNA (see Chapter 5). Unlike nuclear DNA, which in the adult cardiac myocyte has little capacity for replication (see Chapter 6), mitochondrial DNA is capable of replication. Because mechanisms for the repair of free-radical induced damage to mitochondrial DNA are poorly developed, copies of the damaged mitochondrial DNA can accumulate in the failing heart (Sanders, 1995). Antibody-mediated mitochondrial damage may also occur in the failing heart (Schultheiss et al., 1995). The changes in the pattern of energy production in the failing heart, therefore, may represent not only a "reversion to the fetal phenotype," but also mitochondrial damage.

Morphologic evidence for mitochondrial damage in end-stage heart failure is less clear than was once believed. Early reports that mitochondrial volume is decreased in the failing heart (Meerson, 1961; Wollenberger et al., 1962; Page and McCallister, 1973; Anversa et al., 1976, 1979, 1980; Kamereit and Jacob, 1979) have not been confirmed in more recent studies (Kunkel et al., 1987; Hatt, 1988; Schaper et al., 1991; Sabbah et al., 1992; Scholz et al, 1995). There is, however, general agreement that mitochondria are smaller and more numerous in the failing heart. This architectural change may be caused by the mitochondrial gene abnormalities discussed previously.

Creatine Phosphokinase

Decreased levels of creatine phosphokinase, by slowing ADP rephosphorylation by way of the phosphocreatine shuttle, probably play a major role in exacerbating the state of energy starvation in the failing heart (Ingwall et al., 1985; Neubauer et al., 1995; Nascimben et al., 1996). Some compensation for loss of this enzyme in the hypertrophied heart is achieved by an isoform switch that replaces the M isoform of creatine phosphokinase with the B isoform (Meerson and Javick, 1982; Ingwall et al., 1995; Neubauer et al., 1995). Because the B isoform is predominant in the fetal heart, this isoform shift provides another example of the reversion to the fetal phenotype. The affinity of the B isoform of this enzyme for ADP is higher than that of the M isoform, so that this molecular response facilitates ADP rephosphorylation by the phosphocreatine shuttle. Despite this adaptive isoform switch, however, decreased phosphocreatine levels and mitochondrial damage slow ADP phosphorylation and so probably play an important role in limiting energy production in failing cardiac myocytes (Ingwall, 1993).

Consequences of Decreased ATP and Increased ADP Levels

As noted earlier, there are at least three plausible mechanisms by which a decrease in ATP concentration could impair cardiac pumping. Lack of substrate for energy-consuming reactions, the most obvious, is probably not important in the failing heart because normal ATP concentrations are much higher than those needed to saturate these substrate-binding sites. The other mechanisms, a reduction in the allosteric effects of high ATP concentration and reduced free energy of ATP hydrolysis, are more likely to be important in the patient with heart failure.

Binding of ATP to Substrate Sites

The major consequences of energy starvation in the failing heart are probably not caused by a reduced supply of substrate for the many energy-consuming reactions involved in contraction, relaxation, and excitation-contraction coupling. Because the normal cytosolic ATP concentration is 5 to 10 mM, whereas the substrate-binding sites of most ATP-hydrolyzing systems are saturated at ATP concentrations less than 1 µM, except in the dying heart it is unlikely that ATP concentrations decrease to levels below those needed to saturate known energy-consuming reactions.

Reduced Allosteric Effects of ATP

High ATP concentrations exert many allosteric effects. These effects, which do not require that the nucleotide be hydrolyzed, resemble those of a "lubricant" in that ATP accelerates ion pumps, ion exchangers, and passive ion fluxes through membrane channels.

The allosteric effects of ATP, by facilitating the many calcium fluxes involved in both the intracellular and extracellular calcium cycles shown in Figure 3-1, enhance both inotropic and lusitropic function. Even though the calcium fluxes that mediate excitation-contraction coupling are passive (downhill), the ability of high ATP concentrations to accelerate the flux of activator calcium through the calcium channels in the sarcolemma (Kameyama et al., 1986) and sarcoplasmic reticulum (Smith et al., 1986) means that a decrease in ATP concentration could depress contractility. More obvious is the impaired relaxation that is caused by loss of the allosteric effects of ATP that stimulate active (uphill) transport of calcium out of the cytosol by the calcium pump of the sarcoplasmic reticulum (Shigekawa et al., 1978; Nakamura and Tonomura, 1982) and the sodium-calcium exchanger (DiPolo, 1976).

The Na-K ATPase (sodium pump) is also stimulated by an allosteric effect of ATP (Yamaguchi and Tonomura, 1980), so that attenuation of this allosteric effect in an energy-starved heart would increase intracellular sodium concentration. The latter slows calcium extrusion via the sodium/calcium exchanger, which by increasing cytosolic calcium has a positive inotropic effect; this effect, however, impairs relaxation. Sodium pump inhibition also causes intracellular potassium to decrease. This effect is arrhythmogenic because, as discussed earlier, lowering of intracellular potassium depolarizes the resting plasma membrane.

Another important effect of a decrease in ATP levels is loss of an allosteric effect that facilitates dissociation of actin and myosin during diastole (Katz, 1970). Attenuation of this "plasticizing effect" may explain why even a modest decrease of ATP concentration can increase diastolic stiffness in the energy-starved heart.

Reduced Free Energy of ATP Hydrolysis

The functional consequences of energy starvation in the failing heart include a decrease in the free energy of ATP hydrolysis, which is the amount of energy made available by hydrolysis of the terminal phosphate of ATP. The functional consequences of this decrease reflect the surprisingly small "reserve" in the phosphorylation potential of the heart. Even a 15% to 25% reduction in phosphorylation potential, from the value of approximately 60 kJ/mol in the normal heart to between 45 and 50 kJ/mol, can impair ATP-dependent reactions (Kammermeier et al., 1982; Tian and Ingwall, 1996). A decrease in the ATP/ADP ratio, caused mainly by an increase in ADP concentration, appears to reduce the phosphorylation potential to levels that slow both the calcium pump of the sarcoplasmic reticulum (Tian and Ingwall, 1996) and cross-bridge cycling (Tian et al., 1997a, 1997b).

CONCLUSION

The data reviewed in this chapter document a large number of biochemical abnormalities that are seen in the failing heart. Although these many alterations in the processes of energy production, excitation, excitation-contraction coupling, contraction, and relaxation explain most of the clinical manifestations of this syndrome, they do not account for the poor prognosis. In fact, many of these biochemical abnormalities can be viewed as "epiphenomena" that, while real and of immediate significance, are not related to the major problem in these patients, which is the terrible prognosis. To understand the causes of the progressive deterioration of the failing heart, Chapter 4 describes the neurohumoral response, which generates messenger molecules that have profound actions on both cardiac function and clinical prognosis. Chapter 5 carries the discussion of this response to the mediators of an inflammatory reaction that contributes to both clinical disability and deterioration of the failing heart, after which the focus shifts to the molecular mechanisms responsible for the biochemical abnormalities described in this chapter. In this way, the text seeks to integrate the clinical features of this syndrome with the mechanisms responsible for shortening survival, information that is essential in planning therapy for these patients.

BIBLIOGRAPHY

Bers DM (1991). *Excitation-Contraction Coupling and Cardiac Contractile Force.* Kluwer, Dordrecht, The Netherlands.
Hille B (1992). *Ionic Channels of Excitable Membranes.* Sinauer, Sunderland, MA.
Johnson RG, Kranias EG (1998). Cardiac Sarcoplasmic Reticulum Function and Regulation of Contractility. *Ann N Y Acad Sci*, vol. 853.
Katz AM (1992). *Physiology of the Heart,* 2nd ed. Raven Press, New York.
Rüegg C (1992). *Calcium in Muscle Contraction. Cellular and Molecular Physiology*, 2nd ed. Springer, Berlin.
Swynghedauw B (1990). *Cardiac Hypertrophy and Failure.* John Libby, London.

REFERENCES

Allard MF, Henning SL, Wambolt RB, Gransleese SR, English DR, Lopaschuk GD (1997). Glycogen metabolism in the aerobic hypertrophied heart. *Circulation* 96:676–682.
Alpert NR, Gordon MS (1962). Myofibrillar adenosine triphosphatase activity in congestive heart failure. *Am J Physiol* 202:940–946.
Alpert NR, Mulieri LA, Hasenfuss G (1991). Myocardial chemo-energy transduction. In Fozzard H, Haber E, Katz A, Jennings R, Morgan HE, eds. *The Heart and Circulation*, 2nd ed. Raven Press, New York, pp 111–128.
Anand IS, Liu D, Chugh SS, Prahash AJC, Gupta S, John R, Popescu F, Chandrashenkhar Y (1997). Isolated myocyte contractile function is normal in postinfarct remodeled rat heart with systolic dysfunction. *Circulation* 96:3974–3984.
Anderson GL, Morris RG (1978). Role of glycolysis in the relaxation process in mammalian cardiac muscle: comparison of the influence of glucose and 2-deoxyglucose on maintenance of resting tension. *Life Sci* 23:23–31.
Anderson PAW, Allard MF, Thomas GD, Bishop SP, Digerness SB (1990). Increased ischemic injury but decreased hypoxic injury in hypertrophied rat hearts. *Circ Res* 67:948–959.
Anderson PAW, Malouf NN, Oakeley AE, Pagini ED, Allen PD (1991). Troponin T isoform expression in humans. A comparison among normal and failing adult heart, fetal heart, and fetal skeletal muscle. *Circ Res* 69:1226–1233.

Anderson PAW, Grieg A, Mark TN, Malouf NN, Oakeley AE, Ungerleider RM, Allen PD, Kay BK (1995). Molecular basis of human cardiac troponin T isoforms expressed in the developing, adult and failing heart. *Circ Res* 76: 681–686.

Anger M, Lompré A-M, Vallot O, Marotte F, Rappaport L, Samuel J-L (1998). Cellular distribution of Ca^{2+} pumps and Ca^{2+} release channels in rat cardiac hypertrophy-induced by aortic stenosis. *Circulation* 98:2477–2486.

Antz C, Geyer M, Fakler B, Schott MK, Guy HR, Frank R, Ruppersberg JP, Kalbitzer HR (1997). NMR structure of inactivation gates from mammalian voltage-dependent potassium channels. *Nature* 385:272–274.

Anversa P, Loud AV, Vitali-Mazza L (1976). Morphometry and autoradiography of early hypertrophic changes in the ventricular myocardium of adult rat. An electronic microscopic study. *Lab Invest* 35:475–483.

Anversa P, Loud AV, Giocomelli F, Weiner J (1979). Absolute morphometric study of myocardial hypertrophy induced by abdominal aortic stenosis. *Lab Invest* 40:341–349.

Anversa P, Olivetti G, Melissari M, Loud AV (1980). Stereological measurement of cellular and subcellular hypertrophy and hyperplasia in the papillary muscle of adult rat. *J Mol Cell Cardiol* 12:781–795.

Apstein CS, Bing OHL, Levine HJ (1976). Cardiac muscle function during and after hypoxia: effects of glucose concentration, mannitol and isoproterenol. *J Mol Cell Cardiol* 8:627–640.

Apstein CS, Gravino FN, Haudenschild CC (1983). Determinants of a protective effect of glucose and insulin on the ischemic myocardium: effects on contractile function, diastolic compliance, metabolism and ultrastructure during ischemia and reperfusion. *Circ Res* 52:515–526.

Arai M, Matsui H, Periasamy M (1994). Sarcoplasmic reticulum gene expression in cardiac hypertrophy and failure. *Circ Res* 74:555–564.

Arai M, Suzuki T, Nagai R (1996). Sarcoplasmic reticulum genes are upregulated in mild cardiac hypertrophy but downregulated in severe cardiac hypertrophy induced by pressure overload. *J Mol Cell Cardiol* 28:1583–1590.

Aronson RS (1980). Characteristics of action potentials of hypertrophied myocardium from rats with renal hypertension. *Circ Res* 47:443–454.

Awan MZ, Goldspink G (1972). Energetics of the development and maintenance of isometric tension by mammalian fast and slow muscles. *J Mechanochem Cell Motility* 1:97–108.

Bailly P, Bénitah J-P, Mouchoniére M, Vassort G, Lorente P (1997). Regional alterations in the transient outward current in human left ventricular septum during compensated hypertrophy. *Circulation* 96:1266–1274.

Bashore TM, Magorien DJ, Letterio J, Shaffer P, Unverferth DV (1987). Histologic and biochemical correlates of left ventricular chamber dynamics in man. *J Am Coll Cardiol* 9:734–742.

Bennett PB, Valenzuela C, Chen L-Q, Kallen RG (1995). On the molecular structure of the lidocaine receptor of cardiac Na^+ channels. Modification of block by alterations in the α-subunit II-IV interdomain. *Circ Res* 77:584–592.

Berridge M (1993). Inositol trisphosphate and calcium signaling. *Nature* 361:315–325.

Beuckelmann DJ, Näbauer M, Erdmann E (1993). Alterations of K^+ currents in isolated ventricular myocytes from patients with terminal heart failure. *Circ Res* 73:379–385.

Beuve CS, Allen PD, Dambrin G, Rannou F, Marty I, Trouvé P, Bors V, Pavie A, Gandgjbakch I, Charlemagne D (1997). Cardiac calcium channel (ryanodine receptor) in control and cardiomyopathic human hearts: mRNA and protein contents are differentially regulated. *J Mol Cell Cardiol* 29:1237–1246.

Bishop SP, Powell PC, Hasebe N, Shen Y-T, Patrick TA, Hittinger L, Vatner SF (1996). Coronary vascular morphology ion pressure-overload left ventricular hypertrophy. *J Mol Cell Cardiol* 28:141–154.

Bodor GS, Oakeley AE, Allen PD, Crimmins DL, Ladenson JH, Anderson PAW (1997). Troponin I phosphorylation in the normal and failing adult human heart. *Circulation* 96:1495–1500.

Boheler KR, Carrier L, de la Bastie D, Allen PD, Komajda M, Mercadier JJ, Schwartz K (1991). Skeletal actin mRNA increases in the human heart during ontogenic development and is the major isoform of control and failing adult hearts. *J Clin Invest* 88:323–330.

Book C-BS, Moore RL, Semanchik A, Ng Y-C (1994). Cardiac hypertrophy alters expression of Na^+,K^+-ATPase subunit isoforms at mRNA and protein levels in rat myocardium. *J Mol Cell Cardiol* 26:561–600.

Bouvagnet P, Léger J, Dechesne CA, Dureau G, Anoal M, Léger JJ (1985). Local changes in myosin types in diseased human atrial myocardium: a quantitative immunofluorescence study. *Circulation* 72:272–279.

Bricknell OS, Daries PS, Opie LH (1981). A relationship between adenosine triphosphate, glycolysis, and ischemic contracture in the isolated rat heart. *J Mol Cell Cardiol* 13:941–945.

Bugaisky L, Gupta MP, Gupta M, Zak R. (1986) Cellular and molecular mechanisms of cardiac hypertrophy. In Fozzard H, Haber E, Katz A, Jennings R, Morgan HE, eds. *The Heart and Cardiovascular System*, 2nd ed. Raven Press, New York, pp 1621–1640.

Calderone A, Takahashi N, Izzo NJ Jr, Thaik CM, Colucci WS (1995). Pressure- and volume-induced left ventricular hypertrophies are associated with distinct myocyte phenotypes and differential induction of peptide growth factor mRNAs. *Circulation* 92:2385–2390.

Carafoli E (1991). Calcium pump of the plasma membrane. *Physiol Rev* 71:129–153.

Catterall WA (1988). Structure and function of voltage-sensitive ion channels. *Science* 242:50–61.

Catterall WA (1992). Cellular and molecular biology of voltage-gated sodium channels. *Physiol Rev* 72(Suppl): S15–S48.

Cerbai E, Pino R, Pociatti F, Sani G, Toscano M, Maccherini M, Giunti G, Mugelli A (1997). Characterization of the hyperpolarization-activated current I(f) in ventricular myocytes from human failing heart. *Circulation* 95:568–571.

Charlemagne D, Maixent J-M, Preteseille M, Leleivre LG (1986). Ouabain-binding sites and (Na^+,K^+)-ATPase activity in rat cardiac hypertrophy. Expression of the neonatal forms. *J Biol Chem* 261:185–189.

Charlemagne D, Orlowski J, Oliviero P, Rannou F, Sainte Beuve C, Swynghedauw B, Lane LK (1994). Alteration of Na,K-ATPase subunit mRNA and protein levels in hypertrophied rat heart. *J Biol Chem* 269:1541–1547.

Cheng H, Lederer WJ, Cannell MB (1993). Calcium sparks elementary events underlying excitation-contraction coupling in heart muscle. *Science* 262:740–743.

Clapham DE, Ackerman MJ (1997). Ion channels—basic science and clinical disease. *N Engl J Med* 336:1575–1586.

Cunningham ML, Apstein CS, Weinberg EO, Vogel WM, Lorell BH (1990). Influence of glucose and insulin on the exaggerated diastolic and systolic dysfunction of hypertrophied rat hearts during hypoxia. *Circ Res* 66:406–415.

De la Bastie D, Levitsky D, Rappaport L, Mercadier J-J, Marotte F, Wisnewsky C, Brokovich V, Schwartz K, Lompré A-M (1990). Function of the sarcoplasmic reticulum and expression of its Ca^{2+} ATPase gene in pressure-overloaded cardiac hypertrophy in the rat. *Circ Res* 66:554–564.

DeMello WC (1996). Renin-angiotensin system and cell communication in the failing heart. *Hypertension* 27: 1267–1272.

DiPolo R (1976). The influence of nucleotides on calcium fluxes. *Fed Proc* 35:2579–2582.

East T (1958). Failure of the circulation and its treatment. *The Story of Heart Disease.* Dawson and Sons, London, Lecture 4, pp 127–145.

Fabiato A (1983). Calcium-induced release of calcium from the cardiac sarcoplasmic reticulum. *Am J Physiol* 245: C1–C14.

Fabiato A, Fabiato F (1975). Dependence of the contractile activation of skinned cardiac cells on the sarcomere length. *Nature* 256:54–56.

Farhadian F, Contard F, Corbier A, Barrieux A, Rappaport L, Samuel JL (1995). Fibronectin expression during physiological and pathological cardiac growth. *J Mol Cell Cardiol* 27:981–999.

Feinstein MB (1962). Effects of experimental congestive heart failure, ouabain, and asphyxia on the high-energy phosphate content of the guinea pig heart. *Circ Res* 10:333–346.

Feldman AM. Weinberg EO, Ray PE, Lorell BH (1993). Selective changes in cardiac gene expression during compensated hypertrophy and the transition to cardiac decompensation in rats with chronic aortic banding. *Circ Res* 73:184–192.

Fleischer S, Inui M (1989). Biochemistry and biophysics of excitation-contraction coupling. *Ann Rev Biophys Chem* 18:333–364.

Flesch M, Schwinger RHG, Schiffer F, Frank K, Südkamp M, Kuhn-Regnier F, Arnold G, Böhm M (1996). Evidence for functional relevance of an enhanced expression of the Na^+-Ca^{2+} exchanger in failing human myocardium. *Circulation* 94:992–1002.

Furchgott RF, Lee KS (1961). High energy phosphates and the force of contraction of cardiac muscle. *Circulation* 24:416–428.

Gwathmey JK, Copelas L, MacKinnon R, Schoen FJ, Feldman MD, Grossman W, Morgan JP (1987). Abnormal intracellular calcium handling in myocardium from patients with end-stage heart failure. *Circ Res* 61:70–76.

Hardy CJ, Weiss RG, Bottomley PA, Gerstenblith G (1991). Altered myocardial high-energy phosphate metabolites in patients with dilated cardiomyopathy. *Am Heart J* 122:795–801.

Hartmann HA, Tiedeman AA, Chen S-F, Brown AM, Kirsch GE (1994). Effects of III-IV linker mutations on human Na^+ channel inactivation gating. *Circ Res* 75:114–122.

Hatt PY (1988). Morphological approach to the mechanism of heart failure. *Cardiology* 75(Suppl 1):3–7.

Heller L, Stauffer EK (1981). Membrane potentials and contractile events of hypertrophied rat heart muscle. *Proc Soc Exp Biol Med* 166:141–147.

Helmes M, Trombitás K, Granzier H (1996). Titin develops restoring force in rat cardiac myocytes. *Circ Res* 79: 619–626.

Hemwall EL, Duthin V, Houser SR (1984). Comparison of slow response action potentials from normal and hypertrophied myocardium. *Am J Physiol* 246:H675–H682.

Henzi V, MacDermott AB (1992). Characteristics and function of Ca^{2+}- and inositol 1,4,5-trisphosphate-releasable stores of calcium in neurons. *Neuroscience* 46:251–273.

Hewett TE, Grupp IL, Grupp G, Robbins J (1994). Alpha-skeletal actin is associated with increased contractility in the mouse heart. *Circ Res* 74:740–746.

Hibberd MG, Jewell BR (1982). Calcium- and length-dependent force production in rat ventricular muscle. *J Physiol (London)* 329:527–540.

Hille B (1992). *Ionic Channels of Excitable Membranes.* Sinauer, Sunderland, MA.

Hoffman JEI (1987). Transmural myocardial perfusion. *Prog Cardiovasc Dis* 29:429–464.

Hoppe UC, Jansen E, Südkamp M, Beuckelmann DJ (1998). Hyperpolarization-activated inward current in ventricular myocytes from normal and failing human hearts. *Circulation* 97:55–65.

Horisberger JD, Lemas V, Krähenbuhl JP, Rossier BC (1991). Structure-function relationship of Na,K-ATPase. *Annu Rev Physiol* 53:565–584.

Illingworth JA, Christopher W, Ford L, Kobayashi K, Williamson JR (1975). Regulation of myocardial energy metabolism. In Roy P-E, Harris P, eds. *Recent Advances in Studies on Cardiac Structure and Metabolism* 8:271–290.

Ingwall JS (1993). Is cardiac failure a consequence of decreased energy reserve. *Circulation* 87:VII-58–VII-62.

Ingwall JS, Kramer MF, Fifer MA, Lorell BH, Shemin R, Grossman W, Allen PD (1985). The creatine kinase system in normal and depressed human myocardium. *N Engl J Med* 313:1050–1054.

Isacoff EY, Jan YN, Jan LY (1991). Putative receptor for the cytoplasmic inactivation gate in the *Shaker* K+ channel. *Nature* 353:86–90.

Izumo S, Nadal-Ginard B, Mahdavi V (1988). Protooncogene induction and reprogramming of cardiac gene expression produced by pressure overload. *Proc Nat Acad Sci U S A* 85:339–343.

Jacobus WE (1985). Respiratory control and the integration of heart high-energy metabolism by mitochondrial creatine kinase. *Annu Rev Physiol* 47:707–725.

Jacobus WE, Pores IH, Lucas SK, Weisfeldt ML, Flaherty JT (1982). Intracellular acidosis and contractility in the normal and ischemic heart as examined by ^{31}P NMR. *J Mol Cell Cardiol* 14(Suppl 3):13–20.

James J, Robbins J (1997). Molecular remodeling of cardiac contractile function. *Am J Physiol* 273:H21095–H2118.

Jan LY, Jan YN (1992). Tracing the roots of ion channels. *Cell* 69:715–718.

Jan LY, Jan YN (1994). Potassium channels and their evolving gates. *Nature* 371:119–122.

Kagaya Y, Weinberg EO, Ito N, Mochizuki T, Barry WH, Lorell BH (1995). Glycolytic inhibition: effects on diastolic relaxation and intracellular calcium handling in hypertrophied rat ventricular myocytes. *J Clin Invest* 95:2766–2776.

Kamereit A, Jacob R (1979). Alterations in rat myocardial mechanics under Goldblatt hypertension and experimental aortic stenosis. *Bas Res Cardiol* 74:389–405.

Kameyama M, Hescheler J, Hofmann F, Trautwein W (1986). Modulation of Ca current during the phosphorylation cycle in the guinea pig heart. *Pflügers* Arch 407:123–128.

Kammermeier H (1987). Why do cells need phosphocreatine and a phosphocreatine shuttle? *J Mol Cell Cardiol* 19:115–118.

Kammermeier H, Schmidt P, Jüngling E (1982). Free energy change of ATP-hydrolysis: a causal factor of early hypoxic failure of the myocardium? *J Mol Cell Cardiol* 14:267–277.

Katz AM (1964). Heart failure, fundamental mechanisms in myocardial failure. In Andrus EC, Maxwell CH, eds. *The Heart and Circulation,* Vol 1, Research. *FASEB,* Washington, DC, pp 533–537.

Katz AM (1970). Contractile proteins of the heart. *Physiol Rev* 50:63–158.

Katz AM (1992). *Physiology of the Heart,* 2nd ed. Raven Press, New York.

Katz AM (1993). Cardiac ion channels. *N Engl J Med* 328:1244–1251.

Katz AM (1996a). Calcium channel diversity in the cardiovascular system. *J Am Coll Cardiol* 28:522–528.

Katz AM (1996b). Is the failing heart an energy-starved organ? (Editorial). *J Cardiac Failure* 2:267–272.

Katz AM (1998). Selectivity and toxicity of antiarrhythmic drugs: molecular interactions with ion channels. *Am J Med* 104:179–195.

Kellenberger S, Scheur T, Catterall WA (1996). Movement of the Na+ channel inactivation gate during inactivation. *J Biol Chem* 271:30971–30979.

Keung AC (1989). Calcium current is increased in isolated adult myocytes from hypertrophied rat myocardium. *Circ Res* 64:753–763.

Kim HW, Steenaart NAE, Ferguson DG, Kranias EG (1990). Functional reconstitution of the cardiac sarcoplasmic reticulum Ca^{2+}-ATPase with phospholamban in phospholipid vesicles. *J Biol Chem* 265:1702–1709.

Komuro I, Kurabayashi M, Shibazaki Y, Takaku F, Yazaki Y (1989). Molecular cloning and characterization of a Ca^{2+}+Mg^{2+}-dependent adenosine triphosphatase from rat cardiac sarcoplasmic reticulum. Regulation of its expression by pressure overload and developmental stage. *J Clin Invest* 83:1102–1108.

Kostin S, Heleing A, Hein S, Scholz D, Klövekorn W-P, Schaper J (1998). The protein composition of the normal and diseased cardiac myocyte. *Heart Failure Rev* 2:245–260.

Koumi S-I, Backer CL, Arentzen CE (1995). Characterization if inwardly rectifying K+ channel in human cardiac myocytes. Alterations in channel behavior in myocytes isolated from patients with idiopathic dilated cardiomyopathy. *Circulation* 92:164–174.

Kunkel B, Schneider M (1987). Myocardial structure and left ventricular function in hypertrophic and dilative cardiomyopathy and aortic valve disease. In Kaltenbach M, Hopf R, Kunkel B, eds. *New Aspects of Hypertrophic Cardiomyopathy*. Steinkopff Verlag, Darmstadt, pp 15–23.

Lakatta EG, Gerstenblith G, Weisfeldt ML (1997). The aging heart: structure, function and disease. In Braunwald E, ed. *Heart Disease.* WB Saunders, Philadelphia, pp 1687–1703.

Lenhart SE, Schillinger WG, Pieske B, Prestle J, Just H, Hasenfuss G (1998). Sarcoplasmic reticulum proteins in heart failure. *Ann N Y Acad Sci* 853:220–230.

Levitsky DO, Nicoll DA, Philipson KD (1994). Identification of the high affinity Ca^{2+}-binding domain of the cardiac Na+-Ca^{2+} exchanger. *J Biol Chem* 269:22847–22852.

Liao R, Nascimben L, Friedrich J, Gwathmey JK, Ingwall JS (1996). Decreased energy reserve in an animal model of dilated cardiomyopathy. Relationship to contractile performance. *Circ Res* 78:893–902.

Linke WA, Boknik P, Eschenhagen T, Müller FU, Neumann J, Nose M, Jones LR, Schmitz W, Scholz H (1996). Messenger RNA expression and immunological quantification of phospholamban and SR-Ca^{2+}-ATPase in failing and nonfailing human hearts. *Cardiovasc Res* 31:625–632.

Linke WA, Ivemeyer M, Labeit S, Hinssen H, Rüegg JC, Gautel M (1997). Actin-titin interaction in cardiac myofibrils: probing a physiological role. *Biophys J* 73:905–919.

Luo WI, Grupp IL, Harrer J, Ponniah S, Grupp G, Duffy JJ, Doetschman T, Kranias EG (1994). Targeted ablation of the phospholamban gene is associated with markedly enhanced myocardial contractility and loss of β-agonist stimulation. *Circ Res* 75:401–409.

Lytton J, MacLennan DH (1991). Sarcoplasmic reticulum. In Fozzard H, Haber E, Katz A, Jennings R, Morgan HE, eds. *The Heart and Circulation*, 2nd ed. Raven Press, New York, pp 1203–1222.

Marcus ML, Doty DB, Hiratzka LF, Wright CB, Eastham CL (1982). Decreased coronary reserve: a mechanism for angina pectoris in patients with aortic stenosis and normal coronary arteries. *N Engl J Med* 307:1362–1366.

Meerson FZ (1961). On the mechanism of compensatory hypertrophy and insufficiency of the heart. *Cor et Vasa* 3:161–177.

Meerson FZ, Javick MP (1982). Isozyme pattern and activity of myocardial creatine phosphokinase under heart adaptation to chronic overload. *Basic Res Cardiol* 77:349–358.

Mercadier JJ, de la Bastie D, Menasche P, N'Guyen Van Cao A, Bouvenet P, Lorente P, Piwnica A, Slama R, Schwartz K (1987). Alpha-myosin heavy chain isoform and atrial size in patients with various types of mitral valve dysfunction: a quantitative study. *J Am Coll Cardiol* 9:1024–1030.

Mesnard L, Logeart D, Taviaux S, Diriong S, Mercadier J-J, Samson F (1995). Human cardiac troponin T: cloning and expression of new isoforms in the normal and failing heart. *Circ Res* 76:687–692.

Moncman CL, Wang K (1995). Nebulette: a 107 kD nebulin-like protein in cardiac muscle. *Cell Motil Cytoskeleton* 32:205–225.

Morano I, Hädicke K, Grom S, Koch A, Schwinger RHG, Böhm M, Bartel S, Erdmann E, Krause E-G (1994). Titin, myosin light chains and C protein in the developing and failing human heart. *J Mol Cell Cardiol* 26:361–368.

Morano I, Hädicke K, Hasses H, Böhm M, Erdmann E, Schaub MC (1997). Changes in essential myosin light chain isoform expression provide a molecular basis of isometric force regulation in the failing human heart. *J Mol Cell Cardiol* 29:1177–1187.

Näbauer M, Beuckelmann DJ, Erdmann E (1993). Characteristics of transient outward current in human ventricular myocytes from patients with terminal heart failure. *Circ Res* 73:3869–3934.

Nadal-Ginard B, Mahdavi V (1989). Molecular basis for cardiac performance. Plasticity of the myocardium generated through protein isoform switches. *J Clin Invest* 84:1693–1700.

Nagai R, Zarain-Herzberg A, Brandl CJ, Fuji J, Tada M, MacLennan DH, Alpert NR, Periasamy M (1989). Regulation of myocardial Ca^{2+} ATPase and phospholamban mRNA expression in response to pressure overload and thyroid hormone. *Proc Natl Acad Sci U S A* 86:2966–2970.

Nakamura Y, Tonomura Y (1982). The binding of ATP to the catalytic and the regulatory site of Ca^{2+}, Mg^{2+}-dependent ATPase of the sarcoplasmic reticulum. *J Bioeng Biomed* 14:307–318.

Nakao K, Minobe W, Roden R, Bristow MR, Leinwand LA (1997). Myosin heavy chain gene expression in human heart failure. *J Clin Invest* 100:2362–2370.

Nascimben l, Ingwall JS, Pauletto P, Friedrich J, Gwathmey JK, Saks V, Pessina AC, Allen PD (1996). Creatine kinase system in failing and non-failing human myocardium. *Circulation* 94:1894–1901.

Neubauer S, Horn M, Naumann A. Tian R, Laser M, Friedrich J, Gaudron P, Schnackerz K, Ingwall JS, Errl G (1995). Impairment of energy metabolism in intact residual myocardium of rat hearts with chronic myocardial infarction. *J Clin Invest* 95:1092–1100.

Neubauer S, Horn M, Naumann A, Cramer M, Harre K, Newell JB, Peters W, Pabst T, Errl G, Hahn D, Ingwall JS, Kochsiek K (1997). Myocardial phosphocreatine-to-ATP ratio is a predictor of mortality in patients with dilated cardiomyopathy. *Circulation* 96:2190–2196.

Neubauer S, Horn M, Pabst T, Harre K, Stromer H, Bertsch G, Sandstede J, Ertl G, Hahn D, Kochsiek K (1997b). Cardiac high-energy phosphate metabolism in patients with aortic valve disease assessed by 31P-magnetic resonance spectroscopy. *J Invest Med* 45:453–462.

Nguyen T-T T, Hayes E, Mulieri LA, Leavitt BJ, the Keurs HEDJ, Alpert NR, Warshaw DM (1996). Maximal actomyosin ATPase activity and in vitro myosin motility are unaltered in human mitral regurgitation heart failure. *Circ Res* 79:222–226.

Nicoll DA, Longoni S, Philipson KD (1990). Molecular cloning and functional expression of the cardiac sarcolemmal Na^{+}-Ca^{++} exchanger. *Science* 250:469–471.

Nunoki K, Florio V, Catterall WA (1989). Activation of purified calcium channels by stoichiometric protein phosphorylation. *Proc Nat Acad Sci* 86:6816–6820.

Obayashi T, Hattori K, Sugiyama S, Taneka M, Tanaka T, Itoyama S et al (1992). Point mutations in mitochondrial DNA in patients with hypertrophic cardiomyopathy. *Am Heart J* 124:1263–1269.

Owen P, Dennis S, Opie LH (1990). Glucose flux regulates the onset of ischemic contracture in globally underperfused rat hearts. *Circ Res* 66:344–354.

Page E, McCallister LP (1973). Quantitative electron microscopic description of heart muscle cells. Application to normal, hypertrophied and thyroxin-stimulated hearts. *Am J Cardiol* 31:172–181.

Perreault CL, Williams CP, Morgan JP (1993). Cytoplasmic calcium modulation and systolic versus diastolic function in myocardial hypertrophy and failure. *Circulation* 87:VII-31–VII-37.

Peyton RB, Jones RN, Attarian D, Sink JD, van Trigt P, Currie WD, Wechsler AS (1982). Depressed high energy phosphate content in hypertrophied ventricles of animal and man. *Ann Surg* 196:278–283.

Pool PE, Spann JF, Buccino RA, Sonnenblick EH, Braunwald E (1967). Myocardial high energy phosphate stores in cardiac hypertrophy and heart failure. *Circ Res* 21:365–373.

Rauch B, Schultze B, Schultheiss HP (1994). Alteration of the cytosolic-mitochondrial distribution of high-energy phosphates during global myocardial ischemia may contribute to early contractile failure. *Circ Res* 75:760–769.

Reinecke H, Studer R, Vetter R, Holtz J, Drexler H (1996). Cardiac Na^{+}-Ca^{2+} exchange activity in patients with end-stage heart failure. *Cardiovasc Res* 31:48–54.

Remes AM, Hassinen IE, Ikäheimo MJ, Herva R, Hirvonen J, Peuhkurinen KJ (1993). Mitochondrial DNA deletions in dilated cardiomyopathy: a clinical study employing endomyocardial sampling. *J Am Coll Cardiol* 23:935–942.

Roberts JT, Wearn JT (1941). Quantitative changes in the capillary-muscle relationship in human hearts during normal growth and hypertrophy. *Am Heart J* 21:617–633.

Rosen MR, Cohen IS, Steinberg SF (1998). The heart remembers. *Cardiovasc Res* 40:469–482.

Ruth P, Röhrkasten A, Biel M, Bosse E, Regulla S, Meyer HE, Flockerzi V, Hoffman F (1988). Primary structure of the β subunit of the DHP-sensitive calcium channel from skeletal muscle. *Science* 245:1115–1118.

Sabbah HN, Sharov V, Riddle JM, Kono T, Lesch M, Goldstein S (1992). Mitochondrial abnormalities in myocardium of dogs with chronic heart failure. *J Mol Cell Cardiol* 24;1332–1347.

Sack MN, Rader TA, Park S, Bastin J, McCune SA, Kelly DP (1996). Fatty acid oxidation enzyme gene expression is downregulated in the failing heart. *Circulation* 94:2837–2842.

Sanbe A, Tanonaka K, Hanaoka Y, Katoh T, Takeo S (1993). Regional energy metabolism of failing hearts following myocardial infarction. *J Mol Cell Cardiol* 25:995–1013.

Schaper J, Froede R, Hein S, Buck A, Friedl A, Hashizume H, Speiser B, Blesse N (1991). Impairment of myocardial ultrastructure and changes of the cytoskeleton in dilated cardiomyopathy. *Circulation* 83:504–514.

Scheuer J, Buttrick P (1985). The cardiac hypertrophic response to pathologic and physiologic loads. *Circulation* 75(Suppl I, Pt 2):63–68.

Schiaffino S, Reggiani C (1996). Molecular diversity of myofibrillar proteins: gene regulation and molecular significance. *Physiol Rev* 76:371–423.

Schiaffino S, Samuel JL, Sassoon D, Lompré AM, Garner I, Marotte F, Buckingham M, Rappaport L, Schwartz K (1989). Nonsynchronous accumulation of α-skeletal actin and β-myosin heavy chain mRNAs during early stages of pressure-overloaded-induced cardiac hypertrophy demonstrated by in situ hybridization. *Circ Res* 64:937–948.

Scholz J, Hein S, Scholz D, Mollnau H (1995). Multifaceted morphological alterations are present in the failing human heart. *J Mol Cell Cardiol* 27:857–861.

Schröder F, Handrock R, Beuckelmann DJ, Hirt S, Hullin R, Priebe S, Schwinger RHG, Weil S, Herzig S (1998). Increased availability and open probability of single L-type calcium channels from failing compared with non-failing human ventricle. *Circulation* 98:969–976.

Schultheiss H-P, Schulze K, Schauer R, Witzenichler B, Strauer BE (1995). Antibody-mediated imbalance of myocardial energy metabolism. A cause factor of cardiac failure? *Circ Res* 76:64–72.

Schwartz K, de la Bastie K, Mercadier J-J, Swynghedauw B, Lompré A-M (1990). The biochemistry and molecular biology of the sarcomere. In Swynghedauw B, ed. *Cardiac Hypertrophy and Failure*. John Libby, London, pp 105–135.

Schwartz K, Chassagne C, Boehler KR (1993). The molecular biology of heart failure. *J Am Coll Cardiol* 22:30A–33A.

Schwinger RHG, Böhm M, Koch A, Schmidt U, Karczewski P, Bavendiek U, Flesch M, Krause E-G, Erdmann E (1995). Unchanged protein levels of SERCA II and phospholamban but reduced Ca^{2+} uptake and Ca^{2+} ATPase activity of cardiac sarcoplasmic reticulum from dilated cardiomyopathy patients compared with patients with non-failing hearts. *Circulation* 92:3220–3228.

Shigekawa M, Dougherty JP, Katz AM (1978). Reaction mechanism of Ca^{2+}-dependent ATP hydrolysis by skeletal muscle sarcoplasmic reticulum in the absence of added alkali metal salts. I. Characterization of steady state ATP hydrolysis and comparison with that in the presence of KCl. *J Biol Chem* 253:1442–1450.

Shipsey SJ, Bryant SM, Hart G (1997). Effects of hypertrophy on regional action potential characteristics in the rat left ventricle. A cellular basis for T wave inversion? *Circulation* 96:2061–2068.

Small JV, Fürst DO, Thornell L-E (1992). The cytoskeletal lattice of muscle cells. *Eur J Biochem* 208:559–572.

Smith J, Coronado R, Meissner G (1986). Single channel measurements of the calcium release channel from sarcoplasmic reticulum. Activation by calcium and ATP and modulation by magnesium. *J Gen Physiol* 88:573–588.

Smith V-E, Zile MR (1992). Relaxation and diastolic properties of the heart. In Fozzard H, Haber E, Katz A, Jennings R, Morgan HE, eds. *The Heart and Circulation*, 2nd ed. Raven Press, New York, pp 1353–1367.

Smith V-E, Schulman P, Karimeddini MK, White WB, Meeran MK, Katz AM (1985). Rapid ventricular filling in left ventricular hypertrophy. II. Pathological hypertrophy. *J Am Coll Cardiol* 5:869–874.

Solaro RJ, Powers FM, Gao L, Gwathmey JK (1993). Control of myofilament activation in heart failure. *Circulation* 87:VII-38–VII-43.

Studer R, Reinecke H, Bilger J, Eschenahgen T, Böhm M, Hasenfuss G, Just H, Holtz J, Drexler H (1994). Gene expression of the cardiac Na^+-Ca^{2+} exchanger in end-stage human heart failure. *Circ Res* 75:443-453.

Stühmer W, Conti F, Suzuki H, Wang X, Noda M, Yahagi N, Kubo H, Numa S (1989). Structural parts involved in activation and inactivation of the sodium channel. *Nature* 339:597–603.

Suomalainen A, Paetau A, Leinonen H, Majander A, Peltonen L, Somer H (1992). Inherited idiopathic dilated cardiomyopathy with multiple deletions of mitochondrial DNA. *Lancet* 340:1319–1320.

Swain JL, Sabina RL Peyton RB, Jones RN, Wechsler AS, Homes EW (1982). Derangements in myocardial purine and pyrimidine nucleotide metabolism in patients with coronary artery disease and left ventricular hypertrophy. *Proc Natl Acad Sci U S A* 79:655–659.

Sweadner KJ, Herrera VLM, Amato S, Moellmann A, Gibbons DK, Repke KRH (1994). Immunologic identification of Na^+,K^+-ATPase isoforms in myocardium. Isoform change in deoxycortisone acetate-salt hypertension. *Circ Res* 74:669–678.

Swynghedauw B (1986). Developmental and functional adaptation of contractile proteins in cardiac and skeletal muscles. *Physiol Rev* 66:710–771.

Swynghedauw B (1989). Remodeling of the heart in response to chronic mechanical overload. *Eur Heart J* 10:935–943.

Tada M, Katz AM (1982). Phosphorylation of the sarcoplasmic reticulum and sarcolemma. *Annu Rev Physiol* 44:401–423.

ten Eick RE, Whalley D, Rasmussen HH (1992). Connections: heart disease, cellular electrophysiology and ion channels. *FASEB J* 6:2568–2580.

Tian R, Ingwall JS (1996). Energetic basis for reduced contractile reserve in isolated rat hearts. *Am J Physiol* 270: H1207–H1216.

Tian R, Nascimben L, Ingwall JS, Lorell BH (1997a). Failure to maintain a low ADP concentration impairs diastolic function in hypertrophied rat hearts. *Circulation* 96:1313-1319.

Tian R, Christe ME, Spindler M, Hopkins JCA, Halow JM, Camacho SA, Ingwall JS (1997b). Role of MgADP in the development of diastolic dysfunction in the intact beating rat heart. *J Clin Invest* 99:745–751.

Tomaselli GF, Beuckelmann DJ, Calkins HG, Berger RD, Kessler PD, Lawrence JH, Kass D, Feldman AM, Marban E (1994). Sudden cardiac death in heart failure. The role of abnormal repolarization. *Circulation* 90:2534–2539.

Tomita F, Bassett AL, Myerburg RJ, Kimura S (1994). Diminished transient outward currents in rat hypertrophied ventricular myocytes *Circ Res* 75:296–303.

Tritthart H, Luedcke H, Bayer R, Stierle H, Kaufmann R (1975). Right ventricular hypertrophy in the cat—an electrophysiological and anatomical study. *J Mol Cell Cardiol* 7:163–174.

Trombitás K, Granzier H (1997). Actin removal from cardiac myocytes shows that near Z line titin attaches to actin while under tension. *Am J Physiol* 273:C662–C670.

Tsien RW, Tsien RY (1990). Calcium channels, stores, and oscillations. *Annu Rev Cell Biol* 6:715–760.

Tsuchimochi H, Sugi M, Kuro-o M, Ueda S, Takaku F, Furuta S-i, Shirai T, Yazaki Y (1984). Isozymic changes in myosin of human atrial myocardium induced by overload. Immunohistochemical study using monoclonal antibodies. *J Clin Invest* 74:662–665.

Tsutsui H, Tagawa H, Kent RL, McCollam PL, Ishihara K, Nagatsu M, Cooper G IV (1994). Role of microtubules in contractile dysfunction of hypertrophied cardiocytes. *Circulation* 90:533–555.

Wallimann T, Wyss M, Brdiczka D, Nicolay K, Eppenberger HM (1992). Intracellular compartmentation, structure and function of creatine kinase isoenzymes in tissues with high and fluctuation energy demands: the "phosphocreatine circuit" for cellular energy homeostasis. *Biochem J* 281:21–40.

Wangler RD, Peters KG, Marcus ML, Tomanek RJ (1982). Effects of duration and severity of arterial hypertension and cardiac hypertrophy on coronary vasodilator reserve. *Circ Res* 51:10–18.

Weiss JN, Hiltbrand B (1985). Functional compartmentalization of glycolytic versus oxidative metabolism in isolated rabbit heart. *J Clin Invest* 75:436–447.

Weiss JN, Lamp SL (1987). Glycolysis preferentially inhibits ATP-sensitive K^+ channels in isolated guinea pig cardiac myocytes. *Science* 238:67–69.

Wexler LF, Lorell BH, Monomura S-i, Weinberg EO, Ingwall JS, Apstein CS (1988). Enhanced sensitivity to hypoxia-induced diastolic dysfunction in pressure-overload left ventricular hypertrophy in the rat: role of high-energy phosphate depletion. *Circ Res* 62:766–775.

Wicker P, Tarazi RC, Kobayashi K (1983). Coronary blood flow during the development and regression of left ventricular hypertrophy in renovascular hypertensive rats. *Am J Cardiol* 51:1744–1749.

Wier WG, Egan TM, López-López JR, Balke CW (1994). Local control of excitation-contraction coupling in rat heart cells. *J Physiol (London)*. 474:463–471.

Williams RS (1995).Cardiac involvement in mitochondrial diseases and vice versa. *Circulation* 91:1266–1268.

Wit AL, Rosen MR (1991). Afterdepolarizations and triggered activity: distinction from automaticity as an arrhythmogenic mechanism. In Fozzard H, Haber E, Katz A, Jennings R, Morgan HE, eds. *The Heart and Circulation*, 2nd ed. Raven Press, New York, New York, pp 2113–2164.

Wolff MR, Buck SH, Stoker SW, Greaser ML, Mentzer RM (1996). Myofibrillar calcium sensitivity of isometric tension is increased in human dilated cardiomyopathies. Role of altered β-adrenergically mediated protein phosphorylation. *J Clin Invest* 98:167–176.

Wollenberger A, Schulze W (1962). Über das Volumenverhältnis von Mitochiondrien zu Myofibrillen im chronisch überlasteten, hypertrophierten Herzen. *Naturwissenschaften* 7:161–162.

Yamaguchi M, Tonomura Y (1980). Binding of monovalent cations to Na^+,K^+-dependent ATPase purified from porcine kidney. II. Acceleration of transition from a K^+-bound form to a Na^+-bound form by binding of ATP to a regulatory site of the enzyme. *J Biochem (Tokyo)* 88:1377–1385.

Zhang J-F, Randall AD, Ellinor PT, Horne WA, Sather WA, Tanabe T, Schwarz TL, Tsien RW (1993). Distinctive pharmacology and kinetics of cloned neuronal Ca^{2+} channels and their possible counterparts in mammalian CNS neurons. *Neuropharmacology* 32:1075–1088.

4

The Hemodynamic Defense Reaction

The vie constante, *where life manifests itself independently of the external environment [is] characterized by freedom and independence....Here life is never suspended, but flows steadily on apparently indifferent to alterations in its cosmic environment or changes in its material surroundings. Organs, structural mechanisms and tissues all function uniformly....[because] the* milieu intérieur *surrounding the organs, the tissues, and their elements never varies; atmospheric changes cannot penetrate beyond...we have an organism which has enclosed itself in a kind of a hothouse. The perpetual changes of external conditions cannot reach it; it is not subject to them, but is free and independent.*

Claude Bernard (1878)

Claude Bernard, whose eloquent description of the "internal environment" (the *milieu intérieur*) begins this chapter, points out that the constancy of the environment within our bodies is the "primary condition for freedom and independence of existence." The mechanisms that maintain this constancy, called "homeostasis" by Walter Cannon (1932), stabilize the *milieu intérieur* by providing adaptive responses needed to meet the many challenges encountered during our active and sometimes hazardous lives. Under some pathologic conditions, however, the same mechanisms can become maladaptive and may even represent major causes of disability and death. One need only recall that rheumatic heart disease, which as pointed out in Chapter 1 was a major cause of heart failure until the latter half of the 20th century, occurs when the valves of the heart are attacked by antibodies that defend the body against streptococcal infection.

This chapter describes how homeostatic mechanisms that are beneficial in normal individuals establish vicious cycles that contribute to both morbidity and mortality in patients with heart failure. These homeostatic mechanisms, which fall into three classes (Table 4-1), have both adaptive and maladaptive consequences. These are summarized in Table 4-2, which shows that these mechanisms are generally adaptive in the short term and maladaptive over the long term. This duality is also seen for many drugs used to treat heart failure, whose short-term and long-term effects can be quite different, an unex-

TABLE 4-1. *Major elements of the neurohumoral response in heart failure*

I. Hemodynamic defense reaction
A. Salt and water retention
B. Vasoconstriction
C. Cardiac stimulation
II. Inflammation
III. Hypertrophic response

TABLE 4-2. *Neurohumoral response*

Mechanism	Short-term, adaptive	Long-term, maladaptive
Hemodynamic		
Salt and water retention	↑Preload	Edema, anasarca
	Maintain cardiac output	Pulmonary congestion
Vasoconstriction	↑Afterload	↓Cardiac output
	Maintain blood pressure	↑Cardiac energy demand
	Maintain cardiac output	Cardiac necrosis
Increased cardiac	↑Contractility ⎤ Maintain	↑Cytosolic calcium
Adrenergic drive	↑Relaxation cardiac	↑Cardiac energy demand
	↑Heart rate ⎦ output	Cardiac necrosis
		Arrhythmias, sudden death
Inflammatory	"Antiother"	"Antiself"
Macrophages, cytokines,	Antimicrobial	Cardiac cachexia
Free radicals	Attack foreign bodies	Cardiac apoptosis, necrosis
Growth	Adaptive hypertrophy	Maladaptive hypertrophy
Immediate-early gene	↑Sarcomere number	Remodeling
Response, transcription	Maintain cardiac output	↑Energy demand
Factors	↓Load, ↓energy demand	Cardiac necrosis, apoptosis

These compensatory mechanisms, when evoked to meet a short-term challenge, generate an adaptive response. When sustained, as in heart failure, these same mechanisms give rise to maladaptive responses that further reduce cardiac output, and accelerate cell death.

pected finding that has led to a great deal of confusion in this field. It is only over the past decade, with the advent of long-term trials intended to assess different ways to manage this condition, that the clinical importance of this duality has come to be appreciated.

The first homeostatic mechanism listed in Table 4-1, which in this text is referred to as the *hemodynamic defense reaction*, is a neurohumoral response that aids the body in responding to challenges that impair the circulation, notably underfilling of the systemic arterial system or a decrease in blood pressure (Table 4-2, top). In short-term emergencies, this response is adaptive in that it helps the body to meet such challenges as those posed by exercise and blood loss. However, when called upon in a chronic illness such as heart failure, which also causes underfilling of the systemic arterial system, the hemodynamic defense reaction becomes maladaptive and contributes significantly to the long-term problems in these patients.

The second class of homeostatic mechanism that has recently been recognized to operate in heart failure is an *inflammatory reaction* (Table 4-2, middle), which aids the body in responding to invasion by foreign materials, notably infectious organisms, and in eliminating damaged or abnormal cells. Mediators of the inflammatory reaction include the *cytokines*, which also contribute to the wasting (*cachexia*) seen in patients with chronic diseases such as tuberculosis and cancer, and *free radicals*, which destroy bacteria and other foreign material. As is true for the hemodynamic defense reaction, mediators of inflammation appear to play an important maladaptive role in the patient with heart failure. This important topic is examined in Chapter 5.

Over the past decade, a third class of homeostatic mechanism has come to be recognized as playing a crucial role in the patient with heart failure; this is the growth response that causes the failing heart to hypertrophy. It is noteworthy that this mitogenic response is initiated and regulated by many of the signaling molecules that mediate the neurohumoral and inflammatory responses in the failing heart; like the latter, hypertrophy has both adaptive and maladaptive consequences (see Chapters 6-8).

THE HEMODYNAMIC DEFENSE REACTION

The hemodynamic abnormalities in heart failure, as detailed in a brilliant essay by Peter Harris (1983), evoke a neurohumoral response that is virtually the same as that seen in exercise and hemorrhage. Although the initiating mechanisms are very different, Harris points out that the responses to exercise, hemorrhage, and heart failure are all examples of a coordinated "defense reaction" that addresses the challenge caused by altered circulatory hemodynamics. In exercise (Table 4-3), the hemodynamic challenge is to provide the large increase in cardiac output needed to perfuse the active skeletal muscles. Because vasodilatation in the exercising muscles reduces peripheral resistance and so tends to lower blood pressure, the hemodynamic defense reaction plays an essential role in the circulatory adjustments to strenuous exertion. Following hemorrhage, as during exercise, the challenge is to maintain systemic blood pressure; in this setting, often called *hemorrhagic shock*, cardiac output and arterial pressure decrease when blood loss decreases venous return to the heart. In the patient with heart failure, as during exercise, the major challenge is to maintain blood pressure. Hypotension occurs suddenly in other settings, for example, when a large myocardial infarction causes *cardiogenic shock*. A similar state is reached much more slowly in the patient with chronic heart failure, when the damaged heart is unable to pump a normal cardiac output into the arterial system. Although the underlying causes and time courses of these hemodynamic challenges differ markedly, all activate signal transduction cascades whose primary function is to maintain blood pressure and cardiac output.

The most important differences between the physiologic responses to exercise and hemorrhage and the pathologic response in heart failure is in their duration. The hemodynamic defense reaction evoked by exercise rarely lasts more than a few hours, when fatigue requires that the individual rest. In hemorrhage, blood loss either stops and circulating blood volume is restored, generally after a few days, or else the individual dies. In contrast, the hemodynamic abnormalities in heart failure usually persist for the lifetime of the individual. Because the ability of a damaged heart to repair itself is limited, this condition generally worsens because the failing heart deteriorates. Thus, unlike exercise and hemorrhage, in which the neurohumoral response is soon turned off, the underlying problem in chronic heart failure—which is the damaged heart—worsens progressively. Because of this deterioration, the neurohumoral response in heart failure is not merely sustained, but intensifies. The consequences are vividly summarized by Harris (1983):

> Success and survival in the animal kingdom have overwhelmingly depended on physical mobility and strength. To ensure this the body makes use of the neuro-endocrine defense reaction which is also life-saving in injury....When the output of the diseased heart decreases, the body reacts in the way nature has programmed it. It

TABLE 4-3. *Three conditions that evoke the hemodynamic defense reaction*

Condition	Duration	Challenge	Response
Exercise	Minutes/hours	Increase perfusion to exercising muscles	Selective vasoconstriction, cardiac stimulation
Shock	Hours	Loss of vascular volume, hemorrhage	Vasoconstriction, cardiac stimulation, salt and water retention
Heart failure	Lifetime (progressive)	Damage to heart, impaired pumping	Vasoconstriction, cardiac stimulation, salt and water retention

cannot distinguish. But now the neuro-endocrine response persists. Over weeks or months or years the retention of saline threatens the cardiac patient with drowning in his own juice. And every hour of every day he is running for his life.

When viewed from an evolutionary standpoint, it should not be surprising that our bodies are programmed to mount effective and powerful defense reactions during exercise and following blood loss. Traits such as courage and skill in pursuit, which are associated with behavior that requires intense and prolonged exertion, also can lead to hemorrhage, so that an effective hemodynamic defense reaction is of benefit not only to the individual, but also for the species. There is, for example, an obvious advantage for the genetic program to encode adaptive responses that allow large amounts of blood to be delivered to perfuse exercising muscles. Similarly, there are many advantages to mechanisms that allow the injured hunter, the wounded defender of hearth and home, and the woman during childbirth to survive the short-term decrease in vascular filling caused by hemorrhage. Conversely, it may not be entirely inappropriate for the same response to become maladaptive when called upon to compensate for the hemodynamic abnormalities caused by a chronic decrease in cardiac output, as occurs in the patient with heart failure. In this case, an early death not only shortens suffering, but offers advantages to a resource-poor primitive social group by eliminating those individuals unable to recover after irreversible cardiac damage.

MAJOR COMPONENTS OF THE HEMODYNAMIC DEFENSE REACTION

Three components of the hemodynamic defense reaction are of special importance in the patient with heart failure (see Tables 4-1 and 4-2). As summarized in Table 4-2, all provide adaptive short-term support for the circulation during a brief challenge, but all become maladaptive when called upon for long periods in the patient with heart failure.

Salt and water retention, vasoconstriction, and cardiac stimulation, the three major components of the hemodynamic defense reaction, are each mediated by signaling cascades that are controlled by an array of extracellular "messengers." The latter include molecules that act not only on the heart but also on other organs and tissues, including the kidneys, blood vessels, and skeletal muscle. A variety of chemical structures mediate these signals (Table 4-4). These include *peptides* such as angiotensin II, vasopressin (antidiuretic hormone), atrial natriuretic peptide (ANP), endothelin, and the cytokines, that mediate the inflammatory response discussed in Chapter 5. Other classes of signaling molecules that play an important role in the patient with heart failure include *catecholamines*, epinephrine and norepinephrine; aldosterone, a *steroid hormone*; nitric oxide, a *free radical gas*; and the prostaglandins, which are 20 carbon *fatty acids*. These extracellular messengers bind to specific receptors so as to modify intracellular signaling cascades (see Chapter 7).

The many mediators of the hemodynamic defense reaction, although they bind to different receptor classes, can evoke similar, often overlapping responses. In addition to the regulatory effects listed in Tables 4-1 and 4-2, these mediators can also evoke "counterregulatory" responses, which have opposite effects in that they blunt the hemodynamic defense reaction. This intricacy is such that a single extracellular messenger can cause both regulatory and counterregulatory responses by activating different receptor subtypes that produce diametrically opposite effects. Norepinephrine, angiotensin II, vasopressin, and endothelin, for example, all interact with receptor subtypes, some of which cause vasoconstriction, others vasodilatation. To present this panoply of interactions in a clear, coherent, accurate manner is a Herculean challenge. The following provides an overview, giving enough detail to allow the reader to appreciate the background for important developments taking place in the understanding and management of heart failure.

TABLE 4-4. *Some mediators of the neurohumoral response in heart failure*

Mediator	Fluid retention	Vasoconstriction	Cardiac stimulation
Peptide and protein			
Angiotensin II	++	++[a]	+
Arginine vasopressin (ADH)	++[a]	++	+
Atrial natriuretic peptide	−[a]	−	−
Bradykinin	o	−[a]	o
Endothelin	++	++[a]	+
Neuropeptide Y	+	++	−[a]
Catecholamine			
Norepinephrine			
α_1 receptors	++	++	+[a]
α_2 receptors (central)	−	−	−[a]
β receptors	o	−	++[a]
Dopamine	−	−	+[a]
Steroid			
Aldosterone	+[a]	o	o
Fatty acid			
Prostaglandins	+ and −	+ and −*	o
Other			
Nitric oxide (NO)	−	−[a]	−
Agmatine	−	−	−[a]

[a]Indicates the topic in this chapter where each mediator is discussed
++ strong stimulatory effect, + weak stimulatory effect, o effect insignificant or absent, − inhibitory effect

Parallel Actions of Mediators of the Hemodynamic Defense Reaction

Many of the mediators of the neurohumoral response share actions on the kidneys, which causes fluid retention, on the blood vessels, which causes vasoconstriction, and on the heart, which increases contractility (Table 4-5). These parallel effects, which are produced by angiotensin II, vasopressin, endothelin, and norepinephrine, are accompanied

TABLE 4-5. *Signaling molecules*

A. Signaling molecules that play a regulatory role in the hemodynamic defense reaction
  Mediators
    Catecholamines—peripheral effects
    Angiotensin II
    Arginine vasopressin
    Endothelin
  Effects
    Fluid retention by the kidneys
    Vasoconstriction
    Increase cardiac contractility, relaxation, heart rate
    Stimulate cell growth and proliferation
B. Signaling molecules that play a counterregulatory role in the hemodynamic defense reaction
  Mediators
    Catecholamines—central effects
    Atrial natriuretic peptide
    Nitric oxide (NO)
    Bradykinin
    Dopamine
    Agmatine—central effects
  Effects
    Reduce fluid retention by the kidneys
    Vasodilation
    Decrease cardiac contractility, relaxation, heart rate
    Inhibit cell growth and proliferation

by modification of gene expression and promotion of cell growth. How the parallel actions of these many different mediators came about is not clear, but it is amusing to speculate as to how different molecules came to share so many common actions.

The molecules that participate in the hemodynamic defense reaction may first have appeared early during evolution as part of a defense reaction that allowed simple single-celled life forms, called prokaryotes, to survive an environmental change by generating new phenotypes (Katz, 1990a). This primitive means of meeting a challenge by altering gene expression is seen in modern bacteria, which survive such insults as the appearance of an antibiotic by selecting for a phenotype that is resistant to the drug. In these contemporary prokaryotes, this defense reaction operates when a few drug-resistant bacteria appear, and survive and multiply in the new environment. With the evolution of eukaryotes, whose internal environment could be regulated by intracellular, membrane-delimited organelles, and more recently of multicellular life forms able to integrate the functions of different organs, the signaling molecules that contributed to this primitive defense reaction probably came to be used in the more elaborate responses described in this chapter. In this way, perhaps, these diverse signaling molecules became the extracellular messengers that mediate the hemodynamic defense reaction by promoting fluid retention, vasoconstriction, and cardiac stimulation. At the same time, however, these molecules retained their more primitive ability to signal a change in phenotype (see Chapter 6).

Regulatory and Counterregulatory Components of the Hemodynamic Defense Reaction

In addition to initiating the regulatory effects listed in Table 4-5, many of the signaling molecules released in the hemodynamic defense reaction elicit opposite responses that promote diuresis, relax blood vessels, and lessen cardiac stimulation (see Table 4-5). These counterregulatory effects illustrate an important principle in biology: that whenever regulatory signals turn on a process, counterregulatory signals are required to turn the process off. In some cases, a single molecule can generate opposing signals; for example, the voltage-gated ion channels discussed in Chapter 3 respond to membrane depolarization by first opening and then closing the channel pore (Katz, 1993). This ability of a single message first to initiate a response (regulation), and to set into motion other, more slowly developing processes that end the response (counterregulation), prevents runaway signaling. One application of this principle is seen in the water taps commonly found in public washrooms, where flooding is prevented by a system that allows the same "signal" that starts the flow of water to slowly shut off the tap.

In the following discussion, the signaling systems that control fluid retention, vasoconstriction, and cardiac stimulation are reviewed, as are the salient features of the hemodynamic defense reaction. The organization of this discussion is rather arbitrary in that many of these mediators initiate all three responses, and often counterregulatory responses as well. An attempt is made to relate these many messengers to their most important effects, but because this organization often breaks down, a footnote is included in Table 4-4 to help the reader locate discussions of the individual extracellular messengers. Even though it would be simpler to present and discuss a list of these mediators, such an approach seems likely to be as engrossing as a telephone directory.

Virtually all of the extracellular messengers that participate in the hemodynamic defense reaction act when they bind to receptors, generally but not always located on the cell surface. Understanding—and remembering—the many ligand-receptor interactions that are important in patients with heart failure would be relatively simple if each signaling molecule acted through a single class of receptor, and independently of the other mediators. This is not, however, the case. Not only can most of these extracellular messengers bind with high affinity to more than one receptor subtype, but the responses evoked when the same mediator interacts with different receptor subtypes can differ markedly, in some cases opposing one another, which carries the principle of regulation/counterregulation to the molecular level. Furthermore, most of these extracellular signaling molecules modify the actions, and often the production and release, of other mediators of the hemodynamic defense reaction. The resulting molecular heterogeneity provides a striking example of the way that biologic systems coordinate and organize diverse responses to produce a smooth effect (Katz and Katz, 1989). Although useful to the organism and indispensable to the "fine tuning" of responses, these many interactions pose a real impediment to the understanding needed for the optimal management of heart failure. But as the counterintuitive results of many recent clinical trials have shown (see Chapter 9), failure to grasp these principles significantly lowers the quality of care for these patients.

Fluid Retention

Edema, dropsy, anasarca, and dyspnea, which as noted in Chapters 1 and 2 represent the major clinical manifestations of heart failure, are caused when fluid accumulates in the body's tissues. The most important cause of edema formation in these patients is salt and water retention by the kidneys, rather than inability of the failing heart to pump blood out of the veins. This became clear more than 50 years ago when Warren and Stead (1944) noted that weight gain generally preceded a significant increase in venous pressure and appearance of symptoms in early heart failure. An enormous amount of salt and water that can be retained in advanced heart failure is evident when, within several days, diuretic therapy eliminates so much fluid as to cause a weight loss that can exceed 20 kilograms. Harris (1983) notes that fluid accumulation in heart failure is often so dramatic that a visiting Martian could easily conclude that the primary problem in these patient involves the kidneys!

Retention of sodium rather than of water is the major cause of the expanded extracellular fluid volume in heart failure. Although the excess water is more evident in the edematous patient than the increase in total body sodium, it is more correct to view water retention as the result of sodium retention, rather than the other way around. Stated simply, water follows salt. Although water retention can, in some patients, become the more important problem, this occurs most commonly after overly vigorous diuresis in advanced heart failure, when impairment of the body's ability to regulate plasma osmolarity causes excessive water retention. The result is a decrease in serum sodium concentration, called "dilutional hyponatremia." In most heart failure patients, however, sodium retention by the kidneys is the initiating abnormality that causes fluid accumulation.

Mechanisms Responsible for Sodium Retention

Although excess salt intake can contribute to sodium retention in heart failure, the major problem is generally inadequate sodium excretion by the kidneys. It is for this reason that a mainstay of therapy is elimination of sodium using a diuretic; the other approach, restriction of sodium intake, is more difficult because low salt diets are not very palatable, and because strict sodium restriction requires the purchase and preparation of special salt-free foods. The development of safe and effective oral diuretics in the latter half of the 20th century, therefore, revolutionized the therapy of heart failure.

Conceptually, the causes of excess sodium retention by the kidneys are quite simple. Because most of the sodium eliminated in the urine is filtered by the glomeruli, inappropriate sodium retention could occur if too little sodium is filtered to enter the renal tubules, if too much of the filtered sodium is reabsorbed into the plasma by the tubular epithelium, or both. In patients with heart failure, the first mechanism could be explained if the low cardiac output caused a decrease in glomerular filtration rate (GFR) that reduces the amount of sodium entering the renal tubules. The second mechanism, increased sodium reabsorbtion, implies some abnormality that causes too much of the filtered sodium to be transported back into the plasma by the renal tubular epithelial cells. The second of these mechanisms is the major problem in the patient with heart failure.

Early investigators believed that fluid retention in heart failure is due mainly to reduced sodium filtration caused by decreases in renal blood flow and glomerular filtration. It seemed logical that sodium excretion in these patients is reduced by the combination of a low cardiac output, which would decrease renal perfusion, and an elevated venous pressure that slowed the return of blood from the renal circulation. Studies carried out in the 1940s supported this view by demonstrating that renal plasma flow (RPF) and GFR were decreased in advanced heart failure (Merrill, 1946; Mokotoff et al., 1948). However, subsequent measurements showed that resting GFR could be within the normal range in patients with milder heart failure who suffered from fluid retention (Merrill and Cargell, 1948; Heller and Jacobson, 1950) and that sodium excretion could be sharply reduced even when a decrease in cardiac output was barely detectable (Hostetter et al., 1983). Further evidence that fluid retention in heart failure involves more than a simple hemodynamic abnormality was provided by the finding of abnormal blood flow distribution within the kidney (Vander et al., 1958; Kilcoyne et al., 1973; Ichikawa et al., 1984), which indicates that factors acting locally on different regions of the renal vasculature play a major role in the pathogenesis of fluid retention (for reviews, see Hollenberg, 1988, and Raine, 1992).

The most important of the local hemodynamic abnormalities in the kidneys of patients with heart failure is constriction of the efferent arterioles of the glomeruli. Because these arteries carry blood out of the glomerulus, this vasoconstriction increases GFR by increasing intraglomerular pressure; at the same time, this vasoconstrictor response reduces total renal blood flow. The resulting changes in hydrostatic and oncotic pressures within the kidneys promote sodium reabsorbtion by a simple hemodynamic mechanism. The increased glomerular filtration caused by efferent arteriolar vasoconstriction increases the oncotic pressure in fluid that leaves the glomeruli to perfuse the tubules, while at the same time, hydrostatic pressure within the renal tubules is increased. Together, these changes increase reabsorbtion of the tubular fluid. As discussed later, these effects are supplemented by direct stimulation of sodium reabsorbtion by the tubular epithelium.

Mediators of the selective vasoconstrictor response that leads to salt and water retention include norepinephrine, arginine vasopressin, angiotensin II, and endothelin. The effects of these vasoconstrictors are augmented by reduced sensitivity of the renal vasculature to the vasodilator effects of nitric oxide, but are partially offset by counterregulatory effects caused when release of prostaglandins and ANP exert vasodilator effects on the kidneys. In addition to their hemodynamic effects, several of these extracellular messengers act directly on the renal epithelium to cause salt and water retention. Aldosterone, angiotensin II, and norepinephrine all increase tubular sodium reabsorbtion, whereas vasopressin acts on the collecting ducts to promote water reabsorbtion. Together, these signaling molecules cause the salt and water retention responsible for the signs and symptoms of untreated heart failure that were described in Chapter 1.

The following paragraphs outline effects of key mediators of the hemodynamic defense reaction on fluid retention by the kidneys. Detailed discussions of renal blood flow distribution, ion transport, and water reabsorbtion are beyond the scope of this chapter. For complete discussions of these mechanisms, refer to the many texts and reviews describing normal and abnormal renal physiology. The emphasis here is to highlight the role of the extracellular messengers generated by the neurohumoral response in causing fluid in heart failure.

Aldosterone

A major stimulus for sodium retention by the kidneys is provided by increased secretion of aldosterone, a steroid hormone that is produced by the zone glomerulosa of the adrenal cortex. The mechanisms that increase aldosterone secretion in patients with heart failure differ from those that regulate the release of this sodium-retaining hormone in normal individuals (Fig. 4-1). Adrenocorticotropic hormone (ACTH), a pituitary hormone that binds to receptors on adrenal cortical cells to stimulate aldosterone synthesis, regulates the normal diurnal changes in aldosterone secretion. Elevated serum potassium levels also promote aldosterone release, which maintains homeostasis by increasing potassium excretion by the renal tubules. The ability of stress to increase ACTH secretion allows aldosterone to play an important role in restoring fluid volume after hemorrhage.

In heart failure, the mechanisms that stimulate aldosterone release—and therefore sodium retention—differ from the physiologic stimuli described previously and change as this syndrome evolves (Table 4-6). In patients with advanced heart failure, the most important stimulus for aldosterone release is angiotensin II, whose levels are increased when di-

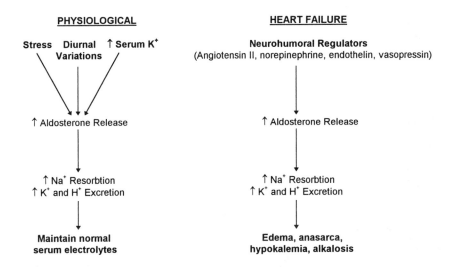

REGULATION OF ALDOSTERONE SYNTHESIS AND RELEASE

FIG. 4-1. Different mechanisms regulate aldosterone synthesis and release in normal individuals and in patients with heart failure. In the former, this steroid serves mainly to maintain normal Na^+ and K^+ levels in the serum, whereas in the patient with heart failure, aldosterone secretion, increased as part of the hemodynamic defense reaction, promotes fluid retention by the kidneys.

TABLE 4-6. *Neurohumoral mediators of salt and water retention in early and late heart failure*

Elevated in early heart failure
  Catecholamines
  Atrial natriuretic peptide
  Arginine vasopressin (antidiuretic hormone)
Elevated mainly after diuretic therapy
  Renin
  Angiotensin II
  Aldosterone

Based on data from Bayliss et al. (1987), Bro-qvist et al. (1989), and Francis et al. (1990).

uretics, which must be used in increasing doses as this illness progresses, activate the renin-angiotensin system. Because circulating levels of angiotensin II do not increase significantly in early, untreated heart failure (Francis et al., 1990), other mediators of the neurohumoral response, notably sympathetic stimulation, vasopressin, and endothelin, probably play the major role in stimulating aldosterone secretion in less seriously ill patients.

Aldosterone acts on the distal tubules both to increase sodium reabsorbtion and to promote the flux of potassium ions into the tubular lumen. The latter, which is accompanied by increased excretion of hydrogen ions, represents an important cause of the hypokalemia and metabolic alkalosis commonly seen in severe heart failure. Drugs that block aldosterone actions (e.g., spironolactone), therefore, not only increase sodium excretion, but also reverse the hypokalemia and alkalosis commonly seen in these patients. Aldosterone also has growth-promoting effects that may contribute to maladaptive hypertrophy by the failing heart (see Chapter 6). Inhibition of this mitogenic effect by spironolactone, an aldosterone receptor blocker that also has a negative inotropic effect (Mügge et al., 1984), may explain recent evidence that it improves survival in patients with severe heart failure (see Chapter 9).

Arginine Vasopressin (Antidiuretic Hormone)

Vasopressin is an octapeptide that, because the human isoform contains an arginine in position 8, is often called *arginine* vasopressin. This hormone is synthesized in the supraoptic and paraventricular nuclei of the hypothalamus, and is stored and released by the posterior pituitary. Vasopressin—as indicated by its name—has a powerful vasoconstrictor action that was discovered when Oliver and Schäfer (1895) injected posterior pituitary extracts into laboratory animals and observed a dramatic elevation in blood pressure. Vasopressin has another important action, to increase the water permeability of the renal collecting ducts. The result is an increase in water reabsorbtion that allows vasopressin to inhibit diuresis, which explains why this peptide is also called antidiuretic hormone (ADH).

The importance of receptor subtypes in determining the responses to the extracellular signaling molecules that mediate the hemodynamic defense reaction is clearly seen in the case of vasopressin, which not only has vasoconstrictor effects but is also a vasodilator. This reflects the existence of two different classes of vasopressin receptor, V_1 and V_2, whose effects are opposite to one another (Fig. 4-2). Binding of vasopressin to the V_1 receptors causes vasoconstriction, whereas activation of the V_2 receptors causes vasodilatation (Walker et al., 1988; Liard, 1989; Gavras, 1990). Although the more important

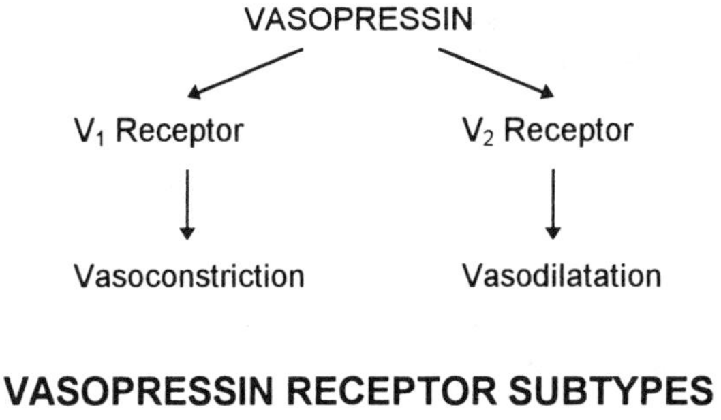

VASOPRESSIN

V₁ Receptor   V₂ Receptor

Vasoconstriction   Vasodilatation

VASOPRESSIN RECEPTOR SUBTYPES

FIG. 4-2. Vasopressin exerts both regulatory vasoconstrictor effects that are mediated by the V₁ receptor, and counterregulatory vasodilator effects that are mediated by V₂ receptors.

effect of vasopressin on blood pressure is the vasoconstriction mediated by the V_1 receptors, the vasodilator response initiated by V_2 receptor activation probably plays a role in the local regulation of renal function.

In normal individuals, the most important physiologic regulator of vasopressin levels is increased plasma osmolarity, which by stimulating osmoreceptors in the hypothalamus, releases this hormone (Fig. 4-3). This physiologic response helps travelers to survive a

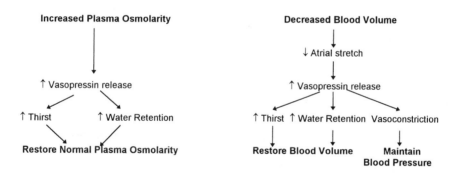

PHYSIOLOGICAL

Increased Plasma Osmolarity

↑ Vasopressin release

↑ Thirst   ↑ Water Retention

Restore Normal Plasma Osmolarity

Decreased Blood Volume

↓ Atrial stretch

↑ Vasopressin release

↑ Thirst   ↑ Water Retention   Vasoconstriction

Restore Blood Volume   **Maintain Blood Pressure**

HEART FAILURE

Excessive Secretion of Neurohumoral Regulators
(Angiotensin II, norepinephrine)

↑ Vasopressin release

↑ Thirst   ↑ Water Retention

Dilutional Hyponatremia

REGULATION OF VASOPRESSIN RELEASE

FIG. 4-3. Vasopressin serves different functions in different settings. Under physiologic conditions, this peptide helps to maintain normal plasma osmolarity and blood volume. Overproduction in heart failure causes a dilutional hyponatremia.

desert crossing, because when a water-deprived individual becomes hemoconcentrated, vasopressin tends to restore normal plasma osmolarity. These adaptive effects occur when vasopressin stimulates hypothalamic osmoreceptors that increase thirst, a response that drives the dehydrated traveler to seek water; at the same time, this peptide increases water reabsorbtion by the kidneys so as to reduce water loss. Normally, these thirst and antidiuretic responses are turned off when plasma osmolarity returns to physiologic levels. The ability of atrial stretch to inhibit vasopressin release also provides an adaptive response by inhibiting thirst and promoting water excretion in response to an expansion of plasma volume. Conversely, the decreased atrial volume following hemorrhage releases vasopressin, which by promoting thirst and retaining water, helps to restore blood volume. Vasopressin release after hemorrhage, and in the severely dehydrated desert traveler, not only helps to normalize blood volume, but because of its vasoconstrictor effect, also maintains blood pressure.

In patients with heart failure, these physiologic control mechanisms are blunted, and often lost (for review, see Francis et al., 1984; Goldsmith and Kubo, 1988; Francis, 1990). As in the case of aldosterone release, vasopressin release in patients with severe heart failure is not under physiologic control. Instead of responding to plasma osmolarity, vasopressin levels come to be determined by the reduced arterial filling (Schreier, 1988) and a central effect of increased levels of angiotensin II (Share, 1979). As heart failure worsens, both of these mechanisms increase vasopressin release, especially after the administration of diuretics (Francis et al., 1985, 1990). These maladaptive responses can be dangerous in severe heart failure, in which inappropriate vasopressin release can increase both thirst and water reabsorbtion by the kidneys to such an extent as to cause a life-threatening dilutional hyponatremia.

Natriuretic Peptides

One of the more startling recent discoveries in cardiology is that the heart is not only a pump but also an endocrine organ. This discovery came about when the density of granules long known to be present in atrial myocardial cells was found to change in response to altered water and electrolyte balance (DeBold, 1979). This observation led to experiments in which the injection of atrial extracts was shown to evoke a powerful natriuretic response (DeBold et al., 1981; for review, see Levin et al., 1998). On a personal note, this discovery explained a phenomenon that had been brought to my attention in 1961 by Paul Wood, the great English cardiologist, and Donald Saunders, then a Cardiology Fellow studying with me at the National Heart Hospital in London (Saunders and Ord, 1962; Wood, 1963). Wood had told us about a patient with paroxysmal supraventricular tachycardia who, during the tachycardia, had massive polyuria even though her cardiac output was very low, as evidenced by cold extremities and small arterial pulses. Saunders, it turned out, had been preparing a case report describing a similar patient, whom he had seen when he was a Medical Resident in South Carolina. I vividly recall our discussing these patients and our speculation that atrial dilatation must, in some way, have signaled the kidneys to initiate a diuresis.

Identification of ANP as the mediator of the diuretic response to atrial dilatation in paroxysmal tachycardia was followed by the finding that ANP levels are elevated in heart failure (Raine et al., 1986; Tikkanen et al., 1989; Francis et al., 1990). The resulting stimulus for diuresis, a counterregulatory effect that inhibits the salt- and water-retaining effects initiated by aldosterone, vasopressin, angiotensin II, and endothelin, is clearly beneficial in these patients, as are the vasodilating actions of ANP that tend to reduce peripheral resistance. Two other natriuretic peptides, BNP and CNP, which have actions similar to those of ANP, were initially identified in the brain (Sudoh et al., 1988, 1990). BNP, unlike ANP, is synthesized by the human ventricle (Yasue et al., 1994), whereas CNP is produced in blood vessels as well as the brain. ANP, in addition to its natriuretic and vasodilator actions, has a negative inotropic effect that is blunted in the failing heart (Tajima et al., 1998). At least three receptor types mediate the natriuretic and vasodilator actions of the natriuretic peptides (Struthers, 1994).

The counterregulatory effects of ANP are attenuated in heart failure (Scriven et al., 1985; Crozier et al., 1986; Cody et al., 1986, Nakamura et al., 1998), in part by other mediators of the hemodynamic defense reaction (DeBona et al., 1989; Redfield et al., 1989). The dominance of the hemodynamic defense reaction in heart failure explains why administration of ANP, which was initially hoped might help alleviate the fluid retention and vasoconstriction in heart failure, has had little impact on clinical management. There is, however, evidence that endogenous ANP can play a significant counterregulatory role in heart failure. This is suggested by the ability of vigorous diuresis to exacerbate renal dysfunction, which may occur when the reduced vascular volume decreases atrial size, and so reduces ANP secretion.

An interesting sidelight of this work is that the gene encoding ANP, which is normally present in fetal but not adult ventricles, is expressed in failing adult human ventricles (Edwards et al., 1988; Takemura et al., 1989; Saito et al., 1989), which provides another example of the reversion of the overloaded heart to the fetal phenotype discussed in Chapter 3. Even more important, from a practical standpoint, is the elevation of plasma levels of all of the natriuretic peptides in heart failure (Mukoyama et al., 1991; Wei et al., 1993; Tsutamoto et al., 1997), due in part to the ability of hemodynamic overloading to stimulate expression of the genes encoding these peptides (Nakagawa et al., 1995). These elevations have recently been suggested to represent a useful means to screen for heart failure in the general population (McDonagh et al., 1998; Clerico et al., 1998; Meada et al., 1998) (see Chapter 9).

Other Mediators of the Renal Response

As already noted, aldosterone, vasopressin, and the natriuretic peptides are not the only molecules that modify renal function in heart failure (see Table 4-4). Activation of the renin-angiotensin and sympathetic nervous systems, along with endothelin, also stimulate the kidneys to expand extracellular fluid volume in these patients. Because angiotensin II, the α_1-adrenergic effects of norepinephrine, and endothelin also have powerful vasoconstrictor effects, these mediators are also discussed.

Vasoconstriction

Increased peripheral vasculature resistance is the second major feature of the hemodynamic defense reaction. This vasoconstrictor response plays an important adaptive short-term role during exercise and following hemorrhage by maintaining arterial pressure needed to perfuse the brain and the heart. However, vasoconstriction becomes maladaptive in patients with heart failure (see Table 4-2) because the increased afterload reduces cardiac output and increases cardiac energy expenditure (see Chapter 3). These effects are especially harmful in patients with severe left ventricular dysfunction, in which increased afterload can impair ejection by the weakened ventricle to such an extent as to reduce aortic pressure. Alleviation of this effect, called "afterload mismatch" (Ross,

1976), explains the apparently paradoxical ability of vasodilators to increase arterial pressure in these patients. Another maladaptive effect of vasoconstriction is to reduce perfusion of the kidney and liver, which can exacerbate the renal and hepatic failure seen in end-stage heart failure.

The most important stimulus for vasoconstriction in heart failure is sympathetic activation (Creager et al., 1986), which releases norepinephrine that binds to peripheral α_1-adrenergic receptors on arteriolar smooth muscle. Other mediators of the vasoconstrictor response include angiotensin II, endothelin, and arginine vasopressin. As was seen in the case of the renal response, however, the neurohumoral response in heart failure includes opposite, counterregulatory, effects; in this case, vasodilation. Mediators of this counterregulatory response include the natriuretic peptides (see above), bradykinin, nitric oxide, dopamine, and some of the prostaglandins, notably PGI_2 (prostacyclin) and PGE_2 (Table 4-7), all of which act directly to relax arteriolar smooth muscle. Binding of norepinephrine to central, preganglionic α_2-receptors also inhibits regulatory neural vasoconstrictor pathways. Sympathetic activation also exerts a vasodilator effect when epinephrine binding to β_2-adrenergic receptors relaxes vascular smooth muscle. In patients with heart failure, however, these counterregulatory effects are overwhelmed by the constrictor response.

Renin-Angiotensin System

The association of left ventricular hypertrophy and hypertension with renal failure, observed by 19th century clinicians (Bright's disease, see Chapter 1) was explained when Tigerstedt and Bergman (1898) found that injection of kidney extracts increased blood pressure. Not illogically, they assumed that these extracts contained a pressor substance, which they named *renin*. It has become clear that renin release by the juxtaglomerular apparatus of the kidneys can explain many of the causal links between Bright's disease, hypertension, and cardiac hypertrophy discussed in Chapter 1. Subsequent research, however, demonstrated that renin is not itself a vasoconstrictor, but instead is a protease that forms an active pressor by catalyzing the hydrolysis of an inactive protein called *angiotensinogen* (Fig. 4-4A). This story became even more complex when it was found that

TABLE 4-7. *Major vasoactive regulators in heart failure*

Vasoconstrictors
  Catecholamine
    Norepinephrine—peripheral α_1-adrenergic stimulation
  Peptide
    Angiotensin II
    Arginine vasopressin
    Endothelin
  Lipid
    Thromboxane A_2
Vasodilator
  Catecholamine
    Norepinephrine—central α_2-adrenergic stimulation
    Epinephrine—β_2-adrenergic stimulation
    Dopamine
  Peptide
    Bradykinin
  Gas
    Nitric oxide (NO), endothelial-derived relaxing factor (EDRF)
  Lipid
    Prostacyclin, prostaglandin E_2

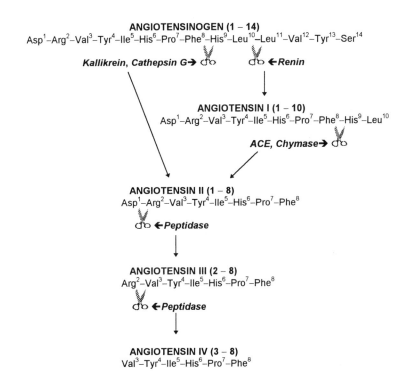

A THE RENIN-ANGIOTENSIN SYSTEM "ORIGINAL VERSION"

B THE RENIN-ANGIOTENSIN SYSTEM "MODERN" VERSION

FIG. 4-4. Activation of the renin-angiotensin system involves a number of proteolytic reactions. **A:** As originally understood, two proteolytic enzymes, renin and angiotensin-converting enzyme, form angiotensin II from its precursor. **B:** Currently, two pathways are known to form angiotensin II from its inactive precursor, and two additional active peptides—angiotensins III and IV—in addition to angiotensin II can be produced by this system.

angiotensin I, the product generated when renin hydrolyzed angiotensinogen, is itself the relatively inactive precursor of yet another proteolytic product, the powerful vasoconstrictor *angiotensin II* (see Fig. 4-4A). These discoveries were made independently by Page and Helmer (1940) in Cleveland, who named the active product angiotonin, and by Braun-Menendez et al. (1940) in Argentina, who chose the name hypertensin—the term *angiotensin*, which was coined 18 years later, represented a compromise (Braun-Menendez and Page, 1958).

Activation of the renin-angiotensin system plays a relatively minor role in the short-term response to exercise but is of greater importance in restoring fluid volume after hemorrhage, which is an adaptive response. In heart failure, however, most of the long-term effects of angiotensin II are maladaptive (Dzau et al., 1983; Francis et al., 1984).

Angiotensin II Formation. The cascade of proteolytic reactions that activates the renin-angiotensin system is much more complex than was initially believed (compare Fig. 4-4A and B). As first described, two enzymatic cleavages convert the inactive precursor angiotensinogen, which contains 14 amino acids, into the active octapeptide angiotensin II. The first, proteolysis by renin, releases the decapeptide angiotensin I. Additional proteolytic reactions, notably that catalyzed by an enzyme generally referred to as angiotensin-converting enzyme (ACE), generates the octapeptide angiotensin II. Angiotensin II can also be released from angiotensin I by chymase (Urata et al., 1990) and synthesized directly from angiotensinogen by the proteolytic actions of kallikrein and cathepsin G (Naveri, 1995) (see Fig. 4-4B). Furthermore, angiotensin II can undergo further proteolysis to generate additional biologically active peptides (for review, see Berk, 1998).

Other Effects of ACE: Breakdown of Bradykinin. Two different proteolytic reactions that are catalyzed by ACE have synergistic effects. In addition to converting angiotensin I to angiotensin II, ACE hydrolyzes and inactivates bradykinin, a counterregulatory peptide that has important vasodilator actions. ACE, therefore, has a dual vasoconstrictor action—it increases the formation of angiotensin II, a vasoconstrictor, and decreases the breakdown of bradykinin, a vasodilator.

Formation of Angiotensin II by Circulating and Tissue Systems. Two parallel systems allow different ACE enzymes to produce angiotensin II. Until recently, attention has focused on the circulating system, in which this peptide is synthesized in the blood. More recently, attention has shifted to the tissue system, in which angiotensin II is formed locally, where it can bind to adjacent cells (paracrine signaling), or to receptors on the same cell that produces this extracellular messenger (autocrine signaling). In the circulating system, renin released into the bloodstream from the kidneys acts on circulating angiotensinogen made in the liver to form circulating angiotensin I; the latter is hydrolyzed mainly by lung ACE to form circulating angiotensin II. In the tissue system, tissue renin produces tissue angiotensin I that is then cleaved to form angiotensin II by tissue ACE. The tissue system, which appears to be most important in the normal heart (van Kats et al., 1998), is activated in failing human hearts (Studer et al., 1994; Zisman et al., 1998). Evidence that these proteolytic reactions can take place in the interstitial fluid, on the plasma membrane, and within cells (Danser and Schlekamp, 1998) provides an additional level of control, and adds an additional level of complexity.

Proteases other than angiotensinogen, notably chymase, can form angiotensin II (Ganten et al., 1976; Dzau, 1988; Lindpainter et al., 1989; Frohlich et al., 1989; Timmermans et al., 1993; Urata and Arakawa, 1998). ACE appears to be most important catalyst in the systemic production of angiotensin II. Although chymase plays a significant role in the normal formation of tissue angiotensin II (Urata et al., 1994), the tissue ACE pathway appears to be more important in the failing human heart (Zisman et al., 1995). Chymase-catalyzed angiotensin II production may play an important role in the growth response that is initiated by this peptide (Urata and Arakawa, 1998).

The two systems that generate angiotensin II appear to serve different functions: systemic ACE is probably most important in regulating vasomotor tone, whereas angiotensin II produced in the tissues exerts local trophic effects that modulate gene expression. In the heart, for example, angiotensin II released by tissue ACE regulates growth and proliferation in both myocytes and nonmyocytes (Baker and Aceto, 1990; Sadoshima and Izumo, 1993). Because circulating and tissue ACE can respond differently to many of the drugs currently used to block the renin-angiotensin system in patients with heart failure, the existence of these different pathways for angiotensin II production offers opportunities for targeted actions that may be of considerable clinical value.

Angiotensin III and IV. Angiotensin II is not the only active peptide generated by the renin-angiotensin system. Two additional biologically active products are formed by further proteolytic cleavage of the octapeptide angiotensin II; these are the heptapeptide angiotensin III and the hexapeptide angiotensin IV (see Fig. 4-4B). Both bind to AT$_1$ receptors to cause vasoconstriction (Garrison et al., 1995; Li et al., 1995, 1997). The ability of these smaller peptides to activate other angiotensin receptor subclasses (Naveri, 1995) raises the possibility that additional effects of these peptides, possibly mediated by still undiscovered angiotensin receptors, might be of clinical importance. At this time, little is known of a possible role for angiotensins III and IV in heart failure.

Angiotensin II Receptor Subtypes. Angiotensin II exerts different regulatory effects when this peptide binds to different receptor subtypes (Rogg, 1990; Murphy, 1991; Mukoyama, 1993; Timmermans et al., 1993; Berk, 1998). The responses initiated by these subtypes not only differ qualitatively, but as is seen for other receptors involved in the neurohumoral response, the responses can oppose one another (Fig. 4-5). Recent drug development, discussed in Chapter 9, has made this once arcane subject of timely interest in the management of heart failure. This is because the two major classes of angiotensin II receptors, designated AT$_1$ and AT$_2$, play different roles in cardiovascular signaling and can be individually targeted for receptor blockade.

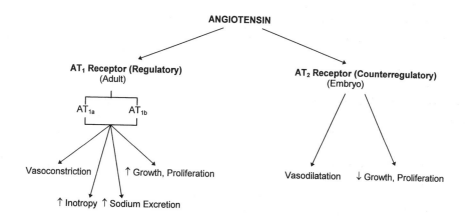

ANGIOTENSIN II RECEPTOR SUBTYPES

FIG. 4-5. Two angiotensin II receptor subtypes exert different effects that, in many cases, oppose one another. The AT$_1$ receptors exert regulatory effects while the effects of AT$_2$ receptor stimulation are generally counterregulatory.

The AT_1 receptors, which predominate in the adult heart, can be viewed as activator (regulatory) receptors; they mediate the vasoconstrictor actions of angiotensin II (Timmermans et al., 1993), increase cardiac contractility (Koch-Weser, 1964; Freer et al., 1976; Kobayashi, 1978; Kass and Blair, 1981; Neyses, 1989; Ikenouchi et al., 1994), cause fibrous tissue and blood vessel proliferation (McEwan et al., 1998), and stimulate cardiac myocyte hypertrophy (see Chapter 6). The AT_1 receptors include at least two "sub-subtypes" called AT_{1A} and AT_{1B}, but it is not clear that both subtypes are found in human hearts (Suzuki et al., 1993). Activation of AT_2 receptors generally has inhibitory (counterregulatory) effects that are opposite to those initiated by AT_1 receptor activation (see Fig. 4-5) (Hein et al., 1995; Ichiki et al., 1995); these include vasodilatation and growth inhibition (Stoll et al., 1995).

The AT_2 receptors can be viewed as a "fetal phenotype" because they play an important role in embryonic development (Zemel et al., 1990) and are the predominant receptor subtypes in fetal rat hearts (Sechi et al., 1992; Everett et al., 1997). During maturation of the rat, the AT_2 receptors are replaced by the AT_1 receptor subtype that predominates in the adult rat heart (Matsubara et al., 1994). A similar transition from AT_2 to AT_1 subtypes has also been found during maturation of the rat aorta (Urata et al., 1989). The growth-promoting response to stretch of isolated neonatal myocytes is accompanied by increased numbers of both AT_1 and AT_2 receptor subtypes (Suzuki et al., 1993; Kijima et al., 1996). Both AT_1 and AT_2 receptor subtypes are found in the adult human heart (Haywood et al., 1997). The AT_2 subtype has been reported to predominate in the hearts of some species; however, the density of these receptor subtypes on cardiac myocytes cannot be estimated with precision because they may be distributed differently among the many cell types in the heart (Kurabayashi and Yazaki, 1997; Regitz-Zagrosek et al., 1998). The density of the AT_1 receptor subtype has been found to be reduced in failing human hearts (Asano et al., 1997; Haywood et al., 1997; Zisman et al., 1998), which decreases the ratio of AT_1 to AT_2 receptor subtypes. These changes represent additional examples of the reversion to the fetal phenotype that accompanies the hypertrophic response of the adult heart.

Downregulation of AT_1 receptors in the failing heart, much like β_1-adrenergic receptor downregulation discussed later in this chapter, blunts some of the maladaptive features of the hemodynamic defense reaction. At the time this text is written, there is much confusion (and controversy) as to the value of AT_1 receptor blockade in improving prognosis in heart failure (see Chapter 9). This uncertainty precludes a clear understanding of the mechanisms and clinical roles of these receptor subtypes and the different intracellular signal transduction cascades that they activate.

Effects of Angiotensin II on Other Mediators of the Hemodynamic Defense Reaction. Like most of the other extracellular messengers described in this chapter, angiotensin II not only acts upon the target organs involved in the hemodynamic defense reaction but also regulates other mediators of the hemodynamic defense reaction. The latter interactions can be of considerable clinical importance. For example, the ability of angiotensin II to stimulate the secretion of aldosterone, vasopressin, catecholamines, and endothelin leads to regulatory amplifications that worsen many of the vicious cycles seen in patients with heart failure. These interlocking responses, which are discussed later in this chapter, make it difficult to predict the long-term effects of drugs that act at any point in these signal transduction cascades.

Endothelin

In the late 1980s, a potent vasoconstrictor was isolated from endothelial cells and, because of its source, was named endothelin (abbreviated ET) (Yanagisawa et al., 1988). It has become clear that members of this class of peptides, which are related to a snake venom called sarafotoxin, can be secreted by many other mammalian cell types. In addition to its vasoconstrictor effects, endothelin exhibits the other properties of a regulator of the hemodynamic defense reaction (see Table 4-5).

There are at least three endothelin isoforms (endothelins 1, 2, and 4) whose production is regulated at two levels. The first, regulation of endothelin *gene expression*, gives rise to protein precursors called *preproendothelins*; the second is *posttranslational (protein) processing*, which, as in the case of the renin-angiotensin system, involves a series of proteolytic reactions that convert preproendothelin first to *proendothelin* (also called "big endothelin") and then to the active peptides (Fig. 4-6) (for review see Kramer et al., 1992). At least three different genes encode the precursors for endothelins 1, 2, and 4, which as described below interact with two different receptor subtypes (A and B), whose relative concentrations vary among different tissues (for review, see Benigni and Remuzzi, 1999).

Expression of the messenger RNA for preproendothelin production is highly regulated, being stimulated by other mediators of the hemodynamic defense reaction (including angiotensin II, vasopressin, and norepinephrine), the cytokine interleukin-1, and several growth factors. Endothelin production is inhibited by the counterregulatory messengers ANP, nitric oxide, and prostaglandins (see Fig. 4-6). Subsequent processing of preproendothelin first forms proendothelin, which is then hydrolyzed by a metalloproteinase called *endothelin converting enzyme* to form endothelin. Chymase, which as noted earlier can convert angiotensin I to angiotensin II, also hydrolyzes proendothelin to form endothelin (Urata and Sarakawa, 1998).

The most important actions of the endothelins on the kidneys and heart resemble those of the other regulatory molecules listed in Table 4-5. As is true for many other regulators, the responses to endothelin depend on the ET isoform and type of ET receptor that is activated (Fig. 4-7). The ET-1 isoform, which appears to be most important in cardiovascu-

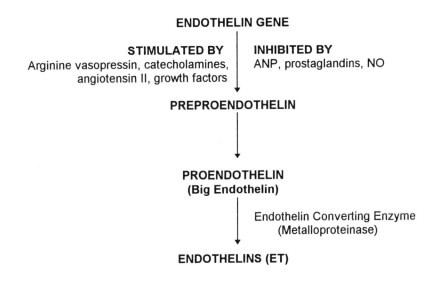

ENDOTHELIN GENE

| **STIMULATED BY** | **INHIBITED BY** |
| Arginine vasopressin, catecholamines, angiotensin II, growth factors | ANP, prostaglandins, NO |

PREPROENDOTHELIN

PROENDOTHELIN
(Big Endothelin)

Endothelin Converting Enzyme
(Metalloproteinase)

ENDOTHELINS (ET)

ENDOTHELIN PRODUCTION

FIG. 4-6. Endothelins are produced by the coordinated regulation of endothelin gene expression and a proteolytic reaction that is catalyzed by a metalloproteinase.

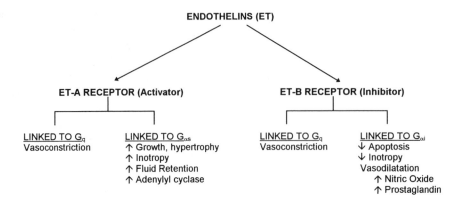

ENDOTHELIN RECEPTOR SUBTYPES

FIG. 4-7. Two endothelin receptor subtypes bind to the different endothelin isoforms with different affinities. Depending on the coupling proteins involved, these receptors exert effects that, in many cases, can oppose one another. Receptor coupling with $G_{\alpha s}$ exerts regulatory effects, whereas those coupled to $G_{\alpha i}$ are generally counterregulatory.

lar regulation, has the highest affinity for ET-A receptors found on vascular smooth muscle. The latter elicit a vasoconstrictor response and so can be viewed as "activator" receptors (much like AT_1). The ET-B receptors, which are found on endothelial cells, release the vasodilators nitric oxide and prostacyclin (DeNucci et al., 1988) and so are inhibitory (much like AT_2). The ability of ET-A receptor activation to induce vasoconstriction is probably mediated by the coupling protein G_q, whereas coupling of ET-A receptors through $G_{\alpha s}$ exerts inotropic, fluid-retaining, and growth-promoting effects. The role of the ET-B receptors is less clear; the latter can mediate a vasoconstrictor response that is probably also mediated by G_q, as well as vasodilator effects that occur when coupling through $G_{\alpha i}$ increases levels of the vasodilators nitric oxide and prostacyclin (Cannan et al., 1996). The latter counterregulatory effects have been reported to predominate in clinical heart failure (Wada et al., 1997). ET-B receptor activation may also inhibit apoptosis (see Chapter 6).

Endothelin-1 levels, like those of the other vasoconstrictors generated in the hemodynamic defense reaction, are increased in patients with heart failure (Margulies et al., 1990; Hiroe et al., 1991; McMurray et al., 1992; Stewart et al., 1992, Cody, 1992; Wei et al., 1994; Kiowski et al., 1995; Pönicke et al., 1998). The most important effects of the elevated ET-1 levels in heart failure are mediated by the ET-A receptor, which causes vasoconstriction, increases myocardial contractility (Suzuki et al., 1989; Ishikawa et al., 1988), stimulates aldosterone secretion (Miller et al., 1989; Cavero et al., 1990; Cozza et al., 1989), inhibits sodium and water excretion by the kidneys (Brooks, 1996; Karet, 1996), and has a growth-promoting effect (Suzuki et al., 1989; Shubeita et al., 1990; Ito et al., 1992, 1994; Levin, 1996; Colucci, 1996, Noll et al., 1996, Ichikawa et al., 1996). The mitogenic effect of endothelin has been suggested to arise from a paracrine action of endothelin-1 that is released from nonmyocytes (Harada et al., 1997) and may play a role in the growth-promoting effects of other mediators of the hemodynamic defense reaction such as adrenergic agonists (Kaburagi et al., 1998).

Recent studies indicate that ET-A receptor blockade improves survival in a rat model of heart failure, probably by inhibiting remodeling (Sasaki et al., 1996; Mulder et al.,

1997; Fraccarollo et al., 1997). The implications of these effects, which are similar to those of the ACE inhibitors, are discussed in Chapter 9, when we consider the importance of maladaptive growth in patients with heart failure.

Nitric Oxide

Vascular endothelium, in addition to producing the vasoconstrictor endothelin, synthesizes a powerful vasodilator (Furchgott and Zawadzki, 1980). Initially called endothelial-derived relaxing factor (EDRF), this physiologic vasodilator is currently known to be nitric oxide (Palmer et al., 1987), a free radical gas whose structural formula is N=O, or more simply NO (for review, see Moncada and Higgs, 1993; Kelly et al., 1996, Ikeda and Shimada, 1997). Nitric oxide is generated by the conversion of L-arginine to L-citrulline in a reaction that is catalyzed by a family of enzymes called *nitric oxide synthase*, generally abbreviated as *NOS*.

Two NOS isoforms are found in the heart. One is a constitutive enzyme called NOS3 or cNOS (the prefix "c" stands for constitutive) that participates in physiologic signaling. The other, which is induced by inflammatory mediators, is called NOS2 or iNOS (where the prefix "i" stands for inducible); this enzyme generates large, toxic amounts of NO (see Chapter 5). A third member of this family, NOS1 or nNOS, is a neuronal enzyme that appears not to be important in cardiovascular regulation. NO exerts many different effects; most simply, these can be divided into those seen at low concentrations, which participate in the hemodynamic defense reaction, and those which reflect the ability of high NO concentrations to generate free radicals during inflammation. As discussed in Chapter 5, the latter may contribute to the progressive deterioration of the failing heart.

Low concentrations of NO are generated when cNOS, the constitutive enzyme, is activated by a variety of receptors (Table 4-8). The low concentrations of NO generated by cNOS serve a counterregulatory role (see Table 4-5). In vascular endothelium, these low NO concentrations serve not only as a physiologic vasodilator but also regulate vascular permeability, platelet aggregation, and oxidative phosphorylation (for review, see Kelly et al., 1996; Kelly and Han, 1997). In working cardiac myocytes and nodal cells, the NO generated by cNOS serves additional functions, including activation of phosphodiesterase inhibitors, which, by increasing cyclic guanine monophosphate (GMP) levels, slows the hydrolysis of cyclic adenosine monophosphate (AMP), thereby augmenting the effects of sympathetic stimulation and causing a weak positive inotropic effect (Prendergast et al., 1997; Preckel et al., 1997; Hare et al., 1998). Different effects of NO are seen at slightly higher concentrations, where NO reduces contractility, inhibits the positive chronotropic and inotropic effects of sympathetic stimulation (Balligand et al., 1993), reduces diastolic stiffness (Paulus et al., 1994), promotes sodium excretion by the kidney (Haynes et al., 1997), and inhibits cell proliferation (Garg and Hassid, 1989). These counterregulatory effects of cNOS-generated NO are a mirror image of those of the regulatory mediators listed in Table 4-5.

TABLE 4-8. *Major isoforms of nitric oxide synthase*

nNOS (NOS1): *Neuronal,* little direct role in cardiovascular regulation.
iNOS (NOS2): *Inducible,* responds to cytokine and endotoxin activation by generating large amounts of NO that participate in inflammation.
cNOS (NOS3): *Constitutive,* responds to activation of a variety of receptors by generating small amounts of NO that participate in the hemodynamic defense reaction, largely as a counterregulatory mediator.

The ability of NO to relax vascular tone is altered in both animal models and human heart failure (Kaiser et al., 1989; Kubo et al., 1991; Elsner et al., 1991; Drexler and Lu, 1992; Katz et al., 1992; Kiuchi et al., 1993; Hirooka et al., 1994), an effect that appears to be due to attenuation of the vasodilator response to NO rather than to reduced NO release (Kubo et al., 1991; Drexler et al., 1991; Kubo et al., 1994; Winlaw et al., 1994; Smith et al., 1994). Many additional effects of cNOS stimulation have been identified in these patients, however, so that the functional significance of NO production in the failing heart remains unclear (Kelly and Han, 1997; Drexler, 1998).

Very different effects of NO are caused when large amounts of this free radical gas are generated by the induction of iNOS. Important inducers of iNOS, discussed in Chapter 5, include cytokines and endotoxins (Moncada et al, 1993). The ability of cytokines such as TNF-α and IL-1β to induce iNOS in cardiac myocytes (Schultz et al., 1995; Balligand et al., 1994) is consistent with evidence that the large amounts of NO synthesized by this enzyme mediate adverse effects of cytokines in the inflammatory response (see Chapter 5).

Bradykinin

Bradykinin and related peptides (kallidins) are vasodilators whose biological actions are mediated by several bradykinin (B) receptors (Mombouli and Vanhoutte, 1992) (Fig. 4-8). Like angiotensin II, kallidins are released from inactive protein precursors, called *kininogens,* by proteolytic enzymes called *kallikreins* (Fig. 4-9) (Carretero and Scicli, 1995). Other parallels between the renin-angiotensin system and the kallikrein-bradykinin system include the existence of both circulating and tissue systems. Bradykinin, the major product of the plasma system, is the octapeptide *Arg-Pro-Gly-Phe-Ser-Pro-Phe-Arg*, whereas kallidin, a closely related vasodilator peptide generated by the tissue system, is lysyl-bradykinin, that is, a nonpeptide that contains an additional N-terminal lysine residue.

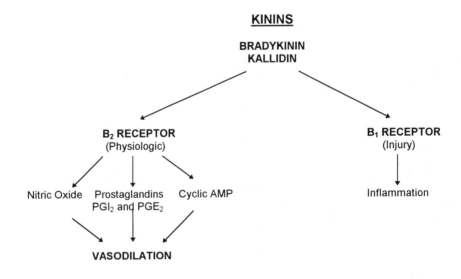

FIG. 4-8. Different kinin receptors mediate different responses to these peptides. The B$_2$ receptors are involved in the circulatory effects; the B$_1$ receptors in the inflammatory response.

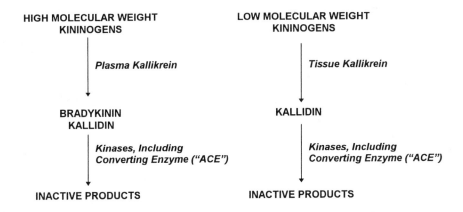

KININ PRODUCTION

FIG. 4-9. Kinins are produced by both plasma and tissue systems. Activation of the plasma system begins with the hydrolysis of high molecular weight kininogens, whereas lower molecular weight kininogens are more important for the tissue system.

Most cardiovascular actions of bradykinin are initiated when this peptide binds to the B_2 kinin receptor. These include an important vasodilator effect, which is mediated by at least three enzymes: *constitutive nitric oxide synthase (cNOS)*, which generates NO (Mombouli and Vanhoutte, 1992; Farhy et al., 1993, Fleming et al., 1994), *phospholipase A_2*, which catalyzes the production of a number of eicosanoids, including the vasodilators prostacyclin and prostaglandin E_2 (Schrör, 1992), and *adenylyl cyclase*, which synthesizes cyclic AMP, another smooth muscle relaxant. Stimulation of NO synthesis by bradykinin may play a role in the inflammatory response discussed in Chapter 5. Bradykinin also inhibits maladaptive growth, an effect whose significance in heart failure remains unclear.

Bradykinin is a substrate for ACE, which is also responsible for the production of angiotensin II (Garrison and Peach, 1990). As a result, ACE inhibitors not only reduce angiotensin II formation but also inhibit the breakdown of bradykinin. These drugs, therefore, have a dual effect to reduce arteriolar tone: they inhibit both the production of the vasoconstrictor angiotensin II and the breakdown of the vasodilator bradykinin. Bradykinin and angiotensin II also have opposing effects on cell growth, so that the ACE inhibitors have an additional synergistic effect: they reduce the formation of a growth promoter (angiotensin II) and inhibit the breakdown of bradykinin, a growth inhibitor. Of clinical importance is the ability of bradykinin to initiate coughing, a sometimes troubling side-effect of treatment with ACE inhibitors.

Adrenomedullin

Adrenomedullin, an extracellular messenger that exerts both counterregulatory and regulatory effects, is a large (52 amino acid) peptide that is secreted by endothelial cells. Levels of adrenomedullin, which has vasodilator (Kitamua et al., 1993), diuretic (Jougasaki et al., 1995a), and positive inotropic effects (Szokodi et al., 1998), are increased in patients with heart failure (Jougasaki et al., 1995b; Nishikimi et al., 1995; Kato et al., 1996; Kobayashi et al., 1996). The clinical importance of these effects, and the potential role of modifying the action of this peptide in patients with heart failure have not yet been established.

Prostaglandins

These polyunsaturated fatty acid derivatives are generated by a family of membrane-associated *cyclooxygenases* (*cox*) enzymes that insert double bonds into arachidonic acid, a 20-carbon fatty acid. Several of the messengers generated by the hemodynamic defense reaction stimulate prostaglandin synthesis; these include norepinephrine, angiotensin II, and vasopressin. Because they are short-lived, prostaglandins generally act locally, gaining access to their target tissues when released from one cell to act on a nearby cell (paracrine effect), or when they bind to receptors on the same cell that released the prostaglandin (autocrine effect). Members of this family exert a variety of effects (for review, see Coleman et al., 1994); some are vasodilators, notably prostacyclin (PGI_2) and prostaglandin E_2 (PGE_2), whereas others, such as thromboxane (TxA_2), cause vasoconstriction. Many also modify platelet function; for example, PGI_2 inhibits platelet aggregation, whereas TxA_2 has a powerful activator effect. Aspirin acetylates, and so irreversibly inhibits cox-1, the platelet cyclooxygenase; the resulting inhibition of platelet function explains why aspirin is so valuable in coronary artery disease. However, aspirin, along with other nonsteroidal antiinflammatory drugs (NSAIDs) that modify prostaglandin metabolism, can interact with the ACE inhibitors that are generally administered to patients with heart failure. The clinical importance of these interactions, however, is not clear (for discussion, see Cleland, 1997).

Some prostaglandins are vasodilators that serve a counterregulatory role in heart failure; these substances mediate the vasodilator effects of bradykinin and possibly of other vasodilators used to treat heart failure. Local effects on the kidneys allow the vasodilator prostaglandins to counteract the sodium-retaining consequences of renal vasoconstriction (Dzau et al., 1984). Other prostaglandins, however, have the opposite effect in that they release the vasoconstrictors norepinephrine and angiotensin II (for review, see Goldsmith and Kubo, 1988). Cyclooxygenase induction may play an important role in mediating an inflammatory response in the failing heart (see Chapter 5; for review, see Wu, 1998). These convoluted effects make it difficult to assess the role of these lipid mediators in heart failure and whether interfering with these pathways would do harm or good. One answer to this latter question has been provided by a large trial in which use of a prostacyclin analogue to treat heart failure had adverse results (Chapter 9).

Stimulation of the Heart

The third major component of the hemodynamic defense reaction is stimulation of the inotropic, lusitropic, and chronotropic properties of the heart (see Table 4-1). The result is an increased cardiac output, brought about by a decrease in end-systolic volume (ESV), a higher end-diastolic volume (EDV), and a more rapid heart rate (HR). Together, these effects modify all three variables in the equation for cardiac output (CO):

$$CO = (EDV - ESV) \times HR \qquad \text{Equation 4.1}$$

Stroke volume (EDV - ESV) is increased both by the lusitropic response, which by facilitating relaxation, increases EDV, and by the inotropic response, which promotes ejection and so reduces ESV. The chronotropic response that increases HR, the third term in Equation 4.1, occurs when sympathetic activation modifies the ion channels so as to accelerate depolarization of the pacemaker cells in the sinus node.

Cardiac stimulation plays an important adaptive role in maintaining tissue perfusion during exercise and following hemorrhage (see Tables 4-2 and 4-3). In both cases, short-term stimulation of the heart helps to maintain cardiac output. Unfortunately, when sustained, cardiac stimulation becomes deleterious, especially in the patient with a damaged or overloaded heart. This fact, however, was far from obvious even a decade ago, when heart failure was generally viewed simply as a hemodynamic syndrome caused by a weakened cardiac pump. It was only after many long-term clinical trials demonstrated that inotropic drugs worsened prognosis that the adverse effects of chronic cardiac stimulation came to be widely appreciated. These topics are discussed in Chapter 3, in which the energetic consequences of cardiac stimulation are discussed, and in Chapters 6 and 7, which discuss the maladaptive growth response of the failing heart.

Autonomic activity is modified greatly in patients with heart failure (for review, see Eckberg, 1997). Activation of the sympathetic nervous system, which plays a major role in the hemodynamic defense reaction, is by far the most important mediator of cardiac stimulation (see Tables 4-4 and 4-5A). Sympathetic stimulation has both regulatory and counterregulatory effects; the former include not only cardiac stimulation but also vaso-constriction and sodium retention by the kidneys. Most of these effects are caused by nor-epinephrine, the most important neurotransmitter released by sympathetic nerve endings. Other neurotransmitters, several of which are discussed in subsequent paragraphs, play a role in stimulating, and in some cases inhibiting, the pumping of the failing heart.

Sympathetic Activation

Several mechanisms allow the hemodynamic defense reaction to activate the sympathetic nervous system (Table 4-9). Most important is the *baroreceptor response* to a decrease in arterial blood pressure and increased rate of pressure increase, which occur during exercise, following hemorrhage, and in patients with heart failure. At least two *neural mechanisms* also contribute to sympathetic stimulation. One, which is initiated in the cerebral cortex, occurs when anticipation of exercise increases heart rate and blood pressure. This can be seen when a dog is placed on a treadmill and the experimenter reaches for the switch that turns on the machine (Rushmer et al., 1959), or when a sprinter hears the starter's gun. Autonomic centers in the brain stem can be stimulated by signals that arise in peripheral tissues, as well as by the baroreceptor reflex already described. These neural mechanisms, in addition to direct effects on sympathetic and parasympathetic tone, can "reset" the arterial baroreceptors so as to increase their sensitivity to further hemodynamic abnormalities. *Metabolic changes*, notably hypoxia, hypercapnia, and acidosis also result in sympathetic activation. These metabolic responses, which are mediated by arterial chemoreceptors, are of minor importance in the neurohumoral response to brief exercise; although they are of more significance during endurance activity and after hemorrhage, their major role is in patients with heart failure (Ponikowski et al., 1997).

TABLE 4-9. *Activators of sympathetic stimulation in the hemodynamic defense reaction*

Hemodynamic
Reduced carotid and aortic baroreceptor stretch.
Nervous
Cortical: anticipation of exercise, stress.
Brain stem: autonomic center activation.
Metabolic
Chemoreceptor activation by hypoxia, hypercapnia, acidosis.

TABLE 4-10. *Major receptor subtypes that mediate actions of norepinephrine*

α_1-Adrenergic receptors
  Smooth muscle contraction—vasoconstriction
  Sodium retention by the kidneys
α_2-Adrenergic receptors
  Central inhibition of sympathetic activity
    Vasodilation
    Cardiac inhibition
β_1-Adrenergic receptors
  Cardiac stimulation—positive inotropy, lusitropy, and chronotropy
β_2-Adrenergic receptors
  Smooth muscle relaxation—vasodilatation

Sympathetic stimulation increases the release of catecholamines, mainly epinephrine from the adrenal medulla, and far more important, norepinephrine from sympathetic nerve endings on the heart and blood vessels.

The norepinephrine released at peripheral sympathetic nerve endings, as noted in Table 4-5, has several important regulatory effects. Binding to α_1-adrenergic receptors on blood vessels evokes a powerful vasoconstrictor response that increases total peripheral resistance and, in the renal circulation, causes local changes that promote sodium retention (Table 4-10). The cardiac actions of norepinephrine, which are normally mediated by β_1-adrenergic receptors, increase inotropy, lusitropy, and chronotropy. A very different response occurs when norepinephrine binds to preganglionic α_2-adrenergic receptors in the central nervous system, where the catecholamine causes a counterregulatory response that inhibits sympathetic outflow (Tables 4-10 and 4-11).

The major hemodynamic effects initiated when norepinephrine binds to peripheral adrenergic receptors are discussed in the following paragraphs; the signal transduction systems activated by adrenergic receptors are outlined in Chapter 7.

Sympathetic Overactivity in Heart Failure. Although tachycardia has long been recognized to occur in heart failure (see Chapter 1), the first direct evidence for sympathetic activation in these patients was the finding of elevated plasma norepinephrine levels (Chidsey et al., 1962) and increased urinary excretion of catecholamines (Chidsey et al.,

TABLE 4-11. *Central and peripheral effects of three receptor systems*

α_2-Adrenergic receptors
  Central effects (counterregulatory)
    Inhibit sympathetic outflow
  Peripheral effects (regulatory)
    Vascular smooth muscle: vasoconstriction
Imidazoline receptors
  Central effects (counterregulatory)
    Inhibit sympathetic outflow
  Peripheral effects (counterregulatory)
    Heart: inhibit norepinephrine release
    Atria: promote atrial natriuretic peptide (ANP) release
Dopaminergic receptors[a]
  Central effects (counterregulatory)
    Inhibit sympathetic outflow
  Peripheral effects (counterregulatory)
    Vascular smooth muscle: vasodilatation

[a]High dopamine concentrations exert regulatory effects by stimulating cardiac β receptors and, when converted to norepinephrine, by activating α_1-adrenergic receptors in vascular smooth muscle.

1965). Two quite different mechanisms could explain these findings. The first is impaired reuptake of norepinephrine into the sympathetic nerve endings, from which this catecholamine is released, a process that normally removes it from adrenergic receptors so as to turn off the signal. The second is increased norepinephrine release. Increased norepinephrine levels in the blood and urine of patients with heart failure, therefore, could be due to excess release, impaired uptake, or both. Some impairment of norepinephrine reuptake has been found in heart failure, but the major abnormality appears to be excessive release (Hasking et al., 1986; Eisenhofer et al., 1996; Davis et al., 1988, Meredith et al., 1993). Measurements that show an increased rate of discharge in the peripheral sympathetic nerves of these patients provides direct proof of sympathetic overactivity in heart failure (Leimbach et al., 1986; Ferguson et al., 1990).

A role for excessive sympathetic activity in determining the poor prognosis in heart failure is suggested by a strong correlation between the extent of elevation of plasma norepinephrine and reduced survival (Levine et al., 1982; Cohn et al., 1984; Francis et al., 1993). This correlation, however, cannot distinguish between cause-effect and effect-cause; that is, whether elevated norepinephrine levels are lethal or whether, instead, the severity of the illness determines the extent to which norepinephrine levels are elevated. Both probably are correct. It is likely that the more severe the impairment of cardiac function, the greater will be the neurohumoral response. Conversely, "toxic" effects of high catecholamine levels have been known for almost a century (for review, see Raab, 1943, 1953; Mueller at al., 1977). These are seen clinically in pheochromocytoma, a catecholamine-secreting adrenal tumor, in which heart failure can develop when excessive β-adrenergic stimulation of the heart causes a necrotizing cardiomyopathy (Scott et al., 1988; Behrana et al., 1989). Recent clinical trials provide further evidence that sympathetic overactivity exerts long-term maladaptive effects in patients with heart failure. These trials are discussed in Chapter 9, which reviews the adverse effects of β-adrenergic agonists and phosphodiesterase inhibitors on survival, and the beneficial effects of long-term treatment with β-adrenergic blockers.

Adrenergic Receptor Subtypes. Almost 50 years ago, Ahlquist (1948) postulated that two classes of receptor mediated the cellular actions of norepinephrine: *α-adrenergic receptors,* which are responsible for the vasoconstrictor effects of sympathetic stimulation, and *β-adrenergic receptors,* which cause both vasodilation and cardiac stimulation (see Table 4-10). This insight, it turns out, actually understates the complexity of this aspect of cellular control in that it has become clear that both α- and β-adrenergic receptors include several subclasses. As in the case of the V_1 and V_2, AT_1 and AT_2, and ET-A and ET-B receptors, this diversity allows norepinephrine to initiate both regulatory and counterregulatory responses. This signaling diversity, as discussed in Chapter 9, has become of considerable practical importance in the clinical management of heart failure.

α-Adrenergic Receptors. The cardiovascular effects of the two major classes of α-adrenergic receptors, $α_1$ and $α_2$, differ markedly (for review, see Kern, 1999). The $α_1$ receptors, which include at least three subtypes (Graham et al., 1996), are located on peripheral tissues including the heart (Noguchi et al., 1995) and vascular smooth muscle, whose function they regulate directly. Although some $α_2$ receptors are found in peripheral tissues, where their actions resemble those of the $α_1$ receptors, the more important $α_2$ receptors are found in the vasomotor centers of the brain stem and on postsynaptic adrenergic neurons, where binding of norepinephrine to $α_2$ receptors *inhibits* sympathetic outflow (see Table 4-11). The central effects of $α_2$-adrenergic activation are, therefore, counterregulatory. One consequence of this rather confusing arrangement is to appreciate that vasodilatation can be achieved both by peripheral α_1-adrenergic blockers and central α_2-adrenergic agonists.

α_1-adrenergic receptors. In addition to their major role as direct mediators of the vasoconstrictor response to sympathetic stimulation (see above), α_1 receptors mediate a positive inotropic effect on the heart (Skomedal et al., 1985; Endoh and Blinks, 1988); this cardiac response, however, is generally minor, and in some species absent. In humans, although α_1-adrenergic receptor activation increases contractility, the inotropic response is weak and, in the human ventricle where the density of α_1-adrenergic receptors is low, of little clinical significance (for review, see Lee, 1993). Activation of α_1-adrenergic receptors by norepinephrine provides a powerful stimulus for myocardial hypertrophy in neonatal cardiac myocytes (Simpson, 1993, see Chapter 7), but this effect is less marked in the adult human heart.

There is not yet agreement whether α_1-adrenergic receptor density is unchanged or increased in the failing heart (Bristow et al., 1988; Vago et al., 1989; Steinfath et al., 1992; Bristow and Gilbert 1995), nor is it known whether human cardiac α_1 receptors play an important role in regulating either contractility or gene expression in clinical heart failure. The role of α-adrenergic receptors in heart failure is further complicated by the presence of α_2 receptors in the human heart; because these are on presynaptic fibers whose major effect is tonic inhibition of norepinephrine release, α_2 blockade can increase contractility indirectly (Parker et al., 1995). It is likely that the major effects of α_1-adrenergic receptors in heart failure do not involve the heart, but instead occur when vasoconstriction increases peripheral resistance and promotes fluid retention by the kidney.

α_2-adrenergic receptors. The most important cardiovascular effects of the α_2-adrenergic receptors are centrally mediated. In the vasomotor centers of the lower brain stem, α_2 adrenergic receptor activation inhibits sympathetic outflow and so is counterregulatory (see Table 4-11). This elaborate control system is made even more complex by the existence of α_2 receptor subtypes. In the mouse, α_2-adrenergic receptor blockade can cause both hypotensive (α_{2a}-adrenergic receptors) and hypertensive (α_{2b}-adrenergic receptors) effects (MacMillan et al., 1996), whereas in humans, the hypotensive effects of α_2-adrenergic receptor stimulation are dominant (Parker et al., 1995). Another counterregulatory signal transduction system, whose central effects are mediated by *imidazoline receptors,* also responds to α_2-adrenergic agonists by inhibiting sympathetic outflow. The potential importance of these overlapping control mechanisms in the treatment of heart failure lies in the potential for development of new drug molecules "targeted" to activate or block specific counterregulatory receptors or receptor subtypes. The possibility that such drugs can improve prognosis in patients with heart failure is currently being examined (Chapter 9).

β-Adrenergic Receptors. Of three known β-adrenergic receptor subtypes, two (β_1 and β_2) play an important role in cardiovascular regulation. The most important actions of the third subtype, β_3 receptors, is to regulate gastrointestinal motility and lipolysis; in the heart, these receptors exert a negative inotropic effect that may be coupled by G_i and do not interact with either β_1 or β_2 receptor blockers (Krief et al., 1993). The β_2 receptors normally predominate in vascular smooth muscle, where they mediate a relaxing effect of norepinephrine; this counterregulatory effect, however, is overwhelmed by the constrictor effects of α_1-adrenergic receptor activation. The most important subtype in the heart is the β_1-adrenergic receptor, which in humans normally constitutes 70% to 80% of the β-adrenergic receptors. As is seen in the case of many other mediators of the neurohumoral response, binding of the same agonist to different receptors can produce different effects. This appears to be true of the heart's β-adrenergic receptors, where different

responses can be attributed to functional compartmentation of cyclic AMP (Zhou et al., 1997). In the rat, increased inotropy and lusitropy are mediated mainly by cardiac β_1 receptors, whereas the cardiac β_2 receptor subtype acts preferentially to increase the opening of plasma membrane calcium channels (Xiao and Lakatta, 1993; Xiao et al., 1994, 1995). Similar differences in the effects of these β-adrenergic receptor subtypes are found in the human heart, although these appear to be less marked than in the rat (Bristow et al., 1989).

β-adrenergic receptor downregulation. Attenuation of the myocardial response to norepinephrine represents one of the most dramatic counterregulatory changes in patients with heart failure (Table 4-12). This occurs when chronic sympathetic stimulation inhibits β-receptor synthesis and reduces the ability of β receptors to respond to the stimulatory effects of norepinephrine, changes once referred to as "tachyphylaxis." The most important mechanism responsible for this attenuation is β receptor *downregulation,* which reduces the number of receptors available to bind to norepinephrine, and an increase in the levels of G_i, a coupling protein that mediates the counterregulatory effects of muscarinic stimulation. The following discussion focuses on the effects of chronic stimulation of the β receptors themselves; changes further "downstream" in these signal transduction cascades are discussed in Chapter 7.

The loss of sensitivity to the inotropic, lusitropic, and chronotropic effects of norepinephrine is both adaptive and maladaptive in the failing heart; it is beneficial because it reduces the deleterious effects of chronic β-adrenergic stimulation, but at the same time cardiac stimulation is blunted so that cardiac output is reduced. Recent clinical trials have shown that, over the long term, the beneficial effects of attenuating the responsiveness of the failing heart to β-adrenergic stimulation far outweigh what turn out to be short-term deleterious effects (Chapter 9).

Downregulation of β-receptors in the failing heart is selective in that the number of β_1 receptors decreases markedly, whereas there is little or no change in the β_2 receptor subtype (Bristow et al., 1986, Böhm et al., 1989; Steinfath et al., 1992; for review see, Broode, 1991). The mechanism responsible for selective downregulation of the β_1 subtype is not known, but has been suggested to occur because sympathetic nerve terminals are closer to the β_1 receptors (Hawthorn and Broadley, 1982). Two mechanisms allow prolonged sympathetic stimulation to downregulate the β-adrenergic receptors: reduced receptor synthesis and receptor inactivation (see Table 4-12). The latter is brought about by a sequence of three steps: inactivation of receptors by phosphorylation, internalization of the phosphorylated receptors, and proteolytic digestion of the internalized receptors (Hausendorff et al., 1990). The first two steps are reversible, but the final step of proteolytic digestion can be reversed only by synthesis of new receptors, a process that is slowed in the failing heart.

TABLE 4-12. *Attenuation of the myocardial response to norepinephrine*

I. Reduced synthesis of β receptors
II. β-Receptor downregulation
   1. Inactivation of β receptors by phosphorylation
     Reversible by dephosphorylation
   2. Internalization of phosphorylated β receptors
     Reversible by return to plasma membrane
   3. Proteolytic digestion of internalized β receptors
     Irreversible, new receptors must be resynthesized (but see I)
III. "Downstream" changes in signal transduction

Reduced β Receptor Synthesis: Levels of the mRNA that encode β-adrenergic receptors, especially the β_1 receptor, are reduced in the failing heart (Ungerer et al., 1993; Ping and Hammond, 1994; Ihl-Vahl et al., 1996). This change probably decreases β_1-receptor gene expression and so slows the synthesis of new β_1-receptors. This is especially important in the failing heart, in which β_1-receptors are being destroyed at an increased rate.

Inactivation of β Receptors by Phosphorylation: Phosphorylation, the first of three steps by which chronic sympathetic stimulation reduces the number of active receptors (see Table 4-12), is catalyzed by an enzyme commonly called β-adrenergic receptor kinase (βARK), which is a member of a class of enzymes called G-protein receptor kinases (GRK) (for review, see Lefkowitz, 1993), which allows βARK-catalyzed phosphorylation to provide a negative feedback in which cyclic AMP produced when norepinephrine activates β receptors attenuates the response to norepinephrine. This counterregulatory step is readily reversed when cyclic AMP levels decrease and the β-adrenergic receptors become dephosphorylated by a phosphoprotein phosphatase.

Inactivation of β-adrenergic receptors by βARK involves a cofactor, called *arrestin,* which prevents the phosphorylated receptor from activating its intracellular signal transduction cascade. Although arrestin expression appears not to change in the failing heart (Ungerer et al., 1994), increased synthesis of βARK in these patients (Ungerer et al., 1993; Ping et al., 1997) provides an additional contribution to the coordinated negative feedback that, by inactivating β-adrenergic receptors, reduces the neurohumoral drive to these hearts.

Internalization of Phosphorylated β Receptors: The second step in receptor inactivation occurs when phosphorylated β receptors become detached from the plasma membrane and move into the cell interior. This reversible process, called *internalization,* renders the receptors inaccessible to the β-adrenergic agonists that impinge on the extracellular surface of these membranes. The phosphorylated receptors remain internalized until they are either destroyed or, after the receptors are dephosphorylated, they return to the plasma membrane in a step that resensitizes the cell to β-adrenergic agonists. If exposure to elevated norepinephrine levels is prolonged, as in the failing heart, dephosphorylation and return of the receptors to the cell surface becomes impaired. In this setting, the internalized receptors are destroyed in the third, and this time irreversible, step in downregulation.

Proteolytic Digestion of Internalized Receptors: The final step in receptor inactivation occurs when internalized β receptors are digested by lysosomal proteases. Unlike phosphorylation and internalization, this mechanism is irreversible, so that restoration of normal sensitivity to norepinephrine requires synthesis of new receptors. As already noted, however, β_1 receptor synthesis is reduced in the failing heart.

Together, the mechanisms responsible for β_1 receptor downregulation help protect the failing heart from the adverse effects of sustained sympathetic stimulation. The adaptive nature of this response has become clear in recent clinical trials, described in Chapter 9, which have shown that circumventing these protective mechanisms—for example, by using phosphodiesterase inhibitors to increase cellular levels of cyclic AMP—worsens prognosis in patients with heart failure. Conversely, β-adrenergic blocking agents, which like β receptor downregulation reduces cyclic AMP production, improve long-term outcome.

Parasympathetic and Purinergic Mechanisms

Two signaling systems that exert counterregulatory effects appear to be modified in heart failure. The first are parasympathetic mechanisms, which are mediated when acetylcholine binding to muscarinic receptors inhibits cyclic AMP production. There is some evidence, but not universal agreement, that parasympathetic tone (Eckberg et al., 1971; Binkley et al., 1991; Nolan et al., 1992) and the number of muscarinic receptors and G_i, which mediate vagal signals (Vatner et al., 1996; Le Guludec et al., 1996), are increased in heart failure. Purinergic receptors, which are stimulated by adenosine and have actions that parallel those of muscarinic receptors, do not, however, appear to be upregulated in the failing heart (Hershberger et al., 1991).

Central Mechanisms

Activation of the sympathetic nervous system, while the most important neural component of the neurohumoral defense reaction, is not the only centrally mediated signaling system that plays a role in heart failure. At least three other neural systems participate in this response; as discussed briefly in the following paragraphs, these produce both regulatory and counterregulatory effects.

Imidazoline Receptors. Because of its similarity to the central α_2-adrenergic system discussed in the preceding section, it is logical to describe the recently discovered imidazoline signaling system at this point (Table 4-13). The endogenous agonist of the imidazoline system is *agmantine*, a derivative of arginine (for review, see Regunathan and Reis, 1996), which binds to a class of receptors called imidazoline receptors. This system, which includes at least two receptor subtypes, I-1 and I-2, is found in both the nervous system and peripheral tissues.

The central imidazoline receptors operate much like central α_2-adrenergic receptors in that agonist binding to presynaptic imidazoline receptors in the brain stem inhibits sympathetic outflow (Dotenwill et al., 1994; Yu and Frishman, 1996). The parallels between these two counterregulatory systems are highlighted by the fact that several α_2-adrenergic receptor agonists also bind to and activate central imidazoline receptors.

In addition to the central imidazoline receptors, peripheral receptors are found in several tissues including the heart, where they inhibit norepinephrine release (Likungu et al., 1996). Imidazoline receptors in the atria release ANP, and so promote natriuresis and diuresis (Mukkadam-Daher et al., 1997). Peripheral imidazoline receptors are also found on human vascular smooth muscle, where they exert an antiproliferative action (Regunathan and Reis, 1997). The many counterregulatory effects of this newly discovered system suggest that imidazoline receptor agonists might be of value in the management of heart failure, a possibility that, as discussed in Chapter 9, is being investigated.

Dopamine and Dopaminergic Receptors. Dopamine, which is a precursor of norepinephrine in its biosynthesis from tyrosine, is a catecholamine that has both central and peripheral effects that are mediated by several classes of dopamine (DA) receptor (for review, see Civelli et al., 1993). At low concentrations, dopamine interacts preferentially with DA_1 receptors that relax smooth muscle; the resulting vasodilatation exerts a counterregulatory effect by lowering peripheral resistance and dilating renal blood vessels.

TABLE 4-13. *Counterregulatory effects of imidazoline receptor activation*

Central effects: inhibit sympathetic outflow
Peripheral effects
   Heart: inhibit norepinephrine release
   Atria: promote atrial natriuretic peptide (ANP) release
   Vascular smooth muscle: antiproliferative

The latter promotes sodium excretion, as does the ability of dopamine to inhibit aldosterone secretion (Krishna et al., 1985). Activation of DA_2 receptors in the brain stem, like the α_2-adrenergic and imidazoline receptors, have counterregulatory effects that inhibit sympathetic outflow (see Table 4-11).

Higher dopamine concentrations, however, have opposite effects. These regulatory responses, which are seen after exogenous administration of large amounts of this catecholamine, enhance the hemodynamic defense reaction by three mechanisms. At high concentrations, dopamine can stimulate β_1-adrenergic receptors, release epinephrine from sympathetic nerve endings in the heart, and become converted to norepinephrine, its natural product. At still higher concentrations, dopamine cross-reacts with peripheral α_1 receptors to cause vasoconstriction. The physiologic role of dopamine, however, is probably confined to the counterregulatory actions of the low concentrations already described.

Neuropeptide Y. Levels of neuropeptide Y, a vasoconstrictor peptide that is released by sympathetic nerve endings along with norepinephrine, are increased by the hemodynamic defense reaction (Grundemar and Hakanson, 1994) and in patients with heart failure (Maisel et al., 1989; Feng et al., 1994; for review, see Francis, 1997). In addition to direct vasoconstrictor actions, which are mediated by Y1 and Y2 receptors in blood vessels, neuropeptide Y potentiates the vasoconstrictor effects of other extracellular messengers, including α_1-adrenergic agonists and angiotensin II, and inhibits acetylcholine release from parasympathetic nerve ending in the heart. These effects of neuropeptide Y, like the cardiac effects of β-adrenergic agonists, appear to be reduced in heart failure (Feng et al., 1996). Neuropeptide Y also has central, counterregulatory actions that inhibit both norepinephrine and renin release. Unlike most of the other vasoconstrictors that participate in the neurohumoral response (see Table 4-5), the actions of neuropeptide Y on the heart appear to include both negative chronotropic and inotropic effects.

TIMING OF APPEARANCE OF MEDIATORS OF THE HEMODYNAMIC DEFENSE REACTION

The many mediators of the neurohumoral response described herein do not appear at the same time in patients with heart failure (see Table 4-6). Sympathetic activation, probably the first of these compensatory mechanisms to be mobilized, is seen in patients who have mild left ventricular dysfunction and few, if any, symptoms, whereas secretion of atrial natriuretic peptide and arginine vasopressin occur somewhat later (Francis et al., 1990; Grassi et al., 1995). It came as somewhat of a surprise that activation of the powerful renin-angiotensin system, which has many interactions with the other mediators of the hemodynamic defense reaction, occurs relatively late in the natural history of this syndrome (Bayliss et al., 1987; Broqvist et al., 1989; Francis et al., 1990). Although plasma norepinephrine, ANP, and vasopressin are elevated in patients with mild left ventricular dysfunction who have neither signs nor symptoms of heart failure, the most dramatic increase in plasma renin levels comes later, often after initiation of diuretic therapy (Francis et al., 1990).

INTERACTIONS AMONG THE MEDIATORS OF THE HEMODYNAMIC DEFENSE REACTION

The surrealistic picture generated by attempts to diagram the interactions between the most important mediators of the hemodynamic defense reaction is shown in Fig. 4-10,

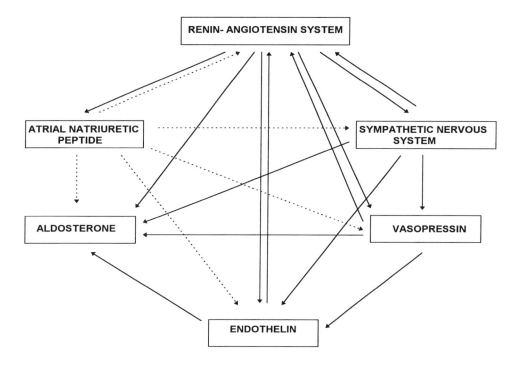

SOME INTERACTIONS AMONG NEUROHUMORAL MEDIATORS

FIG. 4-10. Some of the interactions between some of the key mediators of the hemodynamic defense reaction. Stimulation is depicted by solid arrows, inhibition by dotted arrows. Not all known interactions between these mediators are shown in this illustration, and many important mediators of the neurohumoral response are omitted, along with many counterregulatory interactions. Furthermore, the interactions depicted here do not necessarily apply to all species or to all individuals in one species. The major purpose in providing this illustration is to provide an overview of the complexity of these interactions.

which illustrates yet another level of complexity in this topic. Figure 4-10, which summarizes some of the many reported interactions between the mediators of the neurohumoral response, is neither complete nor entirely accurate; the reason is that the data used to construct this figure were obtained in various animal models as well as patients with heart failure, and some of these interactions are unconfirmed. The point of the figure, however, is not the accuracy of its details, but the overall pattern, which shows a remarkable interplay between the many mediators of this response.

Why do the interactions between the different mediators of the neurohumoral response exhibit such a dazzling intricacy? One explanation is that this interplay evolved to allow the many mediators of this response to be "fine tuned" to meet a variety of minor short-term stresses such as a change in body position or change in blood flow distribution such as occurs after a meal. These minor adjustments resemble the small changes in steering and acceleration needed to drive an automobile on a modern expressway. In emergency situations, such as escape from a predator or massive hemorrhage, these same mechanisms interact and are amplified to generate a powerful coordinated response—much like that of the driver who must swerve to avoid an obstacle that appears unexpectedly on the highway. This need to deal with a sudden, overwhelming emergency and yet to "stay on the road" probably explains how release of most of these mediators came to be controlled by levels of other mediators. Although interactions that amplify the neurohumoral response are valuable, for example the ability of sympathetic stimulation to promote the release of angiotensin II, aldosterone, endothelin, and arginine vasopressin (see Fig. 4-10), mechanisms are also needed to prevent "runaway signaling." The latter is made possible by the ability of these neurohumoral mediators to evoke counterregulatory effects. The resulting array of complex interlocking pathways yields a web such as shown that in Figure 4-10.

The web of interactions shown schematically in Figure 4-10 adds to the challenge in providing rational, mechanistically guided therapy of the individual patient with heart failure. In practical terms, it is important to appreciate the interactions between the many neurohumoral mediators because the drugs used to treat heart failure generally modify both circulatory hemodynamics and the hemodynamic defense reaction. As a result, treatment can both amplify and attenuate many of the interactions shown in Figure 4-10. These interactions vary from patient to patient, a fact that precludes a rigid "care path" approach to therapy, where a step-by-step series of therapeutic actions is set out by a committee of experts. Because the almost inevitable progression of this complex and deadly syndrome changes the "substrate," therapy must be evaluated continually in an iterative manner. This subject is discussed again in Chapter 9, where the iterative processes needed to optimize care of these patients is discussed.

THE GRAND DESIGN

Francis and McDonald (1997) note that many of the mediators of the hemodynamic defense reaction discussed in this chapter can be viewed in terms of a "grand design [that] seems to be to maintain intravascular volume and sufficient perfusion pressure to vital organs." This statement, which echoes the evolutionary overview provided by Peter Harris (1983), defines a valuable set of guidelines for understanding heart failure that is summarized in Table 4-14. Although these mediators share important actions—notably the ability to cause fluid retention, vasoconstriction, and cardiac stimulation—there are subtle and important differences between them. Within this "grand design," for example, sympathetic stimulation acts on the heart and blood vessels to provide a rapid response that maintains blood pressure and cardiac output, whereas the slower activation of the renin-angiotensin system has prominent actions on the kidney, both direct and indirect, that promote sodium retention. These are complemented by the actions of vasopressin that promote water retention (see Table 4-14). However, all of the mediators of the neurohumoral response can be both beneficial and deleterious in patients with heart failure. These variations occur not only because several of these mediators exert counterregula-

TABLE 4-14. *Major actions of key systems that participate in the hemodynamic defense reaction*

Sympathetic nervous system
  Rapid, short-term vasoconstriction and cardiac stimulation—maintains blood pressure and cardiac output
Renin-angiotensin system
  Long-term sodium retention and vasoconstriction—increases blood volume
Arginine vasopressin
  Long-term water retention and vasoconstriction—increases blood volume

---

Modified from Francis and McDonald (1997).

tory effects that are partly offset by regulatory responses evoked by the other mediators, but also because a given response can be helpful or harmful, depending on its intensity and the specific situation in which it is evoked.

CONCLUSION

The important role played by the hemodynamic defense reaction in patients with heart failure represents both a challenge and an opportunity. The challenge is to understand—and predict—the effects of therapy on the interlocking effects of the many mediators of this response. Thus, a drug that alters one component of this response can be expected to perturb other components, if not directly, then almost certainly indirectly. Perturbing these interactions can have different short-term and long-term consequences, which makes it difficult to predict the clinical response when a specific drug is given to an individual patient. Managing heart failure, therefore, is not simple. Overall goals must be clearly set out, and achievable end-points of therapy identified (see Chapter 10).

The complexity of the hemodynamic defense reaction provides opportunities to improve the care of patients with heart failure. These opportunities lie in the ability of thoughtfully designed, carefully monitored therapy to "fine tune" the neurohumoral response so as to maximize benefits and minimize harm. It is already apparent, for example, that renin inhibitors, ACE inhibitors, and possibly steroid and angiotensin II (AT) receptor blockers, have different roles in the management of heart failure. Renin inhibitors, so far, have proven less useful in heart failure than ACE inhibitors, which inhibit angiotensin II formation. Clinical trials, discussed in Chapter 9, clearly show that ACE inhibitors are more valuable in treating heart failure than other vasodilators, a beneficial effect that has made these drugs standard therapy for this syndrome. Partly because the results of clinical trials comparing different AT receptor blockers are controversial, it remains unclear whether the beneficial effects of ACE inhibitors are due to inhibition of angiotensin II formation, inhibition of bradykinin breakdown, or both. Clearly, at all levels, while much is known, even more remains to be learned. As we move through what can be viewed as a Kuhnian paradigmatic shift, from managing hemodynamics to improving prognosis, much is being added to our ability to improve both well-being and outcome in these patients.

BIBLIOGRAPHY

Berne RM, Levy MN, eds (1993). *Physiology*, 3rd ed. Mosby, St. Louis.

Braunwald E, Ross J Jr, Sonnenblick EH, eds (1976). *Mechanisms of Contraction of the Normal and Failing Heart,* 2nd ed. Little Brown, Boston.

Braunwald EH, ed (1997). *Heart Disease. A Textbook of Cardiovascular Medicine,* 5th ed. WB Saunders, Philadelphia.

Cohn JN, ed (1988). *Drug Treatment of Heart Failure.* ATC, Secaucus, NJ.

Fozzard H, Haber E, Katz AM, Jennings R, Morgan HE, eds (1992). *The Heart and Cardiovascular System*, 2nd ed. Raven Press, New York.

Frishman WH, Sonnenblick EH, eds (1996). *Cardiovascular Pharmacology.* McGraw Hill, New York.

Gilman AG, Rall TW, Nies AS, Taylor P, eds (1990). *Goodman and Gilman's The Pharmacological Basis of Therapeutics,* 8th ed. Pergamon, New York.

Gwathmey JK, Briggs GM, Allen PD, eds (1994). *Heart Failure. Basic Science and Clinical Aspects.* Marcel Dekker, New York.

Hosenpud JD, Greenberg BH, eds (1994). *Congestive Heart Failure. Pathophysiology, Diagnosis, and Comprehensive Approach to Management.* Springer, New York.

Laragh JH, Brenner BM, eds (1990). *Hypertension. Pathophysiology, Diagnosis, and Management.* Raven Press, New York.

McCall D, Rahimtoola SH, eds (1995). *Heart Failure.* Chapman & Hall, New York.

Poole-Wilson PA, Colucci WS, Massie BM, Chatterjee K, Coats AS, Eds. *Heart failure. Scientific Principles and Clinical Practice.* Churchill Livingstone, New York.

Sasayama S, Ross J Jr, Brutsaert D (1996). *Heart Failure: New Insight into Mechanisms and Management.* Churchill Livingstone, Tokyo.

Schlant RC, Alexander RW, O'Rourke RA, Roberts R, Sonnenblick EH, eds (1994). *Hurst's The Heart,* 8th ed. McGraw Hill, New York.

Willerson JT, Cohn JN, eds (1995). *Cardiovascular Medicine.* Churchill Livingstone, New York.

REFERENCES

Ahlquist RP (1948). A study of the adrenotropic receptors. *Am J Physiol* 153:586–600.

Asano K, Dutcher DL, Port JD, Minobe WA, Tremmel KD, Roden RL, Bohlmeyer TJ, Bush EW, Jenkin MJ, Abraham WT, Raynolds MV, Zisman LS, Perryman MB, Bristow MR (1997). Selective downregulation of the angiotensin II AT_1-receptor subtypes in failing human ventricular myocardium. *Circulation* 95:1193–1200.

Baker KM, Aceto JF (1990). Angiotensin II stimulation of protein synthesis and cell growth in chick heart cells. *Am J Physiol* 259:H610–H618.

Balligand J-L, Kelly RA, Marsden PA, Smith TW, Michel T (1993). Control of cardiac muscle cell function by an endogenous nitric oxide signaling system. *Proc Natl Acad Sci U S A* 90:347–351.

Balligand J-L, Ungureanu-Longrois D, Simmons WW, Pimental D, Malinski TA, Kapturczak M, Taha Z, Lowenstein CJ, Davidoff AJ, Kelly RA, Smith TW, Michel T (1994). Cytokine-inducible nitric oxide synthase expression in cardiac myocytes. *J Biol Chem* 269:27580–27588.

Bathon JM, Proud D (1991). Bradykinin antagonists. *Annu Rev Pharmacol Toxicol* 31:129–162.

Bayliss J, Norell M, Canepa-Anson R, Sutton G, Poole-Wilson P (1987). Untreated heart failure: clinical and neuroendocrine effects of introducing diuretics. *Br Heart J* 80:329–342.

Behrana A, Haselton P, Leen CIS, et al (1989). Multiple extra-adrenal paragangliomas associated with catecholamine cardiomyopathy. *Eur Heart J* 10:182–185.

Benigni A, Remuzzi C (1999). Endothelin antagonists. *Lancet* 353:133–138.

Berk BC (1998). Angiotensin II receptors and angiotensin II-stimulated signal transduction. *Heart Failure Rev* 3:87–99.

Bernard C (1878). *Leçons sur les phénomènes de la vie communs aux animaux et aux vegetaux.* Translation by Fulton JF. Balliée, Paris.

Binkley PF, Nunziata E, Nelson SD, Cody RJ (1991). Parasympathetic withdrawal is an integral component of autonomic imbalance in congestive heart failure: demonstration in human subjects and verification in a paced canine model of ventricular failure. *J Am Coll Cardiol* 18:464–472.

Böhm M, Pieske B, Schnabel P, Schwinger R, Kemkes B, Klövekorn W-P, Erdmann E (1989). Reduced effect of dopexamine in force of contraction in the failing human heart despite preserved β_2-adrenoreceptor subpopulation. *J Cardiovasc Pharmacol* 14:545–559.

Bousquet P, Feldman J, Schwartz J (1984). Central cardiovascular effects of alpha adrenergic drugs: difference between catecholamines and imidazolines. *J Pharmacol Exp Ther* 230:232–236.

Braun-Menendez E, Page IH (1958). Suggested revision of nomenclature—angiotensin. *Science* 127:242.

Braun-Menendez E, Fasciolo E, Leloir JC, Muñoz JM (1940). The substance causing renal hypertension. *J Physiol (Lond)* 98:283–298.

Bristow MR, Gilbert EM (1995). Improvement on cardiac myocyte function by biological effects of medical therapy. A new concept in the treatment of heart failure. *Eur Heart J* (Suppl F)16:20–31.

Bristow MR, Hershberger RE, Port JD, Minobe W, Rasmussen R (1989). β_1 & β_2 Adrenergic receptor mediated adenylate cyclase stimulation in non-failing and failing human ventricular myocardium. *Mol Pharmacol* 35:295–303.

Bristow MR, Minobe W, Rasmussen R, Hershberger RE, Hoffman BB (1988). Alpha-1 adrenergic receptors in the nonfailing and failing human heart. *J Pharmacol Exp Ther* 247:1039–1045.

Broode O-E (1991) β_1- and β_2-adrenoreceptors in the human heart: properties, function, and alterations in chronic heart failure. *Physiol Rev* 43:203–242.

Brooks DP (1996). Role of endothelin in renal function and dysfunction. *Clin Exp Pharmacol Physiol* 23:3445–3448.

Broqvist M, Dahlström U, Karlberg BE, Karlsson E, Marklund T (1989). Neuroendocrine response in acute heart failure and the influence of treatment. *Eur Heart J* 10:1075–1083.

Cannan CR, Burnett JJ, Lerman A (1996). Enhanced coronary vasoconstriction to endothelin-B receptor activation in experimental congestive heart failure. *Circulation* 93:646–651.

Cannon WB (1932). *The Wisdom of the Body.* WW Norton, New York.

Carretero OA, Scicli AG (1990). Kinins as regulators of blood flow and blood pressure. In Laragh JH, Brenner BM, eds. *Hypertension. Pathophysiology, Diagnosis, and Management.* Raven Press, New York, pp 805–817.

Cavero PG, Miller WL, Heublein DM, Margulies KB, Burnett JC Jr (1990). Endothelin in experimental congestive heart failure in the anesthetized dog. *Am J Physiol* 259:F312–317.

Chidsey CA, Harrison DC, Braunwald E (1962). Augmentation of plasma norepinephrine response to exercise in patients with congestive heart failure. *N Engl J Med* 267:650–654.

Chidsey CA, Braunwald E, Morrow AG (1965). Catecholamine excretion and cardiac stress of congestive heart failure. *Am J Med* 39:442–451.

Civelli O, Buznow JR, Grandy DK (1993). Molecular diversity of the dopamine receptors. *Annu Rev Pharmacol Toxicol* 32:281–307.

Cleland JGF (1997). Anticoagulant and antiplatelet agents. In Poole-Wilson PA, Colucci WS, Massie BM, Chatterjee K, Coats AS, eds. *Heart Failure. Scientific Principles and Clinical Practice.* Churchill Livingstone, New York, pp 759–773.

Clerico A, Iervasi G, Del Chicca MG, Emdin M, Maffei S, Nannipieri M, Sabatino L, Forini F, Manfredi C, Donato L (1998). Circulating levels of cardiac natriuretic peptides (ANP and BNP) measured by highly sensitive and specific immunoradiometric assays in normal subjects and in patients with different degrees of heart failure. *J Endocrinol Invest* 21:170–179.

Cody RJ (1992). The potential role of endothelin as a vasoconstrictor substance in congestive heart failure. *Eur Heart J* 13:1573–1578.

Cody RJ, Atlas SA, Laragh JH, Kubo SH, Covit AB, Ryman KS, Shaknovich A, Pondolfino K, Clark M, Camargo MJE, Scarborough RM, Lewicki JA (1986). Atrial natriuretic factor in normal subjects and heart failure patients. Plasma levels and renal hormonal and hemodynamic responses to peptide infusion. *J Clin Invest* 78:1362–1374.

Cohn JN, Levine TB, Olivari MT, Garberg V, Lura D, Francis GS, Simon AB, Rector T (1984). Plasma norepinephrine as a guide to prognosis in patients with chronic congestive heart failure. *N Engl J Med* 311:819–823.

Coleman RA, Smith WL, Naruyima S (1994). International Union of Pharmacology Classification of prostanoid receptors: properties, distribution, and structure of the receptors and their subtypes. *Pharmacol Rev* 46:205–229.

Colucci W (1996). Myocardial endothelin. Does it play a role in myocardial failure? *Circulation* 93:1069–1072.

Cozza EN, Gomez-Sanchez CE, Foecking MF, Chiou S (1989). Endothelin binding to cultured calf adrenal zona glomerulosa cells and stimulation of aldosterone secretion. *J Clin Invest* 84:1032–1035.

Creager MA, Faxon DP, Cutler SS, et al (1986). Contribution of vasopressin to vasoconstriction in patients with congestive heart failure: comparison with the renin-angiotensin system and the sympathetic nervous system. *J Am Coll Cardiol* 7:758–765.

Crozier IG, Nicholls MG, Ikram H, Espiner EA, Gomez HJ, Warner J (1986). Haemodynamic effects of atrial peptide infusion in heart failure. *Lancet* 2:1242–1245.

Danser AHJ, Schalekamp MADH (1998). Generation and localization of angiotensin II in the heart. *Heart Failure Rev* 3:109–117.

Davis D, Baily R, Zelis R (1988). Abnormalities in systemic norepinephrine kinetics in human congestive heart failure. *Am J Physiol* 254:E760–E766.

DeBold AJ (1979). Heart atria granularity. Effects of changes in water-electrolyte balance. *Proc Soc Exp Biol Med* 161:508–511.

DeBold AJ, Borenstein HB, Veress AT, Sonnenberg H (1981). A rapid and potent natriuretic response to intravenous infection of atrial myocardial extracts in rats. *Life Sci* 28:89–94.

DeBona GF, Herman PJ, Sawin JJ (1989). Neural control of renal function in edema-forming states. *Am J Physiol* 254:R1017–R1024. Drexler H, Lu W (1992). Endothelial dysfunction of hindquarter resistance vessels in experimental heart failure. *Am J Physiol* 262:H1640–H1645.

De Nucci G, Thomas R, D'Orleane-Juste P, Antones E, Waldeer C, Warner TD, Vane JR (1988). Pressor effects of circulating endothelin are limited by its removal in the pulmonary circulation and by the release of prostacyclin and endothelium-derived relaxing factor. *Proc Nat Acad Sci U S A* 85:9797–9800.

Dontenwill M, Tibirica E, Greney G, Bennai FD, Feldman J, Stutzman J, Bricca G, Belcourt A, Bousquet P (1994). Role of imidazoline receptors in cardiovascular regulation. *Am J Cardiol* 74:3A–7A.

Drexler H (1998). Endothelium as a therapeutic target in heart failure. *Circulation* 98:2652–2655.

Drexler H, Hayoz D, Munzel T, Hornig B, Just H, Brunner HR, Zelis R (1992). Endothelial function in chronic heart failure. *Am J Cardiol* 69:1596–1601.

Dzau VJ (1988). Cardiac renin-angiotensin system. Molecular and functional aspects. *Am J Med* 84(Suppl A):22–27.

Dzau VJ (1993). Vascular renin-angiotensin system and vascular protection. *J Cardiovasc Pharmacol* 22(Suppl 5):S1–S9.

Dzau VJ, Hollenberg NK, Wiliams GH (1983). Neurohumoral mechanisms in heart failure. Role in pathogenesis, therapy and drug tolerance. *N Engl J Med* 310:347–352.

Dzau VJ, Packer M, Lilly LS, et al (1984). Prostaglandins in severe congestive heart failure. Relation to activation of the renin-angiotensin system and hyponatremia. *N Engl J Med* 310:347–352.

Eckberg DL (1997). Baroreflexes and the failing heart. *Circulation* 96:4133–4137.

Eckberg DL, Drabinsky M, Braunwald E (1971). Defective cardiac parasympathetic control in patients with heart disease. *N Engl J Med* 258:877–883.

Eisenhofer G, Friberg P, Rundqvist B, Quyyumi AA, Lambert G, Kaye DM, Kopin IJ, Goldstein DS, Esler MD (1996). Cardiac sympathetic nerve function in congestive heart failure. *Circulation* 93:1667–1676.

Elsner D, Muntze A, Kromer E, Reigger GAJ (1993). Systemic vasoconstriction induced by inhibition of nitric oxide synthesis is attenuated in conscious dogs with heart failure. *Cardiovasc Res* 25:438–440.

Endoh M, Blinks JR (1988). Actions of sympathomimetic amines on Ca^{2+} transients and contractions of rabbit myocardium: reciprocal changes in myofibrillar responsiveness to Ca^{2+} mediated through α- and β-adrenoreceptors. *Circ Res* 62:247–265.

Everett AD, Fisher A, Tufro-McReddie A, Harris M (1997). Developmental regulation of angiotensin type 1 and 2 receptor gene expression and heart growth. *J Mol Cell Cardiol* 29:141–148.

Farhy RD, Carretero OA, Ho K-L Scicli AG (1993). Role of kinins and nitric oxide in the effects of angiotensin converting enzyme inhibitors on neointima formation. *Circ Res* 72:1202–1210.

Feng QP, Hedner T, Andersson B, Lundberg JM, Waagstein F (1994). Cardiac neuropeptide Y and noradrenaline balance in patients with congestive heart failure. *Br Heart J* 71:261–267.

Feng QP, Sun XY, Hedner T (1996). Cardiovascular responses and interactions of neuropeptide Y in rats with congestive heart failure. *Blood Pressure* 5:312–318.

Ferguson DW, Berg WJ, Sanders JS (1990). Clinical and hemodynamic correlates of sympathetic nerve activity in normal humans and patients with heart failure; evidence form direct microneurographic recordings. *J Am Coll Cardiol* 16:1125–1134.

Fleming I, Hecker R, Busse R (1994). Intracellular alkalinization induced by bradykinin sustains activation of the constitutive nitric oxide synthase in endothelial cells. *Circ Res* 74:1222–1226.

Fraccarollo D, Hu K, Galuppo P, Gaudron P, Ertl G (1997). Chronic endothelin receptor blockade attenuates progressive ventricular dilatation and improves cardiac function in rats with myocardial infarction. Possible involvement of myocardial endothelin system in ventricular remodeling. *Circulation* 96:3963–3973.

Francis GS (1990). Neuroendocrine activity in congestive heart failure. *Am J Cardiol* 66:33D–39D.

Francis GS (1997). Vasoactive Hormone Systems. In Poole-Wilson PA, Colucci WS, Massie BM, Chatterjee K, Coats AS, eds. *Heart Failure. Scientific Principles and Clinical Practice.* Churchill Livingstone, New York, pp 215–234.

Francis GS, McDonald KM (1995). Neurohumoral mechanisms in heart failure. In McCall D, Rahimtoola SH, eds. *Heart Failure.* Chapman & Hall, New York, pp 91–116.

Francis GS, Siegel R, Goldsmith SR, et al (1985). Acute vasoconstrictor response to intravenous furosemide in patients with chronic congestive heart failure. *Ann Int Med* 103:1–6.

Francis GS, Benedict C, Johnstone DE, Kirlin PC, Nicklas J, Liang C-s, Kubo SH, Rudin-Toretsky E, Yusef S (1990). Comparison of neuroendocrine activation in patient with left ventricular dysfunction with and without congestive heart failure. A substudy of the studies of left ventricular dysfunction (SOLVD). *Circulation* 82:1724–1729.

Francis GS, Cohn JN, Johnson G, Rector TS, Goldman S, Simon A, for the V-HeFT VA Cooperative Studies Group (1993). Plasma norepinephrine, plasma renin activity and congestive heart failure: relations to survival and the effects of therapy in V-HeFT II. *Circulation* 87:VI-40–VI-48.

Francis GS, Goldsmith SR, Levine TB, Olivari MT, Cohn JN (1984). The neurohumoral axis in congestive heart failure. *Ann Intern Med* 101:370–377.

Freer RS, Pappano A, Peach MJ, Bing KT, McLean MJ, Vogel SM, Sperelakis N (1976). Mechanism for the positive inotropic effect of angiotensin II on isolated cardiac muscle. *Circ Res* 39:178–183.

Frohlich ED, Iwata T, Sasaki O (1989). Clinical and physiologic significance of local tissue renin-angiotensin systems. *Am J Med* 87(Suppl 6B):19S–23S.

Furchgott RF, Zawadzki JV (1980). The obligatory role of endothelial cells in the relaxation of arterial smooth muscle by acetylcholine. *Nature* 288:373–376.

Ganten D, Hutchinson JS, Schelling P, Ganten U, Fischer H. The iso-renin angiotensin systems in extrarenal tissue. *Clin Exp Pharmacol Physiol* 3:103–126.

Garg UC, Hassid A (1989). Nitric oxide-generating vasodilators and 8-bromo-cyclic guanosine monophosphate inhibit mitogenesis and proliferation of cultured rat vascular smooth muscle cells. *J Clin Invest* 83:1774–1777.

Garrison JC, Peach MJ (1990). Renin and angiotensin. In Goodman AG, Rall TW, Nies AS, Taylor P. *The Pharmacological Basis of Therapeutics*, 8th ed. Pergamon Press, New York, pp 749–763.

Gavras H (1990). Pressor systems in hypertension and congestive heart failure. Role of vasopressin. *Hypertension* 16:587–593.

Goldsmith SR, Kubo SH (1988) Pathophysiology of heart failure: peripheral vascular factors and neurohormonal mechanisms. In Cohn JN, ed. *Drug Treatment of Heart Failure.* ATC, Secaucus, NJ, pp 149–178.

Graham RM, Perez DM, Hwa J, Piascik MT (1996). α_1-Adrenergic receptor subtypes. Molecular structure, function, and signaling. *Circulation* 78:737–749.

Grassi G, Seravalla G, Cattaneo BM, Lanfranchi A, Vailatis S, Giannattasio C, Del Bo A, Sala C, Bolla GB, Pozzi M (1995). Sympathetic activation and loss of reflex sympathetic control in mild congestive heart failure. *Circulation* 92:3206–3211.

Grundemar L, Hakanson R (1994). Neuropeptide Y effector systems: perspectives for drug development. *Trends Pharmacol Sci* 15:153–159.

Hall JM (1992). Bradykinin receptors: pharmacological properties and biological roles. *Pharmacol Ther* 56:131–190.

Harada M, Itoh H, Nakagawa O, Ogawa Y, Miyamoto Y, Kuwahara K, Ogawa E, Igaki T, Yamashita J, Masuda I, Yoshimasa J, Masuda I, Yoshimasa T, Tanaka I, Saito Y, Nakao K (1998). Significance of ventricular myocytes and nonmyocytes interaction during cardiocyte hypertrophy. Evidence for endothelin-1 as a paracrine hypertrophic factor from cardiac nonmyocytes. *Circulation* 96:3737–3744.

Hare JM, Givertz MM, Creager MA, Colucci WS (1998). Increased sensitivity to nitric oxide synthase inhibition in patients with heart failure. Potentiation of β-adrenergic inotropic responsiveness. *Circulation* 97:161–166.

Harris P (1983). Evolution and the cardiac patient. *Cardiovasc Res* 17:313–319, 373–378, 437–445.

Hasking GJ, Esler MD, Jennings JL, et al (1986). Norepinephrine spillover to plasma in patients with congestive heart failure. Evidence of increased overall and cardiorenal sympathetic nervous activity. *Circulation* 73:615–621.

Hausendorff WP, Caron MG, Leftkowitz RJ (1990). Turning off the signal: desensitization of β-adrenergic receptor function. *FASEB J* 2881–2889.

Hawthorn MH, Broadley KJ (1982). Evidence from use of neuronal uptake inhibition that beta$_1$ adrenoreceptors, but not beta$_2$ adrenoreceptors, are innervated. *J Pharm Pharmacol* 34:664-666.

Haynes WG, Hand MF, Dockrell ME, Lee MR, Hussein A, Benjamin N, Webb DJ (1997). Physiological role of nitric oxide in regulation of renal function in humans. *Am J Physiol* 273:F364–F371.

Haywood GA, Gullestad L, Katsuya T, Hutchinson HG, Pratt RE, Horiuchi M, Fowler MB (1997). AT$_1$ and AT$_2$ receptor gene expression in human heart failure. *Circulation* 95:1201–1206.

Hein L, Barsh GS, Pratt RE, Dzau VJ, Kobilka BK (1995). Behavioural and cardiovascular effects of disrupting the angiotensin II type-2 receptor gene in mice. *Nature* 377:744–747.

Heller BI, Jacobson WE (1950). Renal hemodynamics in heart disease. *Am Heart J* 39:188–204.

Hershberger RE, Feldman AM, Bristow MR (1991). A$_1$-adenosine receptor inhibition of adenylate cyclase in failing and nonfailing human ventricular myocardium. *Circulation* 83:1343–1351.

Hiroe M, Hirata Y, Fujita N, Umezawa S, Ito H, Tsujino M, Koike A, Nogami A, Takamoto T, Marumo F (1991). Plasma endothelin-1 levels in idiopathic dilated cardiomyopathy. *Am J Cardiol* 68:759–761.

Hirooka Y, Imaiziumi T, Tagawa t, Shiramoto M, Endo T, Ando S, Takeshita A (1993). Effects of L-arginine on impaired acetylcholine-induced and ischemic vasodilatation of the forearm in patients with heart failure. *Circulation* 90:658–668.

Hollenberg NK (1988). The role of the kidney in heart failure. In Cohn JN, ed. *Drug Treatment of Heart Failure*. ATC, Secaucus, NJ, pp 105–125.

Hostetter TH, Pfeffer JM, Pfeffer MA, Dworkin LD, Braunwald E, Brenner BM (1983). Cardiorenal hemodynamics and sodium excretion in rats with myocardial infarction. *Am J Physiol* 245:H98–H103.

Ichikawa I, Pfeffer JM, Pfeffer MA, Hostetter TH, Brenner BM (1984). Role of angiotensin II in the altered renal function of congestive heart failure. *Circ Res* 55:669–675.

Ichikawa K-I, Hidai C, Okuda C, Kimata S-I, Matsuoka R, Hosada S, Quertermous T, Kawana M (1996). Endogenous endothelin-1 mediates cardiac hypertrophy and switching of myosin heavy chain gene expression in rat ventricular myocardium. *J Am Coll Cardiol* 27:1286–1291.

Ichiki T, Labosky PA, Shiota C, Okuyama S, Imagawa Y, Fogo A, Nimura F, Ichikawa I, Hogan BLM, Inagami T (1995). Effects on blood pressure and exploratory behaviour of mice lacking angiotensin II type-2 receptor gene. *Nature* 377:748–750.

Ihl-Vahl R, Eschenhagen T, Kübler W, Marquetant R, Nose M, Schmitz W, Scholz H, Strasser R (1996). Differential regulation of mRNA specific for β$_1$- and β$_2$-adrenergic receptors in human failing hearts. Evaluation of the absolute cardiac mRNA levels by two independent methods. *J Mol Cell Cardiol* 28:1–10.

Ikeda U, Shimada K (1997). Nitric oxide and cardiac failure. *Clin Cardiol* 20:837–841.

Ikenouchi H, Barry WH, Bridge JHB, Weinberg EO, Apstein CS, Lorell BH (1994). Effects of angiotensin II on intracellular Ca^{2+} and pH in isolated beating rat hearts loaded with the indicator indo-1. *J Physiol (Lond)* 480:203–215.

Ishikawa T, Yanagisawa M, Kurihara H, Goto K, Masaki T (1988). Positive inotropic effects of novel potent vasoconstrictor peptide endothelin on guinea pig atria. *Am J Physiol* 255:H970–973.

Ito H, Hirata M, Hiroe M, Tsulino M, Adachi S, Takamoto T, Nitta M, Taniguchi K, Marumo F (1992). Endothelin-1 induces hypertrophy with enhanced expression of muscle-specific genes in cultured neonatal rat cardiomyocytes. *Circ Res* 69:209–215.

Ito H, Hiroe M, Hirata M,Fujisaki H, Adachi S, Akimoto H, Ohta Y, Marumo F (1994). Endothelin ET$_A$ receptor antagonist blocks cardiac hypertrophy induced by hemodynamic overload. *Circulation* 89:2198–2203.

Jougasaki M, Wei C-M, Aarhus LL, Heublein DM, Sandberg SM, Burnett JC Jr (1995a). Renal localization and actions of adrenomedullin: a natriuretic peptide. *Am J Physiol* 268:F6576–F663.

Jougasaki M, Wei C-M, McKinley LJ, Burnett JC Jr (1995b). Elevation of circulating and ventricular adrenomedullin I human congestive heart failure. *Circulation* 92:286–289.

Kaburagi S, Hasegawa K, Morimoto T, Araki M, Sawamura T, Masaki T, Sasayama S (1999). The role of big endothelin converting enzyme-1 in the development of α$_1$-adrenergic-stimulated hypertrophy in cultured neonatal rat cardiac myocytes. *Circulation* 99:292–298.

Kaiser L, Spickard RC, Olivier NB (1989). Heart failure depresses endothelium-dependent responses in canine femoral artery. *Am J Physiol* 256:H962–H967.

Karet FE (1996). Endothelin peptides and receptors in human kidney. *Clin Sci* 91:267–273.

Kass RS, Blair ML (1981). Effect of angiotensin II on membrane current in cardiac Purkinje fibers. *J Mol Cell Cardiol* 13:797–809.

Kato J, Kobayashi K, Etoh T, Tanaka M, Kitamura K, Imamura T, Koiwaya Y, Kangawa K, Eto T (1996). Plasma adrenomedullin concentration in patients with heart failure. *J Clin Endocrinol Metab* 81:180–183.

Katz AM (1990a). Angiotensin II: Hemodynamic regulator or growth factor? *J Mol Cell Cardiol* 22:739–747.

Katz AM (1990b). Cardiomyopathy of overload. A major determinant of prognosis in congestive heart failure. *N Engl J Med* 322:100–110.

Katz AM (1993). Cardiac ion channels. *N Engl J Med* 328:1244–1251.

Katz AM, Katz PB (1989). Homogeneity out of heterogeneity. *Circulation* 79:712–717.

Katz SD, Biasucci L, Sabba C, Strom JA, Jondeau G, Balvao M, Solomon S, Nikolic SD, Foreman R, Lejemtel TH (1992). Impaired endothelium-mediated vasodilatation in the peripheral vasculature of patients with congestive heart failure. *J Am Coll Cardiol* 19:918–925.

Kelly RA, Balligand J-L, Smith TW (1996). Nitric oxide and cardiac function (mini review). *Circulation* 79:363–380.

Kelly RA, Han X (1997). Nitrovasodilators have (small) direct effects on cardiac contractility. Is this important? *Circulation* 96:2493–2495.

Kern MJ (1999). Appreciating α-adrenergic receptors and their role in ischemic left ventricular dysfunction. *Circulation* 99:468–471.

Kijima K, Matsubara H, Murasawa S, Maruyama K, Mori Y, Ohkubo N, Komuro I, Yazaki Y, Inada M (1996). Mechanical stretch induces enhanced expression of angiotensin II receptor subtypes in neonatal rats cardiac myocytes. *Circ Res* 79:887–897.

Kilcoyne MM, Schmidt DH, Cannon PJ (1973). Intrarenal blood flow in congestive heart failure. *Circulation* 47:786–797.

Kiowski W, Sütsch H, Hunziker P, Müller P, Kim J, Oechslin E, Schmitt R, Jones R, Bertel O (1995). Evidence for endothelin-1-mediated vasoconstriction in severe chronic heart failure. *Lancet* 346:732–736.

Kitamura K, Kanagawa K, Kawamoto M, Ichiki Y, Nakamura S, Matsuo H, Eto T (1993). Adrenomedullin: a novel hypotensive peptide isolated from human pheochromocytoma. *Biochem Biophys Res Commun* 192:553–560.

Kiuchi K, Sato N, Shannon RP, Vatner DE, Morgan K, Vatner SF (1993). Depressed beta-adrenergic receptor and endothelium mediated vasodilatation in conscious dogs with heart failure. *Circ Res* 73:1013–1023.

Kobayashi K, Kitamura K, Etoh T, Nagamoto Y, Takenaga M, Ishikawa T, Imamura T, Koiwaya Y, Kanagawa Ito T (1993). Increased plasma adrenomedullin levels in chronic congestive heart failure. *Am Heart J* 131:994–998.

Kobayashi M, Furukawa Y, Chiba S (1978). Positive chronotropic and inotropic effects of angiotensin II in the dog heart. *Eur J Pharmacol* 50:19–25.

Koch-Weser J (1964). Myocardial actions of angiotensin. *Circulation Res* 14:337–344.

Kramer BK, Nishida M, Kelly RA, Smith TW (1992). Endothelins: myocardial actions of a new class of cytokines. *Circulation* 85:350–356.

Krief S, Lönnqvist F, Raimbault S, Baude B, Van Spronsen A, Arner P, Strosberg AD, Ricquier D, Emorine LJ (1993). Tissue distribution of β3-adrenergic receptor mRNA in man. *J Clin Invest* 91:344–349.

Krishna GG, Danovitch GM, Beck FW, Sowers JR (1985). Dopaminergic mediation of the natriuretic response to volume expansion. *J Lab Clin Med* 105:214–218.

Kubo SH, Rector TS, Bank AJ, Willams RE, Heifetz SM (1991). Endothelial vasodilation is attenuated in patients with heart failure. *Circulation* 84:1589–1596.

Kubo SH, Rector TS, Bank AJ, Tschumperlin LK, Raij L, Brunsvold N, Kraemer MD (1994). Lack of contribution of nitric oxide to basal vasomotor tone in heart failure. *Am J Cardiol* 74:1133–1136.

Kurabayashi M, Yazaki Y (1997). Downregulation of angiotensin receptor type 1 in heart failure. A process of adaptation or deterioration? *Circulation* 95:1104–1107.

recordings for increased central sympathetic outflow in patients with heart failure. *Circulation* 73:615–621.

Lee HR (1993). α1-adrenergic receptors and heart failure. In Gwathmey JK, Briggs GM, Allen PD, eds. *Heart Failure. Basic Science and Clinical Aspects.* Marcel Dekker, New York, pp 211–234.

Lefkowitz RJ (1993). G-Protein coupled receptor kinase. *Cell* 74:409–412.

Le Guludec D, Cohen-Solal A, Delforge J, Delahaye N, Syrota A, Merlet P (1997). Increased myocardial muscarinic receptor density in idiopathic dilated cardiomyopathy. An in vivo PET study. *Circulation* 96:3416–3422.

Leimbach WN, Wallin BG, Victor RG, Aylward PE, Sundlöf G, Mark AL (1986). Direct evidence from intraneural Levin ER (1996). Endothelins. *N Engl J Med* 333:356–362.

Levin ER, Gardner DG, Samson WK (1998). Natriuretic peptides. *N Engl J Med* 339:321–328.

Levine TB, Francis GS, Goldsmith SR, Simon AB, Cohn JN (1982). Activity of the sympathetic nervous system and renin angiotensin system assessed by plasma hormone levels and their relationship to hemodynamic abnormalities in congestive heart failure. *Am J Cardiol* 49:1659–1664.

Li Q, Zhang L, Pffafendorf M, van Zweiten PA (1995). Comparative effects of angiotensin II and its degradation products angiotensin III and angiotensin IV in rat aorta. *Br J Pharmacol* 116:2963–2970.

Li Q, Zhang L, Pffafendorf M, van Zweiten PA (1997). Comparative vasoconstrictor effects of angiotensin II, III, and IV in human isolated saphenous vein. *J Cardiovasc Pharmacol* 29:451–456.

Liard J-F (1989). Peripheral vasodilatation induced by a vasopressin analogue with selective V2-agonism in dogs. *Am J Physiol* 256:J1621–J1626.

Likungu J, Molderings GJ, Gothert M (1996). Presynaptic imidazoline receptors and alpha 2-adrenoreceptors in the human heart: discrimination by clonidine and moxonidine. *Naunyn-Schmiedebergs Arch Pharmacol* 354:689–692.

Lindpainter K, Jin M, Wilhelm M, Toth M, Ganten D (1989). Aspects of molecular biology and biochemistry of the cardiac renin-angiotensin system. *Br J Clin Pharmacol* 27:159S–165S.

MacMillan LB, Hein L, Smith MS, Piascik MT, Limbird, LE. (1996). Central hypotensive effects of the α2-adrenergic receptor subtype. *Science* 273:801–803.

Maeda K, Tsutamoto T, Wada A, Hisanaga T, Kinoshita M (1998). Plasma brain natriuretic peptide as a biochemical marker of high left ventricular end-diastolic pressure in patients with symptomatic left ventricular dysfunction. *Am Heart J* 135:825–832.

Maisel AS, Scott NA, Motulsky HJ, Michel MC, Boublik JH, Rivier JE, Ziegler M, Allen RS, Brown MR (1989). Elevation of plasma neuropeptide Y levels in congestive heart failure. *Am J Med* 86:43–48.

Margulies KB, Hildebrand FL Jr, Lerman A, Perrella MA, Burnett JC Jr (1990). Increased endothelin in experimental heart failure. *Circulation* 82:2226–2230.

Matsubara H, Kanaskai M, Murasawa S, Tsukaguchi Y, Nio Y, Inada M (1994). Differential gene expression and regulation of angiotensin II receptor subtypes in rat cardiac fibroblasts and cardiomyocytes in culture. *J Clin Invest* 93:1592–1601.

McMurray JJ, Ray SG, Abdullah I, Dargie HJ, Morton JJ (1992). Plasma endothelin in chronic heart failure. *Circulation* 83:1374–1379.

McDonagh TA, Robb SD, Murdoch DR, Morton JJ, Ford I, Morrison CE, Tunstall-Pedoe H, McMurray JJ, Dargie HJ (1998). Biochemical detection of left-ventricular systolic dysfunction. *Lancet* 351:9–13.

McDonald KM, Garr MD, Carlyle PF, Francis GS, Hauer K, Hunter DW, Parrish T, Stillman A, Cohn JN (1995). The relative effects off alpha₁ adrenoreceptor blockade, converting enzyme inhibitor therapy and angiotensin II subtype I receptor blockade on ventricular remodeling in the dog. *Circulation* 90:3034–3036.

McEwan PE, Gray GA, Sherry L, Webb DJ, Kenyon CJ (1998). Differential effects of angiotensin II on cardiac cell proliferation and intramyocardial perivascular fibrosis in vivo. *Circulation* 98:2765–2774.

Meredith IT, Eisenhofer G, Lambert GW, Dewor EM, Jennings GL, Esler MD (1993). Cardiac sympathetic nervous activity in congestive heart failure: evidence for increased neuronal norepinephrine release and preserved neuronal uptake. *Circulation* 88:136–145.

Merrill AJ (1946). Edema and decreased renal blood flow in patients with chronic congestive heart failure: evidence of "forward failure" as the primary cause of edema. *J Clin Invest* 25:389–400.

Merrill AJ, Cargell WH (1948). The effect of exercise on the renal plasma flow and filtration rate of normal and cardiac subjects. *J Clin Invest* 27:272–277.

Mokotoff R, Ross G, Leiter L (1948). Renal plasma flow and sodium reabsorbtion in congestive heart failure. *J Clin Invest* 27:1–9.

Mombouli JV, Vanhoutte PM (1992). Heterogeneity of endothelium-dependent vasodilator effects of angiotensin-converting enzyme inhibitors: role of bradykinin generation during ACE inhibition. *J Cardiovasc Pharmacol* 20(Suppl 9):S974–S982.

Moncada S, Higgs A (1993). The L-arginine-nitric oxide pathway. *N Engl J Med* 329:2002–2012.

Mueller EA, Griffen WST, Wildenthal K (1977). Isoproterenol-induced cardiomyopathy: changes in cardiac enzymes and protection by methyl prednisolone. *J Mol Cell Cardiol* 9:565–578.

Mügge, A, Schmitz W, Scholz H (1984). Negative inotropic effects of aldosterone antagonists in isolated human and guinea pig ventricular heart muscle. *Klin Wochenschr* 62:717–723.

Mukaddan-Dahe S, Lambert C, Gutkowska J (1997). Clonidine and ST-91 may activate imidazoline binding sites in the heart to release atrial natriuretic peptide. *Hypertension* 30:83–87.

Mukoyama M, Hosada K, Suga S, Saito Y, Ogawa Y, Shirakami G, Jougasaki M, Obata K, Yasue H, Kambayashi Y, Inouye K, Imura H (1991). Brain natriuretic peptide (BNP) as a novel cardiac hormone in humans— evidence for an exquisite dual natriuretic peptide system, atrial natriuretic peptide and brain natriuretic peptide. *J Clin Invest* 87:1402–1412.

Mukoyama M, Nkajima M, Horiuchi M, Sasamura H, Pratt RE, Dzau VJ (1993). Expression cloning of type 2 angiotensin II receptor reveals a unique class of seven transmembrane receptors. *J Biol Chem* 268:24359–24362.

Mulder P, Richard V, Derumeaux G, Hogie M, Henry JP, Lallemand F, Compagnon P, Macé B, Comoy E, Letac B, Thuillez C (1997). Role of endogenous endothelin in chronic heart failure. Effect of long-term treatment with an endothelin antagonists on survival, hemodynamics and cardiac remodeling. *Circulation* 96:1976–1982.

Murphy TJ, Alexander RW, Griendling KK, Runge MS, Bernstein KE (1991). Isolation of a cDNA encoding the vascular type-1 angiotensin II receptor. *Nature* 351:233–236.

Nakagawa O, Ogawa Y, Itoh H, Suga S, Komatsu I, Kishimoto K, Yoshimasa T, Nakao K (1995). Rapid translation and early mRNA turnover of brain natriuretic peptide in cardiocyte hypertrophy. Evidence for brain natriuretic peptide as an "emergency" cardiac hormone against ventricular overload. *J Clin Invest* 96:1280–1287.

Nakamura M, Arakawa N, Yoshida H, Makita S, Niinuma H, Hiramori K (1998). Vasodilatory effects of B-type natriuretic peptide are impaired in patients with chronic heart failure. *Am Heart J* 135:414–420.

Naveri L (1995). The role of angiotensin receptor subtypes in cerebrovascular regulation. *Acta Physiol Scand Suppl* 630:1–48.

Neyses L, Vetter H (1989). Actions of atrial natriuretic peptide and angiotensin II on the myocardium: studies in isolated rat ventricular cardiomyocytes. *Biochem Biophys Res Commun* 163:1435–1443.

Nishikimi T, Saito Y, Kitamura K, Ishimitsu T, Eto Y, Kangawa K, Matsuo H, Omae T, Matsuoka H (1995). Increased plasma levels of adrenomedullin in patients with heart failure. *J Am Coll Cardiol* 26:1424–1431.

Noguchi H, Muraoka R, Kigoshi S, Muramatsu I (1995). Pharmacological characterization of α₁-adrenoceptor subtypes in rat heart: a binding study. *Br J Pharmacol* 114:1026–1030.

Nolan J, Flapan AD, Capewell S, MacDonald TM, Neilson JMM, Ewing DJ (1992). Decreased cardiac parasympathetic activity in chronic heart failure and its relation to left ventricular function. *Br Heart J* 67:482–485.

Noll G, Wenzel RR, Lüscher TF (1996). Endothelin and endothelin antagonists: potential role in cardiovascular disease. *Mol Cell Biochem* 157:259–267.

Oliver G, Schäfer EA (1895). On the physiological action of extracts of the posterior pituitary body and certain other glandular organs. *J Physiol (Lond)* 18:277–279.

Packer M (1992). The neurohumoral hypothesis: a theory to explain the mechanism of disease progression in heart failure. *J Am Coll Cardiol* 20:248–254.

Page IH, Helmer OM (1940). A crystalline pressor substance (angiotonin) resulting from the reaction between renin and renin activator. *J Exp Med* 71:29–42.

Palmer RMJ, Ferrige AG, Moncada S (1987). Nitric oxide accounts for the biological activity of endothelium-derived relaxing factor. *Nature* 327:524–526.

Parker JD, Newton GE, Landzberg JS, Floras JS, Colucci WS (1995). Functional significance of presynaptic α-adrenergic receptors in failing and non-failing human ventricle. *Circulation* 92:1793–1800.

Paulus WJ, Vantrimpont PJ, Shah AM (1994). Acute effects of nitric oxide on left ventricular relaxation and diastolic distensibility in humans. Assessment by bicoronary sodium nitroprusside infusion. *Circulation* 89:2070–2078.

Ping P, Hammond HK (1994). Diverse G protein and β-adrenergic receptor mRNA expression in normal and failing porcine hearts. *Am J Physiol* 267:H2079–H2085.

Ping P, Anzai T, Goa M, Hammond HK (1997). Adenylyl cyclase and G protein kinase expression during development of heart failure. *Am J Physiol* 273:H707–H717.

Pönicke K, Vogelsang M, Heinroth M, Becker K, Zolk O, Böhm M, Zerkowski H-R, Brodde O-E (1998). Endothelin receptors in the failing and non-failing human heart. *Circulation* 97:744–751.

Ponikowsi P, Chua TP, Piepoli M, Ondusova D, Webb-Peploe K, Harrington D, Anker SD, Volterrani M, Colombo R, Mazzuero G, Giordano A, Coats AJS (1997). Augmented peripheral chemosensitivity as a potential input to baroreceptor impairment and autonomic imbalance in chronic heart failure. *Circulation* 96:2586–2594.

Preckel B, Kojda G, Schlack W, Ebel D, Kottenberg K, Noack E, Thämer V (1997). Inotropic effects of glyceryl trinitrate and spontaneous NO donors in the dog heart. *Circulation* 96:2675–2682.

Prendergast BD, Sagach VF, Shah AM (1997). Basal release of nitric oxide augments the Frank-Starling response in the isolated heart. *Circulation* 96:1320–1329.

Raab W (1943). The pathogenic significance of adrenaline and related substances in the heart muscle. *Exp Med Surg* 1:188.

Raab W (1953). *Hormonal and Neurogenic Cardiovascular Disorders*. Williams & Wilkins, Baltimore, pp 18–19.

Raine AEG (1992). Renal abnormalities in congestive heart failure. In Fozzard H, Haber E, Katz AM, Jennings R, Morgan HE, eds. *The Heart and Cardiovascular System*, 2nd ed. Raven Press, New York, 1992, pp 1379–1391.

Raine AEG, Erne P, Burgisser E, Muller FB, Bolli P, Burkart F, Buhler FR (1986). Atrial natriuretic peptide and atrial pressure in patients with congestive heart failure. *N Engl J Med* 315:533–538.

Redfield MM, Edwards BS, McGoon MD, Heublein DM, Aarhus LL, Burnett JC Jr (1989). Failure of atrial natriuretic peptide to increase with volume expansion in the dog. *Circulation* 80:651–657.

Regitz-Zagrosek V, Friedel N, Heyman A, Bauer P, Neuss M, Rolfs A, Steffen C, Hildebrandt A, Hetzer R, Fleck E (1995). Regulation, chamber localization, and subtype distribution of angiotensin II receptors in human hearts. *Circulation* 91:1461–1471.

Regitz-Zagrosek V, Neuss M, Graf K, Hsueh WA, Fleck E (1998). Actions of angiotensin II on isolated cardiac fibroblasts. *Heart Failure Rev* 3:87–99.

Regunathan S, Reis DJ (1996). Imidazoline receptors and their endogenous ligands. *Ann Revu Pharmacol Toxicol* 36:511–544.

Regunathan S, Reis DJ (1997). Stimulation of imidazoline receptors inhibits proliferation of human coronary artery vascular smooth muscle cells. *Hypertension* 30:295–300.

Rogg H, Schmid A, DeGasparo M (1990). Identification and characterization of angiotensin II receptor subtypes in rabbit ventricular myocardium. *Biochem Biophys Res Commun* 173:416–422.

Ross J Jr (1976). Afterload mismatch and preload reserve: a conceptual framework for the analysis of ventricular function. *Prog Cardiovasc Dis* 318:255–264.

Rushmer RF, Smith OA Jr, Franklin D (1959). Mechanisms of cardiac control in exercise. *Circ Res* 7:602–627.

Sadoshima J, Izumo S (1993). Molecular characterization of angiotensin-induced hypertrophy of cardiac myocytes and hyperplasia of cardiac fibroblasts. Critical role of the AT_1 receptor subtypes. *Circ Res* 73:413–423.

Saito Y, Nakao K, Arai H, Nishimura K, Okumura K, Obata K, Takemura G, Fujiwara H, Sugawara A, Yamada T, Itoh H, Mukoyama M, Hosada K, Kawai C, Ban T, Yasue H, Imura H (1989). Augmented expression of atrial natriuretic polypeptide gene in ventricle of human failing heart. *J Clin Invest* 83:298–305.

Sakai S, Miyauchi T, Kobayashi M, Yamaguchi I, Goto K, Sugishita Y (1996). Inhibition of the myocardial endothelin pathway improves long term survival in heart failure. *Nature* 384:353–355.

Saunders DE, Ord JW (1962). The hemodynamic effects of paroxysmal supraventricular tachycardia in patients with the Wolff-Parkinson-White syndrome. *Am J Cardiol* 9:223–236.

Schrier RW (1988). Pathogenesis of sodium and water retention in high-output and low-output cardiac failure, nephrotic syndrome, cirrhosis, and pregnancy. *N Engl J Med* 319:1127–1134.

Schrör K (1992). Role of prostaglandins in the cardiovascular effects of bradykinin and angiotensin-converting enzyme inhibitors. *J Cardiovasc Pharm* 20(Suppl 9):S68–S73.

Schultheiss HP, Ullrich G, Schindler M, Schulze K, Strauer BE (1990). The effect of ACE inhibition on myocardial energy metabolism. *Eur Heart J* 11(Suppl B):116–122.

Schultz R, Panas DL, Catena R, Moncada S, Olley PM, Lopaschuk GD (1995). The role of nitric oxide in cardiac depression induced by interleukin-1β and tumor necrosis factor-α. *Br J Pharmacol* 114:27–34.

Scott I, Parkes R, Cameron DP (1988). Pheochromocytoma and cardiomyopathy. *Med J Aust* 148:94–96.

Scriven TA, Burnett JC Jr (1985). Effects of synthetic atrial natriuretic peptides on renal function and renin release in acute experimental heart failure. *Circulation* 72:892–897.

Sechi LA, Griffin CA, Grady EF, Kalinyak JE, Schambelan M (1992). Characterization of angiotensin II subtypes in rat heart. *Circ Res* 71:1482–1489.

Share L (1979). Interrelations between vasopressin and the renin-angiotensin system. *Fed Proc* 38:2267–2271.

Shubeita HE, McDonough PM, Harris AN, et al (1990). Endothelin induction of inositol phosphate hydrolysis, sarcomere assembly, and cardiac gene expression in ventricular myocytes. A paracrine mechanism for myocardial cell hypertrophy. *J Biol Chem* 265:20555–20562.

Simpson P (1993). Nor-epinephrine-stimulated hypertrophy of cultured rat myocardial cells is an alpha-1 adrenergic response. *Am J Physiol* 83:732–738.

Skomedal T, Aass H, Osnes J, Fjeld NB, Klingen G, Langslet A, Semb G (1985). Demonstration of an alpha-adrenoreceptor-mediated inotropic effect of norepinephrine in human atria. *J Pharmacol Exp Ther* 233:441–446.

Steinfath M, Danielsen W, von der Leyden H, Mende U, Meyer W, Neumann J, Nose M, Reich T, Schmitz W, Scholz H, Starbatty J, Stein B, Döring V, Kalmar P, Haverich A (1992). Reduced α_1- and β_2-adrenoreceptor-mediated positive inotropic effects in human end-stage heart failure. *Br J Pharmacol* 105:463–469.

Steinfath M, Lavisky J, Schmitz W, Scholz H, Döring V, Kalmar P (1992). Regional distribution of β_1- and β_2-adrenoceptors in the failing and non-failing human heart. *Eur J Clin Pharmacol* 42:607–612.

Stewart DJ, Cernacek P, Costello KB, Rouleau JL (1992). Elevated endothelin-1 in heart failure and loss of normal response to postural change. *Circulation* 85:510–517.

Stoll M, Steckelings UM, Paul M, Bottari SP, Metzger R, Unger T (1995).The angiotensin AT2-receptor mediates inhibition of cell proliferation in coronary endothelial cells. *J Clin Invest* 95:651–657.

Struthers AD (1994). Ten years of natriuretic peptide research: a new dawn for their diagnostic and therapeutic use? Br Med J 308:1615–1619.

Studer R, Reinecke H, Muller B, Holtz J, Just H, Drexler H (1994). Increased angiotensin-I converting enzyme gene expression in failing human heart. *J Clin Invest* 94:301–310.

Sudoh T, Kangawa K, Minanino N, Matsuo H (1988). A new natriuretic peptide in porcine brain. *Nature* 322:78–81.

Sudoh T, Minanino N, Kangawa K, Matsuo H (1990). C-type natriuretic peptide (CNP): a new member of natriuretic peptide family identified in porcine brain. *Biochem Biophys Res Commun* 168:863–870.

Suzuki J, Matsubara H, Urakami M, Inada M (1993). Rat angiotensin II (type 1A) receptor mRNA regulation and subtype expression in myocardial growth and hypertrophy. *Circ Res* 73:439–447.

Suzuki T, Hoshi H, Mitsui Y (1989). Endothelin stimulates hypertrophy and contractility of neonatal rat cardiac myocytes in a serum-free medium. *FEBS Lett* 268:149–151.

Szokosi I, Kinnune P, Tavi P, Weckström M, T´A2th M, Ruskoaho H (1998). Evidence for cAMP-independent mechanisms mediating the effects of adrenomedullin, a new inotropic peptide. *Circulation* 97:1062–1070.

Tajima M, Bartunek J, Weinberg EO, Ito N, Lorell BH (1998). Atrial natriuretic peptide has different effects on contractility and intracellular pH in normal and hypertrophied myocytes from pressure-overloaded hearts. *Circulation* 98:2760–2764.

Takemura G, Fujiwara H, Korike K, et al (1989). Ventricular expression of atrial natriuretic peptide and its relation with hemodynamics and histology in dilated human hearts. *Circulation* 80:1137–1147.

Tartaglia LA, Ayres TM, Wong GHW, Goeddel (1993). A novel domain within the 55 kd TNF receptor signals cell death. *Cell* 74:845–853.

Tigerstedt R, Bergman PG (1898) Niere und Kreislauf. *Skand Archiv f Physiol* 8:223–271.

Tikkanen I, Fyrhquist F, Metsarinne K, Leidenhius R (1985). Plasma atrial natriuretic peptide in cardiac disease and during infusion in healthy volunteers. *Lancet* 2:66–69.

Timmermans PBMWM, Wong PC, Chiu AT, Herblin WF, Benfield P, Carini DJ, Lee RJ, Wexler RR, Saye JAM, Smith RD (1993). Angiotensin II receptors and angiotensin II receptor antagonists. *Pharmacol Rev* 45:205–251.

Tsitamoto T, Wada A, Maeda K, Hisanaga T, Maeda Y, Fukai D, Ohnishi M, Sugimoto Y, Kinoshita M (1997). Attenuation of compensation of endogenous cardiac natriuretic peptide system in chronic heart failure. Prognostic role of plasma brain natriuretic peptide concentration in patients with chronic symptomatic left ventricular dysfunction. *Circulation* 96:509–516.

Ungerer M, Böhm M, Elce S, Erdmann E, Lohse MJ (1993). Altered expression of β-adrenergic receptor kinase and β_1-adrenergic receptors in the failing human heart. *Circulation* 87:454–463.

Ungerer M, Parruti G, Böhm M, Puzicha M, DeBlasi A, Erdmann E, Lohse MJ (1994). Expression of β-arrestins and β-adrenergic receptor kinases in the failing human heart. *Circ Res* 74:206–213.

Urata H, Arakawa K (1998). Angiotensin II-forming systems in cardiovascular diseases. *Heart Failure Rev* 3:119–124

Urata H, Healy B, Stewart RW, Bumpus FM, Husain A (1989). Angiotensin II receptors in normal and failing human hearts. *J Clin Endocrinol Metab* 69:54–66.

Urata H, Healy B, Stewart RW, Bumpus FM, Husain A (1990). Angiotensin II-forming pathways in normal and failing hearts. *Circ Res* 66:883–890.

Urata H, Hoffmann S, Ganten D (1994). Tissue angiotensin II system in the human heart. *Eur Heart J* 15(Suppl D):68–78.

Vago T, Bevilacqua M, Nobiato G, Baldi G, Chebat E, Bertora P, Baroldi G, Accinni R (1989). Identification of alpha 1-adrenergic receptors on sarcolemma from normal subjects and patients with idiopathic dilated cardiomyopathy: characteristics and linkage to GTP-binding protein. *Circ Res* 64:474–481.

Vander AJ, Marvin RL, Wilde WS, et al (1958). Re-examination of salt and water retention in congestive heart failure. *Am J Med* 25:497–502.

van Kats JP, Danser AHJ, van Meegen JR, Sassen LMA, Verdouw PD, Schalekamp MADH (1998). Angiotensin production by the heart. A quantitative study in pigs with the use of radiolabeled angiotensin infusions. *Circulation* 98:73–81.

Vatner DE, Sato N, Galper JB, Vatner SF (1996). Physiological and biochemical evidence for coordinate increases in muscarinic receptors and Gi during pacing-induced heart failure. *Circulation* 96:102–107.

Walker BR, Childs ME, Adams EM (1988). Direct cardiac effects of vasopressin: role of V_1- and V_2-vasopressinergic receptors. *Am J Physiol* 255:H261–H265.

Warren JV, Stead EA Jr (1944). Fluid dynamics in chronic congestive failure. *Arch Intern Med* 73:138–144.

Wei CM, Heublein DM, Perrella MA, Lerman A, Rodheffer RJ, McGregor CG, Edwards WD, Schaff HV, Burnett JC Jr (1993). Natriuretic peptide system in human heart failure. *Circulation* 88:1004–1009.

Wei CM, Lerman Z, Rodeheffer RJ, McGregor CG, Brandt RR, Wright S, Heublein DM, Kao PC, Edwards WD, Burnett JJ (1994). Endothelin in human congestive heart failure. *Circulation* 89:1580–1586.

Winlaw DS, Smythe GA, Keogh A, Schyoens PM, MacDonald PS (1994). Increased nitric oxide production in heart failure. *Lancet* 344:373–374.

Wood P (1950). *Diseases of the Heart and Circulation.* Eyre and Spottiswoode, London.

Wood P (1963). Polyuria in paroxysmal tachycardia and paroxysmal atrial flutter and fibrillation. *Br Heart J* 25:273–282.

Wu KK (1998). Cyclooxygenase-2 induction in congestive heart failure. Friend or foe? *Circulation* 98:95–96.

Xiao RP, Lakatta EG (1993). β1-Adrenoreceptor stimulation and β2-adrenoreceptor stimulation differ in their effects on contraction, cytosolic Ca^{2+}, and Ca^{2+} current in single rat ventricular cells. *Circ Res* 73:286–300.

Xiao RP, Hohl C, Altschuld R, Jones L, Livingston B, Ziman B, Tantini B, Lakatta EG (1994). β2-adrenoreceptor-stimulated increase in cAMP in rat heart cells is not coupled to changes in Ca^{2+} dynamics, contractility, or phospholamban phosphorylation. *J Biol Chem* 269:19151–19156.

Xiao RP, Ji X, Lakatta EG (1995). Functional coupling of the β2-adrenoreceptor to a pertussis toxin-sensitive G protein in cardiac myocytes. *Mol Pharmacol* 47:322–329.

Yanagisawa M, Kurihara H, Limura S, et al (1988). A novel potent vasoconstrictor peptide produced by vascular endothelial cells. *Nature* 331:411–415.

Yasue H, Yoshimura M, Sumida H, Kikuta K, Kugiyama K, Jougasaki M, Ogawa H, Okumura K, Mukoyama M, Nakao K (1994). Localization and mechanism of secretion of B-type natriuretic peptide in comparison with those of A-type natriuretic peptide in normal subjects and patients with heart failure. *Circulation* 90:195–203.

Yu A, Frishman WH (1996). Imidazoline receptor agonist drugs: a new approach to the treatment of systemic hypertension. *J Clin Pharmacol* 36:98–111.

Zemel S, Millan MA, Feuillal P, Aguilera G (1990). Characterization and distribution of angiotensin II receptors in the primate fetus. *J Clin Endocrinol Metab* 71:1003–1007.

Zhou Y-Y, Cheng H, Bogdanov KY, Hohl C, Altshuld R, Lakatta EG, Xiao RP (1997). Localize cAMP-dependent signaling mediates β2-adrenergic modulation of cardiac excitation-contraction coupling. *Am J Physiol* 273:H1611-H1618.

Zisman LS, Abraham WT, Meixell GE, Vamvakias BN, Quaife RA, Lowes BD, Roden RL, Peacock SJ, Groves BM, Raynolds MV, Bristow MR, Perryman MB (1995). Angiotensin II formation in the intact human heart. Predominance of the angiotensin-converting enzyme pathway. *J Clin Invest* 95:1490–1498.

Zisman LS, Asano K, Dutcher DL, Ferdensi A, Robertson AD, Jenkin M, Bush EW, Bohlmeyer T, Perryman MB, Bristow MR (1995). Differential regulation of cardiac angiotensin-converting enzyme binding sites and AT_1 receptor density in the failing human heart. *Circulation* 98:1735–1741.

5

Neurohumoral Response II: The Inflammatory Response

Who trusted God was love indeed
And love Creation's final law—
Though nature red in tooth and claw
With ravine, shrieked against his creed—

Tennyson, *In Memoriam A.H.H.* 56:13-16

When living organisms first discovered that their neighbors could provide a ready source of food, means evolved to attack and kill other life forms. This, naturally, led to the development of host defenses that enabled organisms to ward off attack, and even better, to turn the tables by killing and eating the attacker! Of course, primitive life forms lacked both tooth and claw—and when injured did not leak hemoglobin-containing fluid; instead, our earliest one-celled ancestors wreaked violence (Tennyson's "ravine") on attackers and prey by secreting noxious chemicals (Beck and Habicht, 1991). The most important signals that regulate this cellular violence are provided by an extended family of peptides, the *cytokines*, which probably sprang from a limited number of ancestral proteins, and possibly only a single protein (Shields et al., 1995). By gene duplication and subsequent divergence, this family has grown to include a variety of signaling peptides (Table 5-1) whose actions include stimulation of both cell growth and cell death, erythrocyte and leukocyte production, and even lactation (Table 5-2). This chapter focuses on the inflammatory cytokines, which can be viewed as coordinating a counterattack as well as a defense. Other members of this family of signaling molecules, the peptide growth factors, are discussed in Chapter 6.

TABLE 5-1. *Members of the cytokine family*

Tumor necrosis factor α
Interleukins 2-7, 9-13
Interferons
Lymphotoxin
Transforming growth factor-β
Growth hormone
Prolactin
Erythropoietin
Thrombopoietin
Leukemia inhibitory factor
Granulocyte colony-stimulating factor

Compiled from Beck and Habicht (1991) and Shields et al. (1995).

TABLE 5-2. *Selected actions of the cytokines*

Initiate signals that cause
  Inflammation
  Cell proliferation
  Cell transformation
  Apoptosis (programmed cell death)
Activate enzymes and pathways involved in signal transduction
  Tyrosine kinases, notably janus kinase (JAK)
  Phospholipases A_2 and C
  Protein kinases A and C
  Stress-activated MAP kinases
Increase levels of intracellular messengers
  Cyclic adenosine monophosphate
  Diacylglycerol
Activate transcription factors
  Signal transducer and activator of transcription (STAT)
  AP-1
  NF-κB
  c-*fos*, c-*jun*
Induce genes that encode
  Nitric oxide synthase (iNOS or NOS2)
  Growth factors: platelet-derived growth factor, granulocyte-macrophage—colony-stimulating factor
  Receptors: epidermal growth factor receptor, interleukin-2 receptor
  Cell adhesion molecules; ICAM-1
  Mediators of inflammation, including other cytokines
  Acute phase and histocompatibility proteins
  Heat shock proteins

Adapted from Vilcek and Lee (1991), Ihle (1995), and Bazzoni and Beutler (1996).

Adaptations of the primitive defense/counterattack mechanism are seen in the *inflammatory response* that attacks invading microorganisms and other foreign materials that enter the body. In addition to providing weapons for this counterattack, many of the signaling molecules that mediate inflammation stimulate reactions that are involved in cell growth and healing. As is seen in the case of the hemodynamic defense reaction, the body is not always wise: sometimes these mechanisms attack "self," rather than "other." For example, the inflammatory response plays a role in the autoimmune diseases and, as discussed in this chapter, also appears to participate in maladaptive responses in patients with heart failure.

IRREVERSIBLE SHOCK

Evidence that cytokines participate in the pathogenesis of cardiovascular disease can be traced back to the 1950s, when it was recognized that delay in fluid replacement following hemorrhage was almost always fatal, even if the late transfusion restored the lost volume. This condition, called "irreversible shock," had been a major problem during World War II, when physicians encountered patients who, because they could not receive prompt transfusion after severe blood loss, generally died. This tragic situation was readily modeled in animals, in whom delayed replacement of lost volume after severe hemorrhage provided only temporary improvement; no matter how much blood was returned to these animals, after several hours of severe hypotension, the added fluid simply flowed out of leaky capillaries into the tissues, blood vessels became relaxed, the heart weakened, blood pressure continued to decline, and the animals died.

Efforts to determine the causes of this fatal outcome led to the identification of several "factors" that lower blood pressure, increase capillary permeability, relax blood vessels, and have a negative inotropic effect on the heart (Opdyke et al., 1946; Wiggers, 1947). Some of these factors were found to be endotoxins (generally lipopolysaccharides) produced by bacteria that multiplied in the poorly perfused bowel and then entered the bloodstream. Administration of bacterial endotoxins could produce cardiovascular abnormalities similar to those seen after prolonged hypotension, including vasodilatation and depression of myocardial contractility (Pope et al., 1945; Gilbert 1960). For these reasons, exogenous toxins appeared to hold the key to understanding the syndrome of irreversible shock. Other studies, however, demonstrated that some of the humoral vasodepressors and negative inotropes that appear in the blood during irreversible shock are produced by the body itself (Shorr et al., 1945; Erdös 1966). Most of these endogenous factors have come to be recognized as members of the cytokine family (Suffrendini et al., 1989; Natanson et al., 1992; Yokoyama et al., 1993; Giroir et al., 1995; Stein et al., 1996). Although cytokine release can be initiated by bacterial endotoxin, these peptides are also released by other stimuli as part of an inflammatory response that is seen in chronic heart failure. This response, however, is more than an attack—or counterattack—because cytokines also stimulate cell growth and proliferation, and so promote repair and healing, which are not illogical accompaniments of a defense reaction.

SYSTEMIC AND LOCAL INFLAMMATORY RESPONSES IN HEART FAILURE

One of the more remarkable features of heart failure to have been recognized in the past decade is that this syndrome is accompanied by an inflammatory response that operates both systemically and locally. The systemic response, which "attacks" tissues throughout the body, plays an important role in causing *cardiac cachexia*, a systemic wasting reaction that is especially severe in end-stage heart failure. This systemic inflammatory response is likely also to be a major cause of the skeletal muscle myopathy in heart failure, which is responsible for the fatigue and muscle weakness that can be troublesome in this syndrome. More recent reports have suggested that this systemic reaction, along with a local inflammatory response in the failing heart, contributes to the myocardial cell death that is responsible for the progressive deterioration of these patients. Limited evidence suggests that stimulation of protein synthesis by locally released inflammatory mediators in the overloaded heart may, at least in its initial stages, provide an adaptive response by promoting hypertrophy (see Chapter 6).

Cardiac Cachexia and the Skeletal Muscle Myopathy of Heart Failure: A Systemic Inflammatory Response

Loss of muscle mass in patients with dropsy, noted by Hippocrates more than 2,500 years ago (see Chapter 1), is recognized to be an important complication of heart failure. Wood (1950), for example, wrote "patients with chronic heart failure usually lose flesh, although loss of weight may be prevented by fluid retention; thus wasting may only be noticed after diuresis; sometimes it is so great as to warrant the term cachexia." As a medical student in the late 1950s, I helped care for a young woman who, shortly before she died of rheumatic mitral insufficiency (which was then inoperable), exhibited the wasting I had come to associate with terminal malignancy. I recall my surprise when the resident told me that cachexia was a common feature of end-stage heart failure. Until recently, however, little attention was paid to the loss of body tissue in these patients, which was often assumed to be caused by a combination of inactivity, inadequate caloric intake, and excessive metabolic demands, sometimes complicated by digitalis-induced nausea and anorexia (Pittman and Cohen, 1964).

It is clear that wasting in heart failure differs from that caused by malnutrition. In the latter, cachexia is due mainly to loss of adipose tissue, whereas in patients with heart failure, the loss is mostly of lean tissue mass (Thomas et al., 1979; Freeman and Roubenoff, 1994). Another possible explanation for the loss of muscle mass in these patients is disuse atrophy, caused by inactivity. However, the skeletal muscle abnormalities caused by disuse differ from the those found in clinical heart failure; for example, the content of the slow skeletal myosin isoform decreases much more in heart failure than after inactivity, while oxidative fiber content decreases more in disuse atrophy (Vescovo et al, 1996). Further evidence that the skeletal muscle myopathy of heart failure is not due entirely to disuse is found in an experimental model of heart failure wherein neither the myosin heavy chain isoform shifts nor loss of oxidative enzymes typical of this myopathy is accompanied by a decrease in locomotor activity of the animals (Simonini et al, 1996). These findings indicate that mechanisms other than starvation and disuse are major causes of cardiac cachexia and the skeletal muscle myopathy that leads to the terrible fatigue so common in heart failure. As discussed in subsequent paragraphs, it seems likely that these abnormalities are due in part to elevated cytokine levels. These inflammatory mediators, long known to cause cachexia and weakness in chronic diseases like malignancy and infection, therefore appear to play an important role in the pathophysiology of heart failure.

The "modern" era in understanding of cardiac cachexia began only a decade ago with the demonstration that circulating levels of tumor necrosis factor α (TNF-α, or cachectin) are elevated in the blood of patients with heart failure (Levine et al., 1990; for review, see Ceconi et al., 1998). This finding has been confirmed and extended by several reports that circulating levels of other cytokines are also elevated in heart failure (McMurray et al., 1991; Dutka et al., 1993; Katz et al., 1994; Matsumori et al., 1994, Testa et al., 1996; Anker et al., 1997a, 1997b; Tsutamoto et al., 1997), and that the extent of these elevations correlates with the severity of symptoms (Testa et al., 1995; Anker et al., 1997a, 1997b). These findings, which represent a significant advance in current understanding of heart failure, are already providing opportunities for the development of new modalities of therapy.

Cardiac Cell Damage: A Local Inflammatory Response

A second feature of the inflammatory response in heart failure, in addition to the systemic response that is involved in the pathogenesis of cachexia and muscle weakness, occurs when cytokines are produced by the myocardium itself. This local response has been found to accompany such inflammatory conditions as viral infections of the heart, cardiac allograft rejection, and myocarditis (Lane et al., 1992; Lange and Schreiner, 1994; Yamada et al., 1994; for relevant symposia proceedings see Kawai and Abelmann, 1987; Sekiguchi and Richardson, 1994; Maisch and Goodwin, 1995). More recent work has demonstrated that TNF-α and other cytokines accumulate in the myocardium after simple hemodynamic overloading.

Elevated levels of cytokines in the hearts of patients with dilated cardiomyopathy, whose clinical picture does not suggest a viral or other infectious etiology, indicate that these inflammatory mediators play a general role in heart failure (Holzinger et al., 1995; Torre-Amione et al., 1996; Habib et al., 1996; Doyama et al., 1996; Satoh et al., 1997). The experimental findings that simple hemodynamic overloading can elevate levels of the mRNA encoding TNF-α within 30 minutes after aortic banding in rat hearts and that, within an hour, TNF-α protein levels increase more than 10-fold in both myocytes and nonmyocytes (Kapadia et al., 1997), indicate that this local inflammatory response is important in virtually all forms of heart failure. Myocardial levels of interleukin-1β (IL-1β), another cytokine, have been found to be increased in a chronic model of pressure overload (Shioi et al., 1997). This cytokine is located mainly within macrophages, which suggests that overload causes the myocardium to release chemotactic and other activating factors that recruit monocytes, which carry this inflammatory mediator to the heart. Yet another inflammatory cytokine, IL-6, is synthesized by the viable cardiac myocytes at the edges of a myocardial infarct (Gwechenberger et al., 1999).

In inflammatory heart diseases like myocarditis, cytokines can be brought to the heart when mononuclear cells are attracted by infectious agents and tissue injury. Although TNF-α is not normally expressed in adult mammalian cardiac myocytes, this cytokine can be produced in hearts that are exposed to endotoxin (Giroir et al., 1992, 1995; Kapadia et al., 1995a, 1995b). The likelihood that cytokines damage the failing heart is supported by the finding that transgenic mice that overexpress TNF-α in their hearts exhibit a dilated cardiomyopathy that has many similarities to clinical heart failure (Kubota et al., 1997; Bryant et al., 1998) and that continuous infusion of TNF-α that achieve levels similar to those seen clinically can cause a dilated cardiomyopathy (Bozkurt et al., 1998).

Taken together, these findings indicate that heart failure is accompanied by a local inflammatory response in which cytokines are produced both by invading monocytes and locally by stressed cardiac myocytes. Although injurious effects of these cytokines may be among the causes of the "Cardiomyopathy of Overload" that contributes to the poor prognosis in heart failure, evidence discussed below suggests that local production of TNF-α and other cytokines may also be protective, at least in the short term.

CYTOKINES

The cytokines, as noted at the beginning of this chapter, are an ancient family of peptides that includes peptide growth factors, prolactin, erythropoietin, transforming growth factor-β (TGF-β), as well as the inflammatory cytokines that are the subject of this chapter (see Table 5-1). The biologic functions of the cytokines, therefore, extend far beyond their participation in inflammation (see Table 5-2). Functional diversity is even seen in the case of a single cytokine; for example, TNF-α can activate members of a family of stress-activated protein kinases that have both growth-promoting effects (Kyriakis et al., 1994; Brenner et al., 1989; Westwick et al., 1994) and the ability to initiate programmed cell death (Tartaglie et al., 1993). The ability of these peptides to activate signal transduction systems that regulate protein synthesis, gene expression, and proliferation, as well as apoptosis (programmed cell death), is consistent with growing evidence that cytokines are involved in both adaptive and maladaptive growth responses in the failing heart. In view of the potential importance of these peptides in the pathogenesis of heart failure, key features of the systems that regulate cytokine production and mediate cytokine actions are reviewed in the following discussion. There are already clues that this information may become important in improving the management of patients with heart failure.

Control of Cytokine Synthesis: NF-κB

Inflammatory cytokines can be produced both by mononuclear cells that are attracted to sites of inflammation and by a variety of cell types, including cardiac myocytes (see earlier discussion). Cytokines are released by proteolytic cleavage of a protein precursor at the plasma membrane. Synthesis of these precursors is regulated by specific transcription factors that activate the genes which encode these peptides.

Among the most important of the transcription factors that regulate cytokine production is NF-κB, which also stimulates the production of additional proteins that participate in immune and inflammatory responses (Fig. 5-1). The latter include *iNOS*, the inducible isoform of nitric oxide synthase, *cyclooxygenase*, which catalyzes prostaglandin synthesis (Wong et al., 1998), and *cell adhesion molecules* (*CAMs*) that attract leukocytes to areas of injury (Barnes and Karin 1997; Stancovski and Baltimore, 1997). In addition to its important role as an integrator of the inflammatory response, NF-κB regulates genes that are involved in cell growth and programmed cell death (Baldwin, 1996; Baeuerle and Baltimore, 1996).

The activity of NF-κB is stimulated by many factors, including endotoxins, mitogens, viral proteins, and the cytokines themselves (Blackwell and Christman, 1997; Israël,

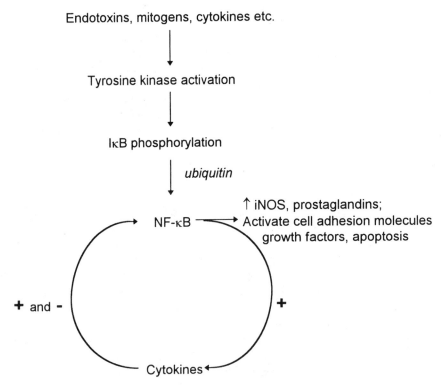

FIG. 5-1. Simulation of cytokine production by endotoxins, mitogens, and other compounds that cause inflammation begins when they activate tyrosine kinases that phosphorylate an inhibitory protein called IκB. In a reaction that involves an additional cofactor called ubiquitin, proteolysis of IκB liberates active NF-κB. The latter is a transcription factor that increases the expression of proteins that synthesize cytokines. The newly formed cytokines can both stimulate and inhibit NF-κB production. NF-κB also increases the synthesis of the inducible isoform of nitric oxide synthase (iNOS), prostaglandins, cell adhesion molecules that attract leukocytes to areas of injury and inflammation, and other mediators that regulate protein synthesis, cell growth, and apoptosis.

1997). The latter activate NF-κB when they bind to their tyrosine kinase receptors. The stimulatory effect of cytokines is indirect, however, because NF-κB is not the substrate for these tyrosine phosphorylations; instead, the substrate for phosphorylation is a protein called IκB. In its dephospho-form, IκB inhibits NF-κB. The ability of phosphorylation to reverse the inhibitory effects of IκB activates NF-κB. This occurs when phosphorylation allows IκB to bind *ubiquitin* in a reaction that leads to IκB proteolysis so as to reverse its inhibition of NF-κB activity. The liberated (activated) NF-κB then translocates to the nucleus, where it stimulates cytokine synthesis (DiDonato et al., 1997; Israël, 1997; Stancovski and Baltimore, 1997) (see Fig. 5-1).

The ability of cytokines to activate NF-κB, and so to increase cytokine synthesis, represents an example of a positive feedback in which a substance stimulates its own production. This amplification, which is commonly seen in biology, initiates a brief but intense burst of cytokine activity. Additional negative feedback loops allow NF-κB to turn off cytokine production so as to prevent runaway signaling (Blackwell and Christman, 1997). Together, these tightly linked control mechanisms can shut down cytokine synthesis shortly after it is activated, even when the stimulating agents remain present (Ye and Young, 1997).

Another mechanism that participates in the control of cytokine production, in addition to the phosphorylation reactions already described, is cleavage of the active peptides from protein precursors at the cell surface. In the case of TNF-α, which is synthesized as a large inactive protein that becomes imbedded in the plasma membrane, the active cytokine is released by proteolysis of its precursor in a reaction that is catalyzed by a metalloproteinase called *TNF-α converting enzyme* (*TACE*) (Black et al., 1997). A role for alterations in this proteolytic reaction in the failing heart has not yet been defined.

Actions of the Cytokines

Many of the actions of the cytokines are mediated by a signal transduction pathway, called the *JAK-STAT pathway* (Fig. 5-2), which is activated when cytokine binding to specific plasma membrane receptors initiates a series of phosphorylation reactions (Vilcek and Lee, 1991; Darnell et al., 1994; Ihle, 1995; Ihle and Kerr, 1995; Bazzoni and Beutler, 1996; Wood et al., 1997; Ransohoff, 1998). This section describes the interactions between the cytokine receptors and the JAK-STAT pathway; the many subsequent steps that are modified by this pathway are discussed in Chapter 7, where the actions of key signal transduction systems are reviewed, notably the stress-activated mitogen-activated protein (MAP) kinases, which appear to play an important role in the failing heart.

Cytokine Receptors

Like most of the extracellular messengers discussed in Chapter 4, cytokines modify cell function when these peptide bind to specific plasma membrane receptors. Cytokine receptors, which are found in almost every cell type, respond to cytokine-binding by activating intracellular signal transduction pathways, most of which activate additional intracellular phosphorylation reactions. Type I receptors, which mediate the effects of inflammatory cytokines, are closely related to the receptors that bind colony-stimulating factors, growth hormone, and prolactin, which as noted in Table 5-1 are also members of the cytokine family. Type II receptors, which bind interferons, play a role in immune reactions.

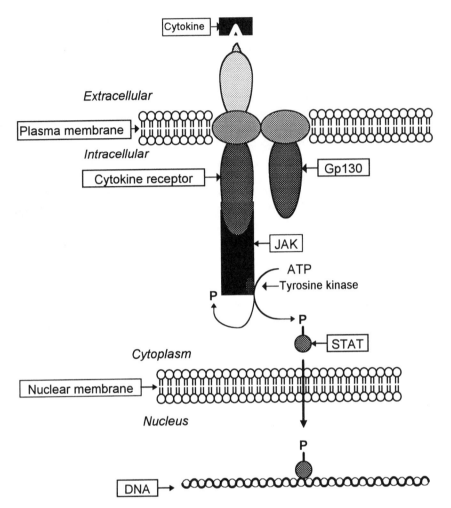

FIG. 5-2. The JAK-STAT pathway, which is activated by cytokine-induced tyrosine phosphorylations, begins when cytokine binding to their specific receptors causes the latter to aggregate. In many cases, these aggregates include an additional protein called gp130, and often additional smaller proteins (not shown). The receptor aggregates then bind members of a family of tyrosine kinases called JAK, which phosphorylate transcription factors called STAT. The activated STATs then move to the nucleus where they bind to regulatory regions of the DNA so as to modify gene expression.

The major effect of cytokine binding to the type I receptors is activation of tyrosine kinases. These enzymes, which phosphorylate tyrosine residues on a variety of proteins, modify subsequent steps in cytokine-activated signal transduction cascades. These include phosphorylation of IκB and the cytokine receptors themselves. An additional protein, called *gp130*, participates in cytokine signaling in many cell types. Like the cytokine receptors, gp130 can be phosphorylated by tyrosine kinases that are activated by cytokine-bound receptors.

Cytokine receptors are specific for individual members of this family of signaling peptides. In some cases, however, a single class of cytokines can bind to more than one receptor; for example, TNF-α binds to both a 55-kD (R1) and a 75-kD (R2) receptor. Cytokine receptors are made up of an extracellular domain that contains the cytokine-binding site, a membrane-spanning segment, and an intracellular (cytoplasmic) domain that transmits cytokine-induced signals to other proteins within the cytosol (Fig. 5-3). The cytokine receptors, which lack intrinsic protein kinase activity, exert their regulatory effects by activating tyrosine kinase reactions further "downstream" in their signaling cascades. The cytoplasmic domain of some cytokine receptors contains a 90 amino acid sequence that, because it stimulates apoptosis (Wallach et al., 1997), is sometimes referred to as a "death domain".

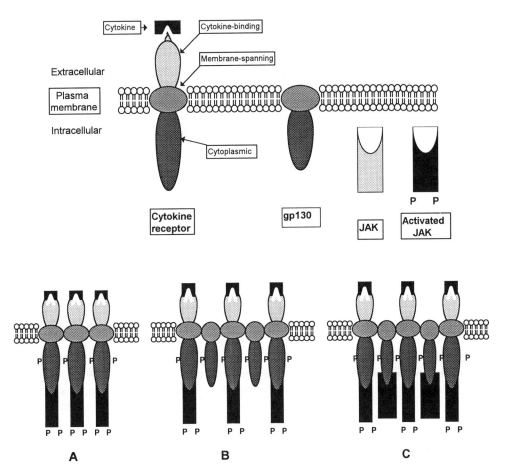

FIG. 5-3. Proteins that participate in cytokine signaling (TOP) include the cytokine receptors, which contain cytokine-binding, membrane-spanning, and cytoplasmic domains; the coupling protein gp130; and the tyrosine kinase enzyme JAK. The latter, in its dephospho-form, is inactive. Cytokine binding causes the receptors to aggregate (bottom), generally in trimers (**A**). In many cases, these aggregates also include gp130 (**B** and **C**). The aggregated receptors (**B**), and in some cases the complexes with gp130 (**C**), bind JAK. When incorporated in these aggregates, JAK can phosphorylate the receptors and, in gp130-containing aggregates, this coupling protein as well. The activated JAKs, which are often autophosphorylated, then phosphorylate additional proteins, notably the STAT class of transcription factors (see Fig. 5-4).

SOLUBLE CYTOKINE RECEPTORS

Although the most important effects of cytokine receptors are mediated by receptor molecules that are bound to the plasma membrane, cytokine receptors are also found in a soluble form. Circulating levels of these soluble receptors, which are quite low in normal individuals, are often elevated in the blood and urine of patients with infectious and autoimmune diseases (for review, see Rose-John and Heinrich, 1994).

Soluble cytokine receptors are produced in two ways. The first, called *shedding*, occurs when limited proteolysis of the membrane-bound receptors releases the extracellular, ligand-binding domain of the receptor molecule. Soluble cytokine receptors can also be synthesized *de novo* from alternatively spliced mRNAs that can encode only the ligand-binding portion of the receptor molecule, and so are able to release soluble peptides that lack the transmembrane and cytosolic parts of the receptor (*differential splicing*). Soluble cytokine receptors often remain able to bind to their specific ligands, although with somewhat reduced affinity, and so can retain biologic activity.

The function of soluble cytokine receptors is not fully understood. They may represent carriers that protect the bound cytokines from proteolytic attack, or they may serve regulatory functions that are similar to those of the complete, membrane-bound receptor. Evidence that soluble cytokine receptors can retain significant activity is found in their ability to form complexes with their ligands that can activate gp130; the latter, as discussed in the next section, is a coupling protein that participates in the intracellular signaling actions of the cytokines. Soluble receptors have also been suggested to block some of the cytotoxic effects of TNF-α (Packer, 1995). The finding that levels of soluble TNF-α receptors are elevated in the blood of heart failure patients (Ferrari et al, 1995; Torre-Amione et al., 1996; Anker et al., 1997c) suggests that the soluble receptors may be of importance in this syndrome.

AGGREGATION REACTIONS INVOLVING THE CYTOKINE RECEPTORS AND gp130

The most important effect of the binding of a cytokine to its receptor is to cause the latter to aggregate, generally as trimers (see Fig. 5-3). In some cases, the active oligomers formed by the cytokine receptors include the coupling protein gp130 (sometimes referred to as the β chain of the cytokine receptor), along with the cytosolic tyrosine kinases discussed later. The aggregation of many cytokine receptors, including the TNF-α receptors, induces conformational changes in the cytoplasmic domains that cause the ligand-bound receptors to activate intracellular tyrosine kinases, which mediate subsequent steps in their signaling cascades (see Fig. 5-3). Some isoforms of gp130, when incorporated into cytokine-receptor aggregates, also bind to and activate tyrosine kinases (Ihle, 1995).

Activated tyrosine kinases catalyze phosphorylation reactions that mediate downstream signaling; these cytokine-activated kinases also phosphorylate the cytokine receptors, gp130, and often the kinases themselves (autophosphorylation). These reactions generally amplify one another, and so provide additional examples of positive feedback loops. Termination of these signals, which is less well understood, may occur when the phosphorylated proteins are dephosphorylated by special phosphatases, or by the action of proteins that directly inhibit other steps in the cytokine-induced phosphorylation pathways (O'Shea, 1997; Endo et al., 1997; Naka et al., 1997; Starr et al., 1997).

Tyrosine phosphorylation is of central importance in most cytokine-mediated cell signaling, although serine and threonine phosphorylations participate in a few of these regulatory mechanisms (Mufson, 1997). The latter, which represents an important "cross over" between two major signal transduction cascades, are especially important in mediating cytokine effects on cell proliferation and survival.

THE JAK-STAT PATHWAY

The most important intracellular mediators of cytokine signaling are a family of intracellular tyrosine kinases generally referred to as *JAK* (see Fig. 5-2). This acronym, which originally stood for "just another kinase" because its function was poorly understood, has been redefined to mean *Janus kinase*. The latter term, which recalls the two-faced Roman god of doorways who looks both outward and inward, was chosen because this enzyme responds to changes in the extracellular environment—binding of cytokines to their receptors in the extracellular medium—by modifying the intracellular environment—phosphorylation of tyrosine moieties in cytosolic substrates. The intricacy of these signaling systems is reflected in the ability of these kinases (hereafter abbreviated JAK) also to phosphorylate cytokine receptors, the coupling protein gp130, and more remarkably, themselves, in phosphorylations that generally provide amplifications within these systems.

Activation of JAK begins when the aggregated cytokine receptors bind this enzyme (see Fig. 5-3). The enhanced catalytic activity may occur when aggregation brings the active sites of different JAK molecules sufficiently near to each other to allow trans-phosphorylations (Ihle, 1995; Ihle and Kerr, 1995), or when conformational changes that accompany these aggregations eliminate an energy barrier in the catalytic reaction (Bazzoni and Beutler, 1996). Further activation of the JAK-receptor aggregate occurs when the activated JAK phosphorylates the intracellular domain of the cytokine receptor, gp130, other JAKs, and additional regulatory proteins that activate intracellular signal transduction cascades (Bazzoni and Beutler, 1996; Ransohoff, 1998).

A major step in cytokine signaling is mediated by a family of transcription factors called *signal transducer and activator of transcription* (*STAT*) (Fig. 5-4) that are sub-

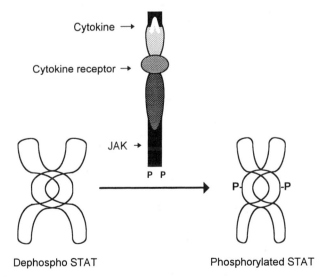

Cytokine →

Cytokine receptor →

JAK →

P P

P-⟨⟩-P

A   Dephospho STAT   Phosphorylated STAT

FIG. 5-4. JAK is a tyrosine kinase that, when phosphorylated in the cytokine receptor complex, mediates cytokine responses by phosphorylating STAT (**A**). *Continued on next page.*

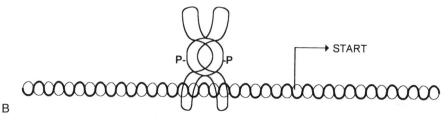

FIG. 5-4. *Continued.* The phosphorylated STAT then translocates to the nucleus where, by binding to a specific DNA sequence, it modifies the ability of the gene to initiate protein synthesis (**B**). The "START" region of the gene marks the point along the DNA strand that separates the regulatory regions (left) from those that encode the protein that is transcribed (right).

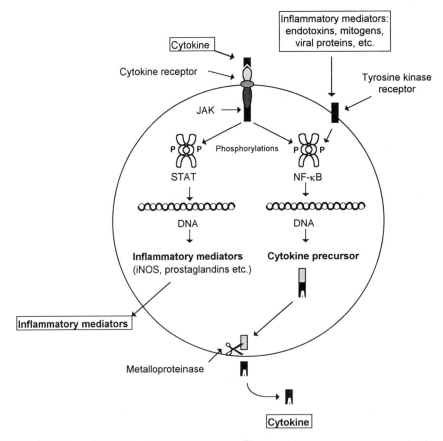

FIG. 5-5. Overview of the actions of the cytokines. The cytokine-receptor complex (top), when it forms the aggregates shown in Figure 5-3, activates the protein kinase JAK. The latter phosphorylates transcription factors of the STAT family (left), which activate genes that produce inflammatory mediators such as iNOS and prostaglandins. Activated JAK, along with other tyrosine kinases that are activated by inflammatory mediators, also catalyzes phosphorylation of the transcription factor NF-κB (right), which increases the production of cytokine precursors. The latter migrate to the plasma membrane where active cytokines are released by members of the family of metalloproteinases. These mechanisms include many additional feedback loops and other regulatory systems not shown in this diagram.

strates for JAK-catalyzed tyrosine phosphorylations. Once phosphorylated, these transcription factors become activated and move to the nucleus where they bind to specific DNA sequences so as to modify gene expression (Fig. 5-5). There are many STATs, which regulate a variety of genes. The specificity of the responses to different cytokines appears to depend on the DNA consensus sequences that bind different isoforms of STAT, rather than the specificity of the JAKs (O'Shea, 1997).

POSSIBLE ADAPTIVE EFFECTS OF TNF-α

The previous discussion has focused on the maladaptive effects of the cytokines, highlighting their possible role in an inflammatory process that contributes to such responses as cardiac cachexia, skeletal muscle weakness and, at a local tissue level, the progressive deterioration of the failing heart. Because these peptides exert so many other biologic effects (see Table 5-2), the possibility that, like the hemodynamic defense reaction discussed in Chapter 4, the cytokines may also participate in adaptive responses must be considered. Support for this interpretation is provided by the ability of cytokines to protect the heart against ischemic injury, possibly by activating the synthesis of enzymes that destroy oxygen free radicals (Nelson et al., 1995; Chandrasekar et al., 1995). Cytokines expressed in ischemic and hypoxic myocardium also inhibit cell damage by increasing the expression of heat shock proteins in cardiac myocytes (Low-Friedrich et al., 1992; Nakano et al., 1996, 1998). The ability of heat shock proteins to inhibit protein denaturation and stabilize cells in response to a variety of stresses, makes it likely that locally produced TNF-α and other cytokines participate in adaptive, as well as maladaptive, responses.

Another potentially beneficial consequence of cytokine production in the overloaded heart is the participation of these inflammatory mediators in signal transduction systems that stimulate cell growth (Palmer et al., 1995; Thaik et al., 1995; Yokoyama et al., 1997; Ono et al., 1998). Such a cytokine-mediated hypertrophic response would provide a beneficial short-term adaptation, although over the long term, stimulation of mitogenic pathways eventually cause harm (see Chapter 8). Thus, although increased cytokine levels initially contribute to an adaptive growth response in the overloaded heart, with time, this response probably becomes maladaptive.

FREE RADICALS AND NITRIC OXIDE

The cytotoxic effects of the cytokines are mediated in part by free radicals. These highly reactive chemical substances have been implicated as causes of ischemic and reperfusion injury (for review, see Reimer and Jennings, 1992), and have been suggested to contribute to the negative inotropic effects of cytokines (Finkel, 1996) as well as the progressive deterioration of the failing heart (Belch et al., 1991). Because cells normally make small amounts of free radicals as byproducts of oxidative phosphorylation, the body has effective defenses that destroy these toxic molecules. Another major source for these reactive compounds is nitric oxide (NO), a free radical gas that is formed by several different nitric oxide synthases. The low concentrations of NO produced by *constitutive nitric oxide synthase* (*cNOS*) mediate physiologic signaling and cause no damage. The much larger amounts of NO that are generated by *inducible nitric oxide synthase* (*iNOS*) can form toxic concentrations of reactive molecules such as nitrogen dioxide and peroxinitrites. These concentration-dependent effects of NO have been divided into three "action phases" (Dugas et al., 1995) that are summarized in Table 5-3.

TABLE 5-3. *Three "action phases" of nitric oxide*

Phase 1: Low nitric oxide (NO) concentrations—intracellular second messenger that activates:
Guanylyl cyclase
Immediate-early gene response
NF-κB
Cytokine production
Antiapoptotic mechanisms
Phase 2: Intermediate NO concentrations—extracellular autocrine and paracrine messenger that regulates:
Vasodilatation
Amplification of NO production by tumor necrosis factor-α
Phase 3: High NO concentrations—toxicity:
Generation of peroxinitrate and other free radicals
DNA alterations
Cell death (apoptosis)

Adapted from Dugas et al. (1995).

In contrast to the low concentrations of NO normally generated within the cytosol, which serve as an intracellular messenger ("phase 1" in Table 5-3), larger amounts diffuse out of cells into the extracellular fluid. Once outside the cell, NO can serve as a messenger that stimulates the cell to modify its own function (autocrine signaling) or to modify the function of nearby cells (paracrine signaling) ("phase 2" in Table 5-3). The most important paracrine effect of NO in the cardiovascular system is to communicate vasodilator signals from the vascular endothelium to smooth muscle, hence the original name: *endothelium-derived relaxing factor* (*EDRF*). As noted, the prooxidant effects of these low and intermediate concentrations of NO are relatively minor and are readily controlled by natural antioxidant systems such as superoxide dismutase, catalase, and glutathione (Dugas et al., 1995).

The actions of NO are quite different when large amounts of this reactive compound are produced in cells that are activated by stimuli such as cytokines and bacterial endotoxin ("phase 3" in Table 5-3). These inflammatory mediators increase the expression of iNOS, the much more active inducible form of nitric oxide synthase (De Belder et al., 1993; Dugas et al., 1995; Thoenes et al., 1996). The large amounts of NO generated by iNOS contribute to the vasodilation and depressed myocardial contractility seen in irreversible shock (Hosenpud et al., 1989; Moncada and Higgs, 1993), activate NF-κB to increase cytokine production, and may contribute a stimulus for cardiac myocyte hypertrophy (Nakamura et al., 1998). Although high NO concentrations can be beneficial by attacking invading organisms, this inflammatory mediator also damages cells and can cause myocardial cell death (Unguranu-Longrois et al., 1995, Stein et al., 1996; Satoh et al., 1997). As previously noted, systemic effects of free radicals produced as the result of cytokine-induced iNOS expression may play an important role in causing cardiac cachexia and possibly the skeletal muscle myopathy of heart failure.

OTHER MEDIATORS OF INFLAMMATORY RESPONSE

In addition to the cytokines, several other mediators activate the inflammatory response. These include kinins, such as bradykinin, histamine, 5-hydroxytryptamine, complement, prostaglandins (Appleton 1994; Appleton et al., 1996; Wong et al., 1998), chemokines (Luster, 1998; Aukurst et al., 1998), and activators of additional stress-related kinases (Kyriakis and Avruch, 1996). Many of these interact with the cytokine system. The role of most other inflammatory mediators in the pathophysiology of heart failure is not well defined and this vast topic is not considered further in this discussion.

CONCLUSION

Evidence that has accumulated over the past decade suggests that both systemic and local inflammation play an important role in heart failure. Best established is a causal link between activation of the systemic inflammatory response and the cardiac cachexia and skeletal muscle myopathy seen in advanced heart failure. An important role for this cytokine-mediated systemic response is suggested by the correlation between the extent of the elevations of circulating inflammatory cytokines and the severity of this syndrome. The appearance of this systemic response probably reflects the fact that, as in other severe chronic diseases, end-stage heart failure evokes what can be viewed as an essentially "mindless" attack on what the body presumes to be an invasion. There are likely to be some short-term benefits of this inflammatory response, but like the hemodynamic defense reaction discussed in Chapter 4, cytokines probably do more harm than good over the long term.

Less clear is the significance of the local inflammatory response, in which cytokines and other mediators of inflammation appear in the failing heart itself. In contrast to the systemic response, in which circulating cytokine levels are elevated mainly in end-stage heart failure, the local response can appear within minutes of an abnormal stress. For example, local elevation of cytokine levels appears to be part of the initial response of the heart to hemodynamic overloading. Although these compounds can exert cytotoxic effects, they also contribute to the hypertrophic response that is of short-term benefit to the overloaded heart. Release of heat shock proteins, another action of locally produced cytokines, also has beneficial effects in the response to injury. From an evolutionary point of view, it is not difficult to understand why the cytokines and other inflammatory mediators evoke a healing response as well as attacking invaders. It makes sense for a primitive defense/counterattack mechanism such as that discussed at the beginning of this chapter to provide for repair and healing of damaged cells. After all, the ideal defense should not only destroy an attacker but also speed recovery from injury.

One potential damaging effect of the local release of cytokines is the ability of many of these peptides to initiate apoptosis. In an organ such as the heart, which is composed of terminally differentiated cells that, because they do not proliferate cannot be replaced, stimuli that lead to programmed cell death represent a disaster. Another harmful effect of the cytokines is related to their ability to induce iNOS, which releases large amounts of NO that contribute to the production of free radicals that damage the failing myocardium.

At this time, knowledge of the role of inflammation in heart failure remains incomplete. One pattern that is emerging from currently available data is that, like the hemodynamic defense reaction (Chapter 4), the inflammatory response may initially be beneficial, but when sustained, becomes deleterious. If this interpretation is correct, efforts to block the effects of cytokines and other inflammatory mediators could provide new approaches to therapy for these patients.

REFERENCES

Anker SD, Clark AL, Kemp M, Salisbury C, Teixeira MM, Hellewell PG, Coats AJS (1997a). Tumor necrosis factor and steroid metabolism in chronic heart failure: possible relation to muscle wasting. *J Am Coll Cardiol* 30: 997–1001

Anker SD, Chua TP, Ponikowski P, Harrington D, Swan JW, Cox WJ, Poole-Wilson PA, Coats AJS (1997b). Hormonal changes and catabolic/anabolic imbalance in chronic heart failure and their importance for cardiac cachexia. *Circulation* 96:526–534.

Anker SD, Coates AJS (1997c). Syndrome of cardiac cachexia. In Poole-Wilson PA, Colucci WS, Massie BM, Chatterjee K, Coats AS, eds. *Heart Failure. Scientific Principles and Clinical Practice.* Churchill Livingstone, New York, pp 261–267.

Appleton I (1994). Wound repair: the role of cytokines and vasoactive mediators. *J Roy Soc Med* 87:500–502.

Appleton I, Tomlinson A, Willoughby DA (1996). Induction of cyclo-oxygenase and nitric oxide synthase in inflammation. *Adv Pharmacol* 35:27–78.

Aukurst P, Ueland T, Müller F, Andreassen AK, Nordøy I, Aas H, Kjekshus J, Simonsen S, Frøland SS, Gullestad L (1998). Elevated circulating levels of C-C chemokines in patients with congestive heart failure. *Circulation* 97:1136–1143.

Baeuerle PB, Baltimore D (1996). NF-κB: ten years later. *Cell* 87:13–20.

Baldwin AS Jr (1996). The NF-κB and IκB proteins: new discoveries and insight. *Annu Rev Immunol* 14:649–681.

Barnes PJ, Karin M (1997). Nuclear factor-κB—a pivotal transcription factor in chronic inflammatory diseases. *N Engl J Med* 336:1066–1071.

Bazzoni F, Beutler B (1996). The tumor necrosis factor ligand and receptor families. *N Engl J Med* 334:1717–1725.

Beck G, Habicht GS (1991). Primitive cytokines: harbingers of vertebrate defense. *Immunol Today* 12:180–183.

Belch JJF, Bridges AB, Scott N, Chopra M (1991). Oxygen free radicals and congestive heart failure. *Br Heart J* 65: 245–248.

Black RA, Rauch CT, Kozlosky CJ, Peschon JJ, Slack JL, Wolfson MF, Castner BJ, Stocking KL, Reddy P, Srinivasan S, Nelson N, Bolani N, Schooley KA, Gerhart M, Davis R, Fitzner JN, Johnson RS, Paxton RJ, March CJ, Cerretti DP (1997). A metalloproteinase that releases tumour-necrosis-factor-α from cells. *Nature* 385:729–733.

Blackwell TS, Christman JW (1997). The role of nuclear factor-κB in cytokine gene regulation. *Am J Respir Cell Mol Biol* 17:3–19.

Boxkurt B, Kribbs SB, Clubb FJ, Michael LH, Didenko VV, Hornsby PJ, Seta Y, Oral H, Spinale FG, Mann DL (1998). Pathophysiologically relevant concentrations of tumor necrosis factor-α promote progressive left ventricular dysfunction and remodeling in rats. *Circulation* 97:1382–1391.

Brenner DA, O'Hara M, Angel P, Chojkier M, Karin M (1989). Prolonged activation of *jun* and collagenase genes by tumour necrosis factor α. *Nature* 337:661–663.

Bryant D, Becker L, Richardson J, Shelton J, Franco F, Peshock R, Thompson M, Giroir B (1998). Cardiac failure in transgenic mice with myocardial expression of tumor necrosis factor α. *Circulation* 97:1375–1381.

Ceconi C, Curello S, Bachetti T, Corti A, Ferrari R (1998). Tumor necrosis factor in congestive heart failure: a new mechanism of disease for the new millennium? *Prog CV Dis* 41:25–30.

Chandrasekar B, Colston JT, Freeman GL (1997). Induction of proinflammatory cytokine and antioxidant enzyme gene expression following brief myocardial ischemia. *Clin Exp Immunol* 108:346–351.

Darnell JE, Kerr IM, Stark GR (1994). JAK-STAT pathways and transcriptional activation in response to IFNs and other extracellular signaling molecules. *Science* 264:1415–1421.

De Belder AJ, Radomski MW, Why HJF, Richardsom PJ, Bucknall CA, Salas E, Martin JF, Moncada S (1993). Nitric oxide synthase activities in human myocardium. *Lancet* 341:84–85.

DiDonato JA, Hayakawa M, Rothwarf DM, Zandi E, Karin M (1997). A cytokine-responsive IκB kinase that activates the transcription factor NF-κB. *Nature* 388:548–554.

Doyama K, Fujiwara H, Fukumoto M, Tanaka M, Fujiwara Y, Oda T, Inada T, Ohtani S, Hasegawa K, Fujiwara T, Sasayama S (1996). Tumor necrosis factor is expressed in cardiac tissues of patients with heart failure. *Int J Cardiol* 54:217–225.

Dugas B, Debré P, Moncada S (1995). Nitric oxide, a vital poison inside the immune and inflammatory network. *Res Immunol* 146:664–670.

Dutka DP, Elborn JS, Delamere F, Shape DJ, Morris GK (1993). Tumour necrosis factor-alpha in severe congestive heart failure. *Br Heart J* 70:141–143.

Endo TA, Masuhara M, Yokouchi M, Suzuki R, Sakamoto H, Mitsui K, Matsumoto A, Tanimura S, Ohtsubo M, Misawa H, Miyazaki T, Leonor N, Taniguchi T, Fujita T, Kanakura Y, Komiya S, Yoshimura A (1997). A new protein containing an SH2 domain that inhibits JAK kinases. *Nature* 387:921–924.

Erdös EG (1966). Hypotensive peptides: bradykinin, kalliden, and eledosin. *Adv Pharmacol* 4:1–90.

Ferrari R, Bachetti T, Confortini R, Opasich C, Febo O, Corti A, Cassani G, Visioli O (1995). Tumor necrosis factor soluble receptors in patients with various degrees of congestive heart failure. *Circulation* 92:1479–1486.

Finkel MS (1996). Effects of proinflammatory cytokines on the mammalian heart. *Heart Failure Rev* 1:203–210.

Freeman LM, Roubenoff R (1994). The nutrition implications of cardiac cachexia. *Nutrition Rev* 52:340–347.

Gilbert RP (1960). Mechanisms of the hemodynamic effects of endotoxin. *Physiol Rev* 40:245–279.

Giroir BP, Horton JW, White JD, McIntyre KL, Lin CQ (1994). Inhibition of tumor necrosis factor prevents myocardial dysfunction during burn shock. *Am J Physiol* 267:H118–H124.

Giroir BP, Johnson JH, Brown T, Allen GL, Beutler B (1992). The tissue distribution of tumor necrosis biosynthesis during endotoxemia. *J Clin Invest* 90:693–698.

Gwechenberger M, Mendoza LH, Youker KA, Frangogiannis NG, Smith W, Michael LH, Entman ML (1999). Cardiac myocytes produce interleukin-6 in culture and in viable border zone of reperfused infarctions. *Circulation* 99:546–551.

Habib FM, Springall DR, Davies GJ, Oakley CM, Yacoub MH, Polak JM (1996). Tumor necrosis factor and inducible nitric oxide synthase in dilated cardiomyopathy. *Lancet* 347:1151–1155.

Holzinger C, Schollhammer A, Imhof M, Reinwald C, Kramer G, Zuckerman A, Wolner E, Steiner G (1995). Phenotypic patterns of mononuclear cells in dilated cardiomyopathy. *Circulation* 92:2876–2885.

Hosenpud JD, Campbell SM, Medelson DJ (1989). Interleukin-1-induced myocardial depression in an isolated beating heart preparation. *J Heart Transplant* 8:460–464.

Ihle JN (1995). Cytokine receptor signalling. *Nature* 377:591–594.

Ihle JN, Kerr IM (1995). Jaks and Stats in signaling by the cytokine receptor superfamily. *Tr Genetics* 11:69–74.

Israël A (1997). IκB kinase all zipped up. *Nature* 388:519–521.

Kapadia S, Lee J, Torre-Amione G, Mann DL (1995a). Endotoxin-induced TNF-α gene and protein expression in adult feline myocardium. *Am J Physiol* 37:H517–H525.

Kapadia S, Lee J, Torre-Amione G, Birdsall HH, Ma TS, Mann DL (1995b). Tumor necrosis factor gene and protein expression in adult feline myocardium after endotoxin administration. *J Clin Invest* 96:1042–1052.

Kapadia S, Oral H, Lee J, Nakano M, Taffet GE, Mann DL (1997). Hemodynamic regulation of tumor necrosis factor-α gene and protein expression in adult feline myocardium. *Circ Res* 81:187–195.

Katz SD, Rao R, Berman JW, Schwarz M, Demopolilos L, Bijou R, LeJemtel TH (1994). Pathophysiological correlates of increased serum tumor necrosis factor in patients with congestive heart failure: relation to nitric oxide-dependent vasodilatation in the forearm circulation. *Circulation* 90:12–16.

Kawai C, Abelmann WH (1987). *Pathogenesis of Myocarditis and Cardiomyopathy. Cardiomyopathy Update 1.* University of Tokyo Press, Tokyo.

Kubota T, McTiernan CF, Frye CS, Slawson SE, Lemster BH, Koretsky AP, Demetris AJ, Feldman AM (1997). Dilated cardiomyopathy in transgenic mice with cardiac-specific overexpression of tumor necrosis factor-α. *Circ Res* 81:627–635.

Kyriakis JM, Avruch J, (1996). Sounding the alarm: protein kinase cascades activated by stress and inflammation. *J Biol Chem* 271:24313–24316.

Kyriakis JM, Bannerjee P, Nikolakaki E, Dal T, Rubie EA, Ahmad MF, Avruch J, Woodgett JR (1994). The stress-activated protein kinase subfamily of c-Jun kinases. *Nature* 369;156–160.

Lane JR, Neumann DA, Lafond-Walker A, Herskowitz A, Rose NR (1992). Interleukin 1 or tumor necrosis factor can promote coxsackie B3-induced myocarditis in resistant B10.A mice. *J Exp Med* 175:1123–1129.

Lange LG, Schreiner GF (1994). Immune mechanisms of cardiac disease. *N Engl J Med* 330:1129–1135.

Levine B, Kalman J, Mayer L, Fillit HM, Packer M (1990). Elevated circulating levels of tumor necrosis factor in severe chronic heart failure. *N Engl J Med* 323:236–241.

Low-Friedrich I, Weisensee D, Mitrou P, Schoeppe W (1992). Cytokines induce stress protein formation in cultured cardiac myocytes. *Basic Res Cardiol* 87:12–18.

Luster AD (1998). Chemokines—chemotactic cytokines that mediate inflammation. *N Engl J Med* 338:436–445.

Maisch B, Goodwin JF (1995). Diagnosis and treatment in dilated heart muscle disease. *Eur Heart J* 16(Suppl O).

Matsumori A, Yamada T, Suzuki H, Matoba Y, Sasayama S (1994). Increased circulating cytokines in patients with myocarditis and cardiomyopathy. *Br Heart J* 72:561–666.

McMurray J, Abdullah I, Dargie HJ, Shapiro D (1991). Increased concentrations of tumour necrosis factor in "cachectic" patients with severe chronic heart failure. *Br Heart J* 66:356–358.

Moncada S, Higgs A (1993). The L-arginine-nitric oxide pathway. *N Engl J Med* 329:2002–2012.

Mufson RA (1997). The role of serine/threonine phosphorylation in hematopoietic receptor signal transduction. *FASEB J* 11:37–44.

Naka T, Narazaki M, Hirata M, Matsumoto T, Minamoto S, Aono A, Nishimoto N, Kajita T, Taga T, Yoshizaki K, Akira S, Kishimoto T (1997). Structure and function of a new STAT-induced STAT inhibitor. *Nature* 387:924–928.

Nakamura K, Fushimi K, Kouchi H, Mihara K, Miyazaki M, Ohe T, Namba M (1998). Inhibitory effects of antioxidants on neonatal rat cardiac myocyte hypertrophy induced by tumor necrosis factor-α and angiotensin II. *Circulation* 98:794–999.

Nakano M, Knowlton AA, Yokoyama T, Lesslauer W, Mann DL (1996). Tumor necrosis factor-α induced expression of heat shock protein 72 in adult feline cardiac myocytes. *Am J Physiol* 270:H1231–H1239.

Nakano M, Knowlton AA, Dibbs Z, Mann DL (1998). Tumor necrosis factor-α confers resistance to hypoxic injury in adult mammalian cardiac myocyte. *Circulation* 97:1392–1400.

Natanson CP, Eichenhotz PW, Danner RL, Eichacker W, Hoffman D, Kuo SM, Banks TJ, MacVioittie TJ, Parrillo JE (1992). Endotoxin and tumor necrosis factor challenges in dogs simulate the cardiovascular profile to human septic shock. *J Exp Med* 169:823–832.

Nelson SK, Wong GH, McCord JM (1995). Leukemia inhibitory factor and tumor necrosis factor induce manganese superoxide dismutase and protect rabbit hearts from reperfusion injury. *J Mol Cell Cardiol* 27:223–229.

Ono K, Shioi T, Furukawa Y, Sasayama S (1998). Cytokine gene expression after myocardial infarction in rat hearts. Possible implication in left ventricular remodeling. *Circulation* 98:149–156.

Opdyke DF, Wiggers CJ (1946). Studies of right and left ventricular activity during hemorrhagic hypotension and shock. *Am J Physiol* 147:270–280.

O'Shea JJ (1997). JAKs, STATs, cytokine signal transduction, and immunoregulation: are we there yet? *Immunity* 7:1–11.

Packer M (1995). Is tumor necrosis factor an important neurohumoral mechanism in chronic heart failure. *Circulation* 92:1379–1382.

Palmer JN, Hartogensis WE, Patten M, Foruin FD, Long CS (1995). Interleukin 1β induces cardiac myocyte growth but inhibits cardiac fibroblast proliferation in culture. *J Clin Invest* 95:2555–2564.

Pittman JG, Cohen P (1964). The pathogenesis of cardiac cachexia. *N Engl J Med* 271:403–409, 453–460.

Pope A, Zamecnik P, Aub JC, Brues AM, Dubos RJ, Nathanson IT, Nutt AL (1945). The toxic factors in experimental traumatic shock. VI. The toxic influence of the bacterial flora, particularly *Clostridium welchii*, in exudates of ischemic muscle. *J Clin Invest* 24:856–863.

Ransohoff RM (1998). Cellular responses to interferons and other cytokines: the JAK-STAT paradigm. *N Engl J Med* 338:616–618.

Reimer KA, Jennings RB (1992). Myocardial ischemia, hypoxia and infarction. In Fozzard H, Haber E, Katz AM, Jennings R, Morgan HE, eds. *The Heart and Cardiovascular System*, 2nd ed. Raven Press, New York, pp 1875–1973.

Rose-John S, Heinrich PC (1994). Soluble receptors for cytokines and growth factors: generation and biological function. *Biochem J* 300:281–290.

Satoh M, Nakamura M, Tamura G, Makita S, Segawa I, Tashiro A, Satodate R, Hiramori K (1997). Inducible nitric oxide synthase and tumor necrosis factor-alpha in myocardium in human dilated cardiomyopathy. *J Am Coll Cardiol* 29:716–724.

Sekiguchi M, Richardson PJ (1994). *Prognosis and Treatment of Cardiomyopathies and Myocarditis. Cardiomyopathy Update 5.* University of Tokyo Press, Tokyo.

Shields DC, Harmoin DL, Nunez F, Whitehead AS (1995). The evolution of haematopoietic cytokine/receptor complexes. *Cytokine* 7:679–688.

Shioi T, Matsumori A, Kihara Y, Inoko M, Iwanaga Y, Yameda T, Iwasaki A, Matsushima K, Sasayama S (1997). Increased expression of interleukin-1β and monocyte chemotactic and activating factor/monocyte chemoattractant protein-1 in the hypertrophied and failing heart with pressure overload. *Circ Res* 81:664–671.

Shorr E, Zweifach BW, Furchgott RF (1945). On the occurrence, sites and modes of origin and destruction, of principles affecting the compensatory vascular mechanisms in experimental shock. *Science* 102:489–498.

Simonini A, Long CS, Dudley GA, Yue P, McElhinny J (1996). Heart failure causes changes in skeletal muscle morphology and gene expression that are not explained by reduced activity. *Circ Res* 79:128–136.

Stancovski I, Baltimore D (1997). NF-κB activation: the IκB kinase revealed? *Cell* 91:299–302.

Starr R, Wilson TA, Viney Em, Murray LJL, Rayner JR, Jenkins BJ, Gonda TJ, Alexander WS, Metcalf D, Nicola NA, Hilton DJ (1997). A family of cytokine-inducible inhibitors of signaling. *Nature* 387:917–921.

Stein B, Frank P, Schmitz W, Scholz H, Thoenes M (1996). Endotoxin and cytokines induce direct cardiodepressive effects in mammalian cardiomyocytes via induction of nitric oxide synthase. *J Mol Cell Cardiol* 28:1631–1639.

Suffrendini AF, Fromm RE, Parker MM, Brenner M, Kovacs JA, Wesley RA, Parrillo JE (1989). The cardiovascular response of normal humans to the administration of endotoxin. *N Engl J Med* 321:280–287.

Testa M, Yeh M, Lee P, Fanelli R, Loperfido F, Berman JW, LEJemtel TH (1996). Circulating levels of cytokines and their endogenous modulators in patients with mild to severe congestive heart failure due to coronary artery disease or hypertension. *Am J Cardiol* 28:964–971.

Thaik CM, Calderone A, Takahashi N, Colucci WS (1995). Interleukin-1β modulates the growth and phenotype of neonatal rat cardiac myocytes. *J Clin Invest* 96:1093–1099.

Thoenes M, Förstermann U, Tracey WR, Bleese NM, Nüssler AK, Scholz H, Stein B (1996). Expression of inducible nitric oxide synthase in failing and non-failing human heart. *J Mol Cell Cardiol* 28:165–169.

Thomas RD, Silverton NP, Burkinshaw L, Morgan DB (1979). Potassium depletion and tissue loss in chronic heart disease. *Lancet* 2:9–11.

Torre-Amione G, Kapadia S, Lee J, Durand J-B, Bies RD, Young JB, Mann DL (1996). Tumor necrosis factor-α and tumor necrosis factor receptors in the failing human heart. *Circulation* 93:704–711.

Tsutamoto T, Hisanaga T, Wada A, Maeda K, Ohnishi M, Fukai D, Mabuchi N, Sawaki M, Kinoshita M (1998). Interleukin-6 spillover in the peripheral circulation increases with the severity of heart failure, and the high plasma level of interleukin-6 is an important prognostic predictor in patients with congestive heart failure. *J Am Coll Cardiol* 31:391–398.

Unguranu-Longrois D, Balligand J-L, Kelly RA, Smith TW (1995). Myocardial contractile dysfunction in the systemic inflammatory response syndrome: role of a cytokine-inducible nitric oxide synthase in cardiac myocytes. *J Mol Cell Cardiol* 27:155–167.

Vescovo G, Serafini F, Tenderini P, Carraro U, Dalla Libera L, Catani C, Ambrosio GB (1996). Specific changes in skeletal muscle myosin heavy chain composition in cardiac failure: differences compared with disuse atrophy as assessed on microbiopsies by high resolution electrophoresis. *Heart* 76:337–343.

Vilcek J, Lee TH (1991). Tumor necrosis factor. New insights into the molecular mechanisms of its multiple actions. *J Biol Chem* 266:7313–7316.

Wallach D, Boldin M, Varfolmeev E, Bayaert R, Vandenabeele P, Fiers W (1997). Cell death induction by receptors of the TNF family: towards a molecular understanding. *FEBS Lett* 410:96–106.

Westwick JK, Weitzel C, Minden A, Karin M, Brenner D (1994). Tumor necrosis factor α stimulates AP-1 activity through prolonged activation of the c-Jun kinase. *J Biol Chem* 269:26936–26401.

Wiggers CJ (1947). Myocardial depression and shock. *Am Heart J* 33:633–650.

Wong SCY, Fukuchi M, Melnyk P, Rodger I, Giaid A (1998). Induction of cyclooxygenase-2 and activation of nuclear factor-κB in myocardium of patients with congestive heart failure. *Circulation* 98:100–103.

Wood P (1950). *Diseases of the Heart and Circulation.* Eyre and Spottiswoode, London, pp 174–175.

Wood TJJ, Haldosen L-A, Sliva D, Sundström M, Norstedt G (1997). Stimulation of kinase cascades by growth hormone: a paradigm for cytokine signaling. *Prog Nucl Acid Res* 57:73–94.

Yamada T, Matumori A, Sasayama S (1994). Therapeutic effect of anti-tumor necrosis factor-α antibody on the murine model of viral myocarditis induced by encephalomyocarditis virus. *Circulation* 89:846–851.

Ye J, Young HA (1997). Negative regulation of cytokine gene transcription. *FASEB J* 11:825–833,

Yokoyama T, Nakano M, Bednarczyk JL, McIntyre BW, Entman M, Mann DL (1997). Tumor necrosis factor α-provokes a hypertrophic growth response in adult cardiac myocytes. *Circulation* 95:1247–1252.

Yokoyama T, Vaca L, Rossen RD, Durante W, Hazarika P, Mann DL (1993). Cellular basis for the negative inotropic effects of tumor necrosis factor-α in the adult mammalian heart. *J Clin Invest* 92:2303–2312.

6

The Hypertrophic Response: Programmed Cell Death

Will I not walk in the footsteps of those who came before me? Indeed I will use their old path, but if I find one that is more appropriate and more level, I will use it. Those who have made investigations before us are not our masters, but our instructors. The truth is open to all; it is not exclusively owned. Much that is true remains to be discovered by future investigators.

Seneca, *Epistle XXXII.11.* Trans. P. B. Katz

Enlargement of the failing heart, which as noted in Chapter 1 was the first compensatory mechanism to have been recognized in this syndrome (see also Katz 1997, 1998), has both beneficial and deleterious effects. Like the hemodynamic defense reaction discussed in Chapter 4, hypertrophy of a damaged or overloaded heart is initially adaptive, but after time, maladaptive effects that accompany cardiac enlargement come to dominate the picture in these patients. The adaptive nature of the hypertrophic response in the overloaded heart was recognized in the 18th century, as were the different patterns of cardiac enlargement that have come to be known as eccentric and concentric hypertrophy. The clinical syndromes and prognostic implications associated with these different forms of hypertrophy were noted almost 200 years ago, and by the end of the 19th century, progressive dilatation of the failing ventricle (currently called "remodeling") was recognized as a major cause of clinical deterioration in patients with heart failure. This surprisingly modern view that hypertrophy could hasten the deterioration of the failing heart was eclipsed in the early decades of the 20th century by the rapid development of cardiac hemodynamics, and pushed further into the background by subsequent advances in cardiovascular surgery. Demonstration that the biochemical and biophysical processes responsible for contraction and relaxation were impaired in the failing heart also drew attention away from the maladaptive consequences of hypertrophy. It has only been during the past decade, when therapy began to consider the poor prognosis in this syndrome, that the focus returned to growth abnormalities in the failing heart, but with new perspectives made possible by developments in molecular biology.

This chapter begins with a general discussion of the regulation of growth and differentiation in the mammalian heart, emphasizing the constraints imposed on the growth response to overload caused by the fact that adult cardiac myocytes are terminally differentiated cells that have little or no ability to divide. A description of the cell cycle (the processes that regulate cell division) is followed by discussions of some of the growth factors that regulate this proliferative response. Different phenotypes of cardiac myocyte hypertrophy are related to concentric and eccentric hypertrophy, and to the progressive dilatation of the failing heart. The chapter concludes with a description of programmed cell death (apoptosis), one way by which the growth response to overload can lead to cell death.

DIFFERENTIATION OF MYOCYTES IN THE NORMAL ADULT HEART

Adult human cardiac myocytes are terminally differentiated cells, which means that these are highly specialized cells that have little or no capacity to proliferate. Terminally differentiated myocardial cells cannot synthesize DNA at a rapid rate, and protein synthesis is relatively slow, with half-lives for several myofibrillar proteins between 1 and 2 weeks (Rabinowitz, 1974). Adult mammalian cardiac myocytes have a limited capacity for mitosis, and when subjected to severe stress, and able to divide. This ability to proliferate, which was well known to the morphologists of the first half of the 20th century (for review, see Rumyantsev, 1977), has recently been rediscovered (Anversa and Kajstura, 1998). However, as discussed in Chapter 8, these attempts at proliferation do not end well. In contrast, the connective tissue cells that provide essential structural support to the heart rapidly synthesize protein and DNA, and are able to undergo cell division, albeit rather slowly. The cells that produce the heart's fibrous matrix normally divide every 80 to 120 days, although this proliferative response can be accelerated by overload and other stresses.

Human cardiac myocytes lose the capacity for healthy cell division shortly after birth, so they are as old as we are; at 65 years old, as I write this chapter, my cardiac myocytes—which so far are working quite well—are also eligible for Medicare! It is not obvious why cardiac myocytes lose their ability to undergo normal cell division, why human hearts become unable to regenerate these vital cells. The answer may be that this restriction keeps these cells focused on their essential task, to contract and relax, without pause, for a lifetime. Withdrawal of cardiac myocytes from the cell cycle may therefore be the price required for the heart to beat approximately 100,000 times a day, 36 million times a year, 2 1/2 billion times over a lifetime of 70 years.

Inability of adult cardiac myocytes to proliferate means that these cells can adapt to a sustained overload only by becoming larger. Because hypertrophy, unlike hyperplasia, does not require that the cell suspend its other activities, this growth response seems well suited for the heart, which must beat continuously to supply nutrients to, and remove wastes from, the other tissues of the body. As noted by Goss (1966): "By giving up the potential for hyperplasia in favor of the necessity for constant function, [the heart, lungs and kidneys] have adapted a strategy that enables them to become hypertrophic to a limited extent while doing their jobs efficiently." Because the heart cannot suspend its pumping to generate new myocytes, the cardiac myocytes formed at the end of embryonic life spend their lifetimes in selfless labor, denied the joys of reproduction and replication. Another "reason" why cardiac myocytes withdraw from the cell cycle may be to avoid hazards associated with proliferation, which include a form of cell death called apoptosis (see later discussion). Much like an individual who chooses a cloistered life, differentiation shelters cells from the programmed cell death that often accompanies cell proliferation.

The heart's withdrawal from the cell cycle can be contrasted with the behavior of a primitive stem cell, which like the queen bee in a hive, does little except generate progeny. The bone marrow stem cell, for example, neither fights infection nor carries oxygen, but instead reproduces continuously to replace worn-out leukocytes and erythrocytes that, while performing these essential functions, are relatively short-lived. Following this analogy, cardiac myocytes are like worker bees, whose only role is to toil for the good of the community. But unlike worker bees, injured or damaged cardiac myocytes cannot be replaced.

TERMINAL DIFFERENTIATION AND WITHDRAWAL FROM THE CELL CYCLE

Terminal differentiation is the process by which cells give up their ability to divide in order to carry out a strictly defined task. Examples of terminally differentiated cells include striated muscle (both skeletal and cardiac), neurons, and mature polymorphonuclear leukocytes. In the latter, renunciation of cell proliferation is so complete that the nuclei have become pyknotic. An even more "extreme" example of terminal differentiation is seen in the mature erythrocyte, which has lost its nucleus to become virtually a bag of hemoglobin. The latter example clearly illustrates the irreversibility of terminal differentiation, a fact that is of considerable importance in understanding the consequences of myocyte death in the failing heart.

Although differentiation is accompanied by the loss of many functions, there is no contradiction between specialization and simplification. Consider, for example, the tapeworm, a highly specialized platyhelminth that has lost virtually all digestive functions in order to live a parasitic existence that depends on the digestive juices of its host. The life of a terminally differentiated cell, like that of the tapeworm, is one of boredom and drudgery; there is no variety, just the same task performed over and over and over. This certainly characterizes the lifetime of work performed by the cardiac myocyte.

Because differentiation and withdrawal from the cell cycle go hand-in-hand, it is not surprising that both are initiated by the same control mechanisms, that the regulatory factors that initiate differentiation also inhibit proliferation. In understanding the maladaptive features of the growth response in the failing heart, it is important to recognize that the growth factors that stimulate hypertrophy also reactivate features of a proliferative response that (as discussed later) are best left dormant. This is due, in part, to the ability of many of the signals that promote cell growth also to initiate the programmed cell death called apoptosis.

Consequences of Overload

The advantages gained by an organ that depends on terminally differentiated cells carry a serious cost; that is, when an excessive load is placed on such an organ, new cells cannot be generated. As the permanent withdrawal of terminally differentiated cells from the cell cycle rules out the option of making additional cells (hyperplasia) to meet a sustained overload, the only compensatory mechanisms that remain are for the cells to work harder, to enlarge (hypertrophy), or both. If myocyte enlargement was a benign process, the hypertrophic response would only be helpful. However, the growth factors that increase cell size create serious problems for the overloaded heart. In the first place, these stimuli disturb the state of terminal differentiation that protects cardiac myocytes from many of the hazards associated with growth. In addition, as discussed in Chapter 3, myocyte hypertrophy creates energetic problems because oxygen diffusion into the core of large fibers can be impaired. Furthermore, the combination of wall thickening and increased intramyocardial tension reduces coronary perfusion, which exacerbates a state of energy starvation that is already a problem in the overloaded heart. As stated more than 30 years ago (Katz and Shaffer, 1966): "... the failing heart is not simply an enlarged version of the normal heart."

Consequences of Myocardial Cell Death

Cell death does not pose a serious challenge in organs made up of proliferating cells—surviving cells divide and their progeny take over for their lost cousins. In an organ made up of terminally differentiated cells, however, when a damaged or "worn out" cell dies, it cannot be replaced. In the case of the kidneys, where cells are lost during normal aging, the considerable reserves of renal function present during youth decrease gradually with age. However, except under extreme conditions, the additional burden placed on surviving renal cells is minimal and, unless the kidneys become diseased, is generally of little importance. In contrast, the impact of cell death in the heart is serious. Because cardiac output must be maintained, loss of functioning myocytes increases the work that must be performed by the surviving myocytes. These increased demands, which go on day and night, at rest, and especially during periods of stress, evoke a growth response that establishes the vicious cycle shown in Table 6-1. This vicious cycle, in which cell death increases overload, which accelerates cell death, which increases overload, and so on, represents a major problem in the patient with heart failure.

Aging

The myocardial cell death that occurs during aging represents an important challenge to the heart, as well as a growing public health and economic problem in the developed world. Because myocyte loss overloads the surviving myocardium, the myocardial changes that accompany normal aging resemble those seen in the overloaded heart. Most ominously, the maladaptive consequences of aging and overload are synergistic in that both contribute to the vicious cycle described in Table 6-1. The problem of myocyte death in the hearts of the elderly is especially serious because loss of vascular compliance that also accompanies aging increases systolic left ventricular systolic wall stress. Because increased wall stress represents a major stimulus for myocyte hypertrophy, the hypertrophic response caused by myocardial cell death is amplified by the greater impedance to ejection caused by stiffening of the blood vessels. It is therefore not difficult to explain the very high prevalence of heart failure in the elderly.

TABLE 6-1. *Consequences of withdrawal from the cell cycle (terminal differentiation)*

1. Cells that die cannot be replaced:
    In tissues with a large reserve, such as the kidneys, a decline in function is "felt" mainly during periods of stress, so that demands on surviving cells are not increased during the resting state until loss of function is severe.
    In the heart, loss of functioning myocytes overloads the surviving myocytes even under resting conditions. Because overload-induced hypertrophy shortens cell survival, the following vicious cycle is established:

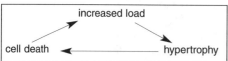

2. The only option by which cells can meet an overload is hypertrophy:
    In tissues where a decline in function is "felt" mainly during periods of stress, such as the kidneys, the stimulus to hypertrophy is initially intermittent and not intense.
    In the heart, where overload increases the work of the myocytes even during rest, the stimulus to hypertrophy is present at all times; because overload-induced hypertrophy shortens cell survival, it establishes the vicious cycle described in 1.

Reversion to the Fetal Phenotype

The terminally differentiated cells of the adult heart express an adult complement of genes that differ from those expressed during fetal life. When growth of adult cardiac myocytes is stimulated by overload, they tend to revert to the phenotypic pattern that existed in the fetal heart. This means that hypertrophy is accompanied by preferential activation of genes that encode protein isoforms normally expressed in embryonic life. The tendency of the overloaded heart to revert to the fetal phenotype can be viewed as an "attempt" to dedifferentiate, so that reactivation of growth in overloaded cardiac myocytes is, in some ways, analogous to Faust's effort to regain his "lost youth." However, the attempt of the overloaded heart to recover its youthful capacity for proliferation, like Faust's bargain with the devil, ends badly, largely because when cardiac myocytes enlarge, they do not last long. Just as Faust had to pay for the temporary restoration of his youthful vigor by spending eternity in Hell, so the hypertrophied heart pays for its increased capacity to work with a shortened cell survival. In accord with a pattern of short-term benefit, long-term harm, the growth response of the overloaded heart, while initially adaptive, eventually becomes maladaptive.

THE CARDIOMYOPATHY OF OVERLOAD

The deleterious consequences of cardiac hypertrophy, in which the effort to grow and dedifferentiate sets into motion processes that shorten cell survival, can be viewed as a "cardiomyopathy of overload" (Katz, 1990, 1994, discussed also in Chapter 8). It is not an exaggeration to state that overload has detrimental effects on the heart that resemble those of a cytotoxic viral infection. This is seen quite clearly in experimental aortic stenosis, in which the hypertrophic response that initially helps these animals to survive the hemodynamic overload leads eventually to progressive cardiac deterioration (Meerson, 1961). Perhaps the most deadly aspect of the cardiomyopathy of overload is acceleration of the vicious cycle shown in Table 6-1, in which stimuli that cause the heart to hypertrophy shorten the lifespan of working myocytes, which further overloads the surviving myocytes, which augments the stimulus to hypertrophy, and so on. In patients with heart failure, this maladaptive response is enhanced by growth-promoting effects of many mediators of the hemodynamic defense reaction, and by actions of several of the inflammatory cytokines. The clinical relevance of the concept of a cardiomyopathy of overload is seen in the results of a number of recent clinical trials, which have shown that unless therapy is directed to attenuating maladaptive growth in the failing heart, this progressive cardiomyopathy has terrible consequences.

AN OVERVIEW OF WHAT IS TO FOLLOW

The following discussion of the mechanisms that regulate cell growth and division begins with a review of the myogenic determinants and other transcription factors that make a heart cell a heart cell. This normal embryonic program, called *myogenesis,* is seen to cause both differentiation, which generates the normal adult phenotype, and withdrawal from the cell cycle, which blocks subsequent cell division. We then turn to the general features of the cell cycle, which in simple prokaryotic organisms operates continuously in what can be viewed as "primitive" or "undifferentiated" growth. Some of the transcription factors and other regulatory elements that control the more complex cell cycle in eukaryotes are described, as are factors that reawaken growth in the terminally differentiated cells of the overloaded heart. This discussion of the control of cell division and protein synthesis is intended as background for understanding the potential role of maladaptive growth in causing the progressive deterioration of the failing heart. After examining different phenotypes that appear in the adult heart, this chapter concludes with a description of programmed cell death, or apoptosis, yet another feature of the maladaptive growth response that, along with necrosis, may play an important role in causing the progressive deterioration of the overloaded heart.

This chapter deals with a vast topic. A major difficulty is that it is not yet known which features of these growth mechanisms cause cell death in the failing heart, nor has the extent of cell death been quantified. Emerging patterns in this important field are likely to help in understanding new approaches for managing patients with heart failure.

MYOGENESIS

As a general rule, cells that divide rapidly are not highly specialized, whereas cells that are specialized divide slowly, if at all. It is not surprising, therefore, that the same stimuli that cause undifferentiated mesodermal precursor cells to become muscle also shut down cell division. These "myogenic" stimuli are provided by several families of transcription factors that bind specific DNA sequences to cause both differentiation into muscle and withdrawal from the cell cycle.

Although both cardiac and skeletal muscle are composed of striated fibers, the processes of myogenesis in these cells differ from one another, as well as from those in

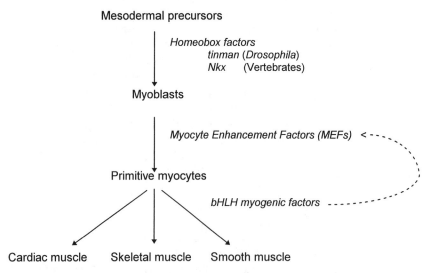

FIG. 6-1. Schematic diagram of myogenesis showing three steps in the transition from an undifferentiated mesodermal cell to differentiated cardiac, skeletal, and smooth muscle. The transcription factors that control the first two steps are similar for these three types of muscle, whereas the final step, which leads to the formation of cardiac, skeletal, and smooth muscle, is governed by different, muscle-specific, factors. This figure is oversimplified in that many of these transcription factors do not act in the strict linear cascade shown here, but instead can interact one with another at a given step; for example, the transition from primitive myocytes to differentiated muscle types is controlled not only by myocyte enhancement factors, but also by basic helix-loop-helix transcription factors (dotted arrow). (Adapted from Fishman and Olson, 1997.)

smooth muscle (for review see Doevendans and van Bilsen, 1996; Firulli and Olson, 1997). Most skeletal muscles arise from somites that appear near the neural tube early in embryonic development, whereas cardiac muscle is derived from anterior lateral plate mesodermal cells that migrate ventrally to form the primitive heart tube. Smooth muscle cells have a more diverse origin, arising from primitive cell types in the neural crest, lateral mesenchyma, and elsewhere. The regulatory factors that control myogenesis in these three muscle types also differ. Common to all are two classes of transcription factors that control the initial steps in myogenesis: the transitions from mesodermal precursors to form myoblasts, and from myoblasts to primitive myocytes (Fig. 6-1).

Homeobox Proteins and Myocyte Enhancer Factors

The two classes of transcription factors that control the initial steps in myogenesis are found in metazoan species ranging from insects and vertebrates (Mably and Liew, 1996; Fishman and Olson, 1997). The first class, which is encoded by *homeobox* genes, regulate the synthesis of proteins that contain highly conserved homeodomains. These homeobox proteins are members of a very important family of transcription factors that coordinate developmental patterning; for example, they program anterior-posterior specializations in the animal body. The homeobox proteins involved in myogenesis include a *drosophila* transcription factor called *tinman* (so named because when it is absent, the fruit fly—like the tin woodman of Oz—has no heart), and the Nkx factors, the vertebrate homologues. Both convert mesodermal precursor cells to primitive myoblasts. The next step in myogenesis is controlled by members of a family of transcription factors called *myocyte enhancer factors* (*MEFs*), which by activating the expression of muscle-specific genes, generate primitive myocytes (see Fig. 6-1).

Members of a quite different class of growth regulators also play an important role in determining dorsal-ventral patterning and left-right asymmetry. These are the peptide growth factors discussed in subsequent paragraphs, whose actions appear to control the looping of the primitive heart tube.

Basic Helix-Loop-Helix Proteins and Other Myogenic Factors

Further specialization into the adult cardiac, skeletal, and smooth muscle phenotypes, the third step in Fig. 6-1, is directed by yet another family of transcription factors. These are basic proteins that, because they contain two α-helices separated by a nonhelical loop, are called *basic helix-loop-helix proteins* (abbreviated *bHLH*). Binding of bHLH myogenic factors to specific DNA consensus sequences favors differentiation and inhibits the cell cycle (Olson, 1993; Sartorelli et al., 1993; Edmondson and Olson, 1993; Chien et al., 1993). As shown in Fig. 6-1, bHLH factors can also interact with the MEFs in controlling earlier "steps" in myogenesis. Different bHLH factors promote the synthesis of the adult muscle protein isoforms characteristic of each specific muscle type; these many bHLH myogenic factors appear and then disappear at different times during embryogenesis. Members of the bHLH family that control cardiac myogenesis are quite different from those that operate in skeletal muscle. Best known of the latter are *MyoD, myogenin, Myf-5,* and *MRF4*. The bHLH myogenic factors that operate in the heart, which include *dHAND* and *eHAND*, are even more complex, in part because different regions of the adult heart, including the right and left ventricles, are derived from specialized "modules." These modules govern the architecture of the many structures found in the mature heart (Mably and Liew, 1996; Lin et al., 1997; Firulli and Olson, 1997) and so are responsible for the appearance of atrial and ventricular myocardium, His-Purkinje fibers, nodal cells, and the many other specialized myocardial cells found in the adult heart.

Heterogeneity of the Myocardium

The cellular composition of the adult heart exhibits a remarkable local heterogeneity, even within a given cardiac structure (for review, see Katz and Katz, 1989). For example, striking differences are found in the electrophysiologic properties of the myocardial cells in different layers of the ventricular wall (Antzelevitch et al., 1991; Di Diego et al., 1996; Anyukhovsky et al., 1996) (Fig. 6-2), and cells containing different myosin isoforms are found intermingled in the atrial myocardium (Sartore et al., 1981; Bouvagnet et al., 1984). The latter produces a pattern so elaborate as to resemble a mosaic, in which different cell types constitute the individual tesserae (the colored stones that pattern a mosaic) (Fig. 6-3). This heterogeneity reflects the operation of "subprograms" of gene regulation, which respond to local factors so as to control expression of different isoforms of specific contractile proteins in different regions of the heart. The peptide growth factors and cell adhesion molecules that probably mediate these local responses are discussed later.

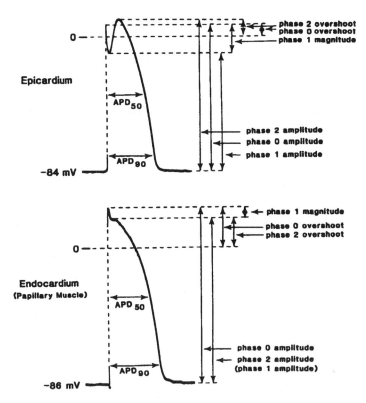

FIG. 6-2. Transmembrane action potentials recorded from a strip of right ventricular epicardium (upper panel) and endocardium (papillary muscle, lower panel). Among the major differences between these layers of the ventricular wall is the much larger dip immediately after the action potential upstroke in the epicardium. (Reprinted from Litovsky and Antzelevitch [1989], by permission of the American Heart Association, Inc.)

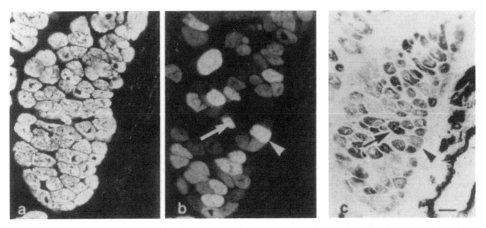

FIG 6-3. Microphotographs of serial sections from the anterior wall of the human right atrium processed for indirect immunofluorescence with two different antiventricular human myosin antibodies (panels a and b), and stained histochemically for myosin ATPase activity (panel c). An antibody that stained all atrial fibers uniformly is shown in panel a, and an antibody that stained certain fibers more strongly than others is shown in panel b. The arrowhead shows a fiber that is highly reactive with the antibody used to stain panel b, but exhibits weak ATPase activity in panel c. The arrow shows a fiber that is weakly reactive with the antibody, but exhibits high ATPase activity. Bar = 20 μ. (Reprinted from Bouvagnet et al. [1984] by permission of the American Heart Association, Inc.)

The interplay between the molecular mechanisms that determine the overall architecture of the heart and the programs and subprograms that regulate local heterogeneities provides a coordinated pattern of growth stimuli that generates the remarkably heterogeneous structure of the adult heart. Although the "master control" is by the myogenic factors outlined in Fig. 6-1, it is the local factors that, in the last analysis, probably have the "final say" in determining the composition of each individual myocyte in the adult heart (Mima et al., 1995).

Clinical Significance

Genetic abnormalities in the myogenic determinants that regulate the subprograms described in the preceding paragraphs may play a role in some clinical cases of dilated cardiomyopathy. Several studies have focused on the actions of a family of zinc-based transcriptional regulators called *LIM*. The latter promote both myogenesis (Arber et al., 1994) and formation of a cytoskeletal protein called *MLP*, which is part of the network of intracellular fibers that provides a scaffolding within cells (Schemeichel and Beckerle, 1994). Transgenic mice deficient in the LIM protein exhibit cytoskeletal disruption and develop a dilated cardiomyopathy that resembles that seen clinically (Arber et al., 1997) as do animals with abnormalities in MEF2, which, along with a bHLH, regulates the expression of another cytoskeletal protein called *desmin* (Kuisk et al., 1996). The relationship between cytoskeletal protein mutations and dilated cardiomyopathies is described further in Chapter 8, which discusses the implications of evidence that up to one third of patients with idiopathic dilated cardiomyopathies have a familial basis for their heart failure.

THE CELL CYCLE

The integrated molecular control system that governs cell proliferation, in which one cell becomes two cells, is often called the *cell cycle*. Much more is involved in this process than *mitosis*, the mechanical separation of two daughter cells, each containing a set of genes duplicated from the mother cell. In addition to the culminating event of cell division, the cell cycle proceeds through of a series of highly regulated and coordinated steps involving cell enlargement, the synthesis of a new complement of DNA, and nuclear division. Each of these steps is regulated by interlocking signaling factors that coordinate the many steps in this vital process.

The antiquity of the cell cycle is evidenced by similarities in the mechanisms that regulate gene expression in organisms that diverged very early in evolution, and by remarkable congruencies in the actions of the molecules that regulate the cell cycle in different species. The ancient origin of these regulatory mechanisms was noted in Chapter 4, which considered the ability of several quite different molecules to evoke similar responses to stress. The catecholamine norepinephrine, as well as the peptides angiotensin II, endothelin, and vasopressin, all increase calcium entry across the plasma membrane, and all cause salt and water retention, vasoconstriction, and positive inotropy. In addition, all regulate gene expression, the most primitive means for adapting to stress. These parallel actions suggest that messenger molecules that stimulated proliferation in early prokaryotes came to be used by the more complex single-celled eukaryotes to fight back—or run away—when attacked. These same messengers were then used by multicellular organisms to mount the coordinated response that, in Chapter 4, was called the "hemodynamic defense reaction."

The Cell Cycle in Prokaryotes

The role played by the cell cycle in responding to stress is seen clearly in prokaryotes, in which cell proliferation allows these primitive living organisms to meet a challenge; as already noted, they literally grow their way out of trouble. These early life forms lack a formed nucleus (hence the name *prokaryote*) and other internal membrane structures, and have little ability to control their internal environment. The DNA in prokaryotic cells is a circular molecule that undergoes replication essentially without interruption, with only brief pauses during cell division. Because the cell cycle is continuously active, prokaryotes can be viewed as growth machines. As each prokaryote represents an independent entity with its own specific complement of expressed genes, rapid selection and proliferation of cells best able to survive an environmental change provide a very effective means to allow a population to adapt to a new challenge. Thus, when a population of prokaryotes encounters a stress, such as a change in the composition of the surrounding sea water, survival is made possible by the ability of a few hardy organisms to replace the population with cells selected for their ability to survive the stress. Even if the vast majority succumb to the perils of the environment, the rapidity of cell cycling allows a few survivors to multiply quickly to fill the ecologic niche.

Bacteria, our modern prokaryotes, illustrate the advantages of rapid growth. Some bacteria can divide every 20 minutes, so that by doubling three times an hour, a single individual can generate more than 4 billion descendants—almost the human population of this planet—in a bit more than 10 hours. At the same time, these rapidly dividing cells undergo genetic diversification, which allows a bacterial population to respond to an environmental change by selecting and reproducing those individuals whose gene products favor survival. This is the basis for the development of antibiotic resistance.

The Cell Cycle in Eukaryotes

In contrast to rapidly proliferating prokaryotes, the cell cycle in the more complex eukaryotic cells is neither continuous nor constant in rate, but instead occurs in spurts. Another difference between prokaryotes and eukaryotes is that in the latter, DNA replication, which is completed before the cell divides, occurs within a membrane-enclosed nucleus (hence the name *eukaryote*, which simply means having a discrete nucleus). The pauses that occur between mitoses are necessary to allow the newly formed eukaryotes to rebuild and reorganize their complex, often highly specialized, internal structure.

The rate of cell cycling varies greatly among eukaryotic cells, with pauses averaging 10 to 20 hours, but often much longer. In the heart, as already noted, cell division ends shortly after birth, after which the pause lasts essentially forever. Control of the cell cycle in these intricately designed cells requires elaborate systems to organize and coordinate the various steps that lead to cell division. As discussed later, growth factors that stimulate overloaded cardiac myocytes to reenter the cell cycle probably play an important role in causing the progressive deterioration of the failing heart.

Polyploidy

Nuclear division (*karyokinesis*) and cell division (*cytokinesis*) are usually coordinated with each other, so that the cell cycle gives rise to daughter cells containing a single nucleus. In some tissues, however, karyokinesis can occur without cytokinesis, giving rise to multinucleate cells. This occurs in the heart, where early in postnatal life, myocardial cell division (cytokinesis) ceases before nuclear division (karyokinesis). In some cells, DNA replication can take place with neither cytokinesis nor karyokinesis, which results in a *polyploid cell* that contains more than two sets of chromosomes. According to Rumyantsev (1977), about 25% of normal adult human cardiac myocytes are diploid and more than half are tetraploid. There are several reports that polyploidy is increased in the hypertrophied heart (Sandritter and Scomazzi, 1964; Kompmann et al., 1966; Grove et al., 1969; Vliegen et al., 1995), especially when the hypertrophy occurs in children (Brodsky et al., 1994). The degree of ploidy also increases with aging (Rumyantsev, 1977; Brodsky et al., 1991). The disproportional increase in DNA in the hypertrophied heart fits with other data that suggest that overload causes some effort at cell division. Following injury to a frog heart, for example, attempts of uninjured myocytes to divide cause these cells to resemble those seen in the overloaded mammalian heart. These changes are described by Rumyantsev (1977) as "dedifferentiative reorganization of cardiac myocytes," in which

> different "attempts" at regeneration were found...such as mitotic and amitotic divisions of myonuclei near sites of lesions, formation of myoblasts, and sprouting of muscle buds from myofiber stumps. All of these manifestations, if found, were generally abortive and not sufficient for regeneration of a considerable part of the destroyed muscle.

A further discussion of the heart's attempts at proliferation is found in Chapter 8.

The similarity of these overload-induced abnormalities to many of the abnormal structural features seen in the failing human heart supports the view that cardiac myocyte hypertrophy represents an unnatural growth response (Katz, 1990, 1994). The following description of key elements and regulators of the cell cycle provides a background to aid in understanding the possible causes of this abnormal growth response.

Phases of the Cell Cycle

The intermittence of cell division in eukaryotes is made possible by a highly regulated cell cycle, which consists of many steps that are controlled by different—but often homologous—families of regulators. The eukaryote cell cycle is generally divided into four phases (Fig. 6-4). Two are active: a phase of DNA replication, called the "*S phase*," and one of cell division, called the "*M phase*." Between these active phases are two "gaps," during which the cells enlarge and carry out their physiologic functions while temporarily suspending most activity that is directly related to cell division. These gaps are the "*G_1 phase*" between M and S, and the "*G_2 phase*" between S and M (see Fig. 6-4). A major regulatory point in the cell cycle occurs late in G_1; this is the *G_1 restriction point,* at which cell cycling stops between "spurts" of cell division (Pardee, 1989). Cells that pass this restriction point become committed to the next cell cycle, which means that cell divi-

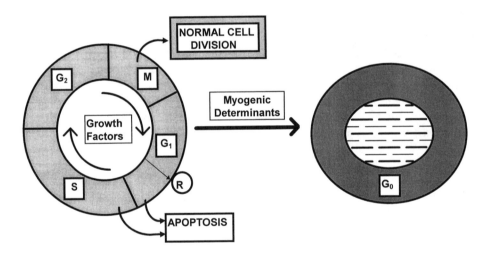

PROLIFERATING　　　　　　　　　　**TERMINALLY DIFFERENTIATED**
FETAL MYOCYTE　　　　　　　　　　　　　**ADULT MYOCYTE**

FIG 6-4. Schematic depiction of the phases of the cell cycle and transition to a terminally differentiated adult cardiac myocyte. Left: The cell cycle, as occurs in the proliferating cells of the embryonic heart, proceeds in a counterclockwise direction. The first "gap" phase, G_1, occurs after mitosis (M). Cells in the G_1 phase can enlarge and carry out their physiologic functions, but from the standpoint of the cell cycle they remain quiescent. Cells in the G_1 phase become committed to the cell cycle when they pass the G_1 restriction point (R). The cell cycle then proceeds though a phase of DNA synthesis (S), a second gap phase (G_2), and normal cell division (M). Cells become susceptible to programmed cell death (apoptosis) late in the G_1 phase and during the S phase. Right: Myogenic determinants cause cells to withdraw from the cell cycle and enter a prolonged quiescent phase, sometimes called G_0, in which they become terminal differentiated, mature adult myocytes.

sion has become independent of *external* stimuli. Once cells are committed to proliferate, each step in the cell cycle remains under the control of interlocked *internal* mechanisms.

In many tissues, including the heart, cells can enter a prolonged quiescent phase during which they cease to divide, and so become "protected" from many stimuli that would otherwise influence gene expression. This quiescent phase of cell proliferation, called G_0, can be viewed as a "side branch" or detour out of the cell cycle (see Fig. 6-4). Use of the term G_0 to describe the quiescent state of the cell cycle in adult cardiac myocytes is not strictly correct because G_0 initially referred to the cell cycle arrest and low metabolic state of serum-depleted cultured cells. A more correct term for the terminally differentiated myocytes of the adult heart might be "permanent arrest in the G_1 phase"; with apologies to the experts, the simpler term G_0 is used throughout this text.

Terminally differentiated cells, such as adult cardiac myocytes, are in this G_0 phase and have virtually no ability to reenter the cell cycle. Thus, even though overload reactivates mechanisms that stimulate cell growth, the terminally differentiated myocytes of the adult heart can make only an abortive attempt to reenter the cell cycle. Unfortunately, such attempts to proliferate turn out badly. The reason is that growth-promoting stimuli that impinge on overloaded cardiac myocytes cannot reverse the transition from G_1 to G_0, and so do not restore the capacity for healthy cell division. Instead, overload initiates a hypertrophic response that, although beneficial in the short-term, shortens the life of the heart (Meerson, 1961). The maladaptive consequences of this effort to reenter the cell cycle indicate that the protection offered by retreat of cardiac myocytes into the quiescent G_0 phase is not absolute. Instead, when cardiac myocytes are stimulated to exit G_0, they undergo an abnormal growth response that I call "cardiomyopathy of overload" (Katz, 1990, 1994). Possible mechanisms responsible for this maladaptive growth response are discussed in Chapter 8.

Cyclins, CDK, and Related Proteins

The cell cycle is controlled by factors that modify the transitions both between and within the phases shown in Fig. 6-4. Most of these factors operate by activating protein kinases that catalyze the phosphorylation of regulatory proteins. The latter include mediators of additional intracellular signaling cascades, and transcription factors that when they bind to specific DNA sequences, modify gene expression. As is true of the interactions between cytokine receptors and JAK, described in Chapter 5, many of these protein kinases are themselves substrates for additional autophosphorylations and cross-phosphorylations that both amplify and inhibit their regulatory effects. Similar patterns are seen in proteins that regulate the cell cycle.

Four classes of protein are central to cell cycle regulation. Two of these, which operate as "matched pairs," are the *cyclin-dependent protein kinases* (*CDK*), and the *cyclins* (Fig. 6-5). The CDKs phosphorylate serine and threonine residues on proteins that control the transitions between the phases of the cell cycle depicted in Fig. 6-4, whereas cyclins regulate CDK activity. The many isoforms of the cyclins and CDKs form pairs in which a given CDK is regulated by a specific cyclin. The CDKs are enzymatically inactive until they bind to their appropriate cyclin, which then partially activates the CDK; however, full activation of the CDKs requires additional factors (see later discussion). The interactions between cyclins and CDKs are analogous to those between the regulatory and catalytic subunits of cyclic AMP-dependent protein kinases (PKA), with which they share structural homologies; however, the regulatory subunit of PKA inhibits kinase activity, whereas cyclins activate CDK.

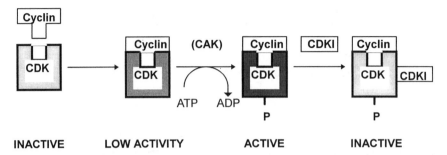

FIG. 6-5. The major regulators of the cell cycle are a class of protein kinases called CDK (cyclin-dependent protein kinases), which, in their basal state, are inactive. Members of the CDK family interact specifically with and are activated by their individual cyclins to form cyclin/CDK pairs. Activation by cyclin, however, is only partial. Full activation requires phosphorylation of the cyclin-bound CDKs by another class of protein kinases called CAK (CDK-activating kinases). Important inactivators of the phosphorylated cyclin/CDK pairs include CDKIs (cyclin dependent kinase inhibitors). Additional regulation (not shown) is effected by phosphatases that dephosphorylate the CDKs, and several additional proteins.

By themselves, cyclins achieve only a partial activation of their corresponding CDKs; as shown in Fig. 6-5, full CDK activity requires the participation of the third family of proteins, called *CDK-activating kinases* (*CAK*). The latter, yet another class of protein kinases, phosphorylate and activate the cyclin–CDK complex (see Fig. 6-5) (Jeffrey et al., 1995: Morgan, 1955). The fourth major family of proteins that regulates the cell cycle are the *cyclin-dependent kinase inhibitors* (*CDKI*) (Nasmyth and Hunt, 1993; Peters, 1994), which help to turn off the cell cycle by inhibiting the active, phosphorylated cyclin/CDK pairs (see Fig. 6-5).

Figure 6-5 provides only an overview of cell cycle regulation. Omitted in this three-step sequence are many additional regulatory reactions, including at least one phosphorylation that inactivates phosphorylated cyclin/CDK pairs, and proteins that regulate various steps in these reactions. The latter include phosphatases that inhibit cell cycling by dephosphorylating CDKs after they are phosphorylated by CAK, and both the peptide growth factors and adhesion molecules that are described later in this chapter.

Cyclin/CDK pairs activate the many steps of the cell cycle; they stimulate cell growth in G_1, promote DNA replication in S, and induce cell division in M. Other cyclin/CDK pairs stimulate the transitions from G_2 to M, and from G_1 to S. Downregulation of a pair that plays a key role in both S and the transition from G_2 to M may stimulate the heart to withdraw from the cell cycle (Yoshizumi et al., 1995). Other cyclins that respond to angiotensin II–stimulated signaling cascades (Sadoshima et al, 1997) may play an important role in the cardiomyopathy of overload. The actions of cyclin/CDK pairs are not limited to cell cycle regulation; some interact with the myogenic determinants discussed earlier and the "pocket" proteins that are described in the following section.

Retinoblastoma Protein and Related Tumor Suppressor ("Pocket") Proteins

Among the most important substrates for cyclin/CDK-catalyzed phosphorylations are members of a family of growth-regulatory proteins whose prototype is the *retinoblastoma protein* (called *pRb* in this text). Children who lack both copies of the retinoblastoma gene exhibit abnormal proliferation of their retinal cells, which undergo malignant transformation and often form metastasizing tumors. In fact, pRb is a general inhibitor of tumorigenesis, as evidenced by the tendency of children with retinoblastoma gene defects to develop osteogenic sarcomas and other malignancies. It is clear that these clinical manifestations are caused by loss of the normal cell cycle inhibition by pRb, which for this reason is often referred to as a *tumor suppressor* (for reviews, see Peeper and Bernards, 1997; Herwig and Strauss, 1997; Dynlacht, 1997; Maioni and Amati, 1997). The tumor suppressor proteins are among the most important regulators of the cell cycle; they are also called "pocket" proteins because their structure includes a pocket that reversibly binds a number of transcription factors (Fig. 6-6). In the heart, the most important member of this family is p107, which is homologous to pRb (Ewen et al., 1993; Gu et al., 1993).

The regulatory actions of the pocket proteins are modulated when phosphorylation and dephosphorylation changes their affinity for binding to transcription factors that regulate cell cycling and gene expression (see Fig. 6-6). In the hypophosphorylated (growth-inhibitory) state, in which few serine and threonine residues are phosphorylated, the pocket proteins bind, and so inactivate, important transcription factors such as E2F. Serine and threonine phosphorylation converts the pocket proteins to their hyperphosphorylated (growth-permissive) state, in which a reduced affinity for these DNA-binding peptides "kicks" E2F out of the pocket. This activates the transcription factors, which become able to regulate specific genes (see later discussion).

Phosphorylation and dephosphorylation of various pocket proteins regulate such important processes as cell division, myogenesis and differentiation (Walsh and Perlman, 1997), and apoptosis (Hertwig and Strauss, 1997; Wang et al., 1997). Their ability to serve as substrates for many different protein kinases allows the pocket proteins to provide a "convergence point" at which a multitude of tyrosine kinase receptors, steroid receptors, and G-protein–coupled receptors all initiate regulatory phosphorylations (reviewed by Bartek et al., 1997). Protein kinases that hyperphosphorylate the pocket proteins include not only the cyclin/CDK pairs that regulate the cell cycle (Ravitz and Wenner, 1997) but also some of the bHLH myogenic factors discussed earlier. One way that these myogenic factors cause differentiation and inhibit cell cycling is by "locking" the pocket proteins in the hypophosphorylated, growth-inhibitory state (Gu et al., 1993; Maione and Amati, 1997). The resulting suppression of cell division is accompanied by other actions of the myogenic factors that stimulate expression of the muscle-specific genes responsible for differentiation of the adult myocyte phenotype. An important way that the myogenic determinants modify the cell cycle is by altering the synthesis of the pocket proteins. This action is seen in the case of MyoD, one of the bHLH myogenic factors important in skeletal muscle differentiation, which inhibits proliferation by increasing expression of the gene that encodes pRb (Martelli et al., 1994). In the heart, where the regulators of myogenesis are different, the major pocket protein, p107, appears to be a less powerful inhibitor of proliferation (Schneider et al., 1994).

The pocket proteins bind a variety of transcription factors and signaling peptides; in addition to those which control the cell cycle, these include tumor viruses, whose oncogenic activity may arise from their ability to sequester these tumor suppressors. Among the most important is a class of transcription factors called E2F, which become inactivated when bound to the hypophosphorylated pocket proteins and, when the pocket proteins are phosphorylated, are released to regulate cell growth and proliferation (see Fig. 6-6).

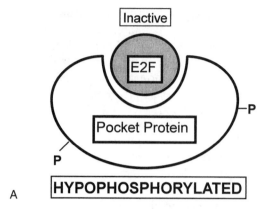

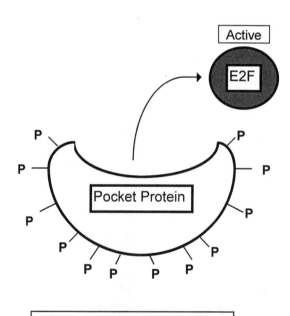

FIG. 6-6. Pocket protein activity is regulated by phosphorylation. In the hypophosphorylated state (**A**), the pocket proteins bind, and so inactivate, transcription factors such as E2F. Phosphorylation of serine and threonine residues in the pocket proteins (**B**) reduces their binding affinity for these transcription factors, which are then released in an active form that regulates gene expression and protein synthesis.

E2F and Related Transcription Factors

There are many different E2Fs, which allows these transcription factors to stimulate expression of genes that encode several proteins that regulate the cell cycle (for reviews, see Hertwig and Strauss, 1997; Bernards, 1997; Ravitz and Wenner, 1997). In the heart, E2F transcription factors repress some of the processes that lead to terminal differentiation. Conversely, in proliferating cells, E2F activates reactions that cause reentry into the cell cycle (Kirshenbaum et al., 1996). In terminally differentiated cardiac myocytes, however, these E2F-mediated reactions can stimulate maladaptive growth.

Binding of E2F by the hypophosphorylated pocket proteins arrests the cell cycle of proliferating cells in the early G_1 phase, and so favors entry into G_0, the quiescent phase where cell cycling stops. Conversely, release of these transcription factors, as occurs when the pocket proteins are phosphorylated by cyclin/CDK pairs, provides a powerful stimulus for growth. Release of one E2F in mid to late G_1 stimulates the cell cycle to proceed beyond the restriction point, thereby committing the cell to DNA synthesis and eventual mitosis. The link between cell growth and cell death, which represents one of the "hazards" of cell cycling, is seen in the ability of some E2Fs to induce apoptosis (Qin et al., 1994; Kirshenbaum et al., 1996), a topic that is considered later.

The interweaving of the many regulatory mechanisms that control cell proliferation is seen in the many different ways that signals induced by E2F can be turned off (Fig. 6-7). In addition to forming a complex with hypophosphorylated pocket proteins, E2F can be inactivated when it is phosphorylated by one of the cyclin/CDK pairs (cyclinA/CDK2) and when this cyclin/CDK pair binds the transcription factor. Yet another layer of regula-

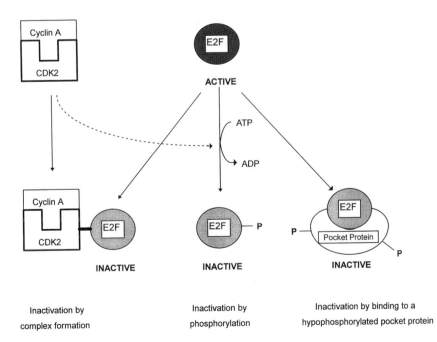

FIG. 6-7. The transcription factor E2F can be inactivated in several ways: when it forms a complex with the cyclin/CDK pair cyclin A/CDK2 (left), by CDK-catalyzed phosphorylation (center), and by binding by a hypophosphorylated pocket protein (right).

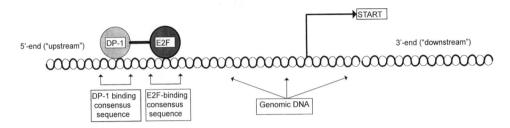

Fig. 6-8. Members of the E2F family of transcription factors bind with high specificity to a sequence of base pairs in the 5′-region of the genomic DNA called an "E2F-binding consensus sequence." E2F-binding to this regulatory region can increase or decrease expression of the protein encoded by the gene. This regulation reflects the ability of E2F to modify replication of the DNA sequence downstream from the "START" region that begins the encoding of the protein transcribed by this gene. E2F often interacts with another family of transcription factors, called DP-1, to form a heterodimer that regulates gene expression.

tion is provided by changes in the rate of synthesis of E2F; for example, levels of the mRNA that encodes E2F are increased late in the G_1 phase of the cell cycle, which suggests that accelerated transcription of the E2F gene amplifies its growth-promoting signal. The ability of E2F transcription factors to form heterodimers with members of another family of transcription factors called DP-1 (Fig. 6-8) illustrates further the elaborate control mechanisms that regulate cell proliferation (for reviews, see Hertwig and Strauss, 1997; Bernards, 1997; Ravitz and Wenner, 1997).

In this discussion of cell cycle regulation, many aspects of this system are not discussed to avoid making the discussion more complex than necessary in keeping the focus on mechanisms that help in understanding how these regulatory mechanisms contribute to the pathophysiology of heart failure.

PEPTIDE GROWTH FACTORS

Our discussion of differentiation, growth, and proliferation has, up to this point, focused on regulatory mechanisms that operate *within cells*, highlighting the roles of the myogenic factors, cyclin/CDK pairs, pocket proteins, and E2F, which control molecular events occurring in the cytoplasm and nucleus. At this point, the focus of this discussion of cell growth shifts across the plasma membrane, from the intracellular control systems to regulatory factors that originate *outside of cells*. As is true of most topics discussed in this chapter, understanding of extracellular signaling mechanisms is expanding rapidly. Because this represents yet another vast topic, the emphasis here is on the general features of a few selected extracellular messengers. This discussion does not focus on the growth factors that are most important in causing the deleterious effects of hypertrophy because the molecular basis for the transition from adaptive to maladaptive hypertrophy, while vitally important, is poorly understood.

The importance of extracellular factors in controlling cell growth in eukaryotes became apparent in early efforts to culture normal mammalian cells in artificial media. Because the media used in these studies lacked factors needed to stimulate proliferation, most of these cultured cells lost their ability to divide, DNA synthesis ceased, and the cell cycle generally came to a halt just before the restriction point in the G_1 phase discussed earlier. Addition of nutrients, vitamins, and trace elements failed to restore the ability of these cultured cells to divide, whereas addition of serum (e.g., fetal calf serum) to artificial media bathing these quiescent cells generally initiated proliferation. The ingredients essential for cell division contained in these sera came to be called "growth factors." In some cases, mammalian cells were found to have become independent of the external factors that normally control cell cycling; because such cells exhibit the uncontrolled growth characteristic of malignancy, they are said to have undergone *malignant transformation.*

Factors that stimulate cell proliferation include a family of extracellular signaling peptides, called *peptide growth factors* (for a recent overview, see Waltenberger, 1997). In addition to regulating the cell cycle, these growth factors exert a multitude of effects on protein synthesis, gene expression, and cell proliferation. Several of these growth factors were first identified through their ability to induce malignant transformations. These peptides, many of which are listed in Table 5-1, are members of the cytokine family; they include platelet-derived growth factor (PDGF), epidermal growth factor (EGF), fibroblast growth factor (FGF), insulin-like growth factor (IGF), vascular endothelial growth factor (VEGF), and transforming growth factor (TGF). Although generally named for the tissues from which they were first isolated, or whose growth they were initially found to stimulate, such terms as "platelet-derived growth factor" or "fibroblast growth factor" do not imply tissue specificity. Instead, like most growth factors, these peptides regulate growth and proliferation in many cell types throughout the body. Key to appreciating the biologic function of the peptide growth factors is that, because they often mediate autocrine and paracrine signaling, most serve as *local* growth regulators.

Growth Factor Receptors and Cell Signaling

Growth factors reach their receptors on the cell surface by way of the extracellular fluid; their source can be distant cells (endocrine signaling), adjacent cells (paracrine signaling), or the same cell that binds the growth factor (autocrine signaling). The cellular effects of the peptide growth factors, like those of the inflammatory cytokines, begin when these peptides bind to membrane receptors. The ligand-bound receptors then form aggregates that activate either of two classes of protein kinase (Table 6-2). In most cases, the substrate for these kinases is the amino acid tyrosine; a major exception is the TGF-β superfamily, which like the cyclin/CDK pairs, generally activate kinases that phosphorylate serine and threonine.

The signaling cascades set into motion when these growth factors interact with their receptors are similar to those initiated by the inflammatory cytokines discussed in Chapter 5. Key to the subsequent steps in these intracellular pathways is a sequence of phosphorylations that is initiated when ligand-bound receptors form aggregates that activate latent protein kinases. There are, however, many differences in the details of these pathways. For example, the receptors that bind inflammatory cytokines can form both trimers,

TABLE 6-2. *Major receptor types and protein kinases activated by peptide growth factors*

Receptors that activate *tyrosine kinases*
  Ligands: PDGF, EGF, FGF, IGF, VEGF
Receptors that activate *serine/threonine kinases*
  Ligands: the TGF family

  PDGF, Platelet-derived growth factor; EGF, epidermal growth factor; FGF, fibroblast growth factor; IGF, insulin-like growth factor; VEGF, vascular endothelial growth factor; TGF, transforming growth factor.

as in the case of TNF-α, or dimers, as in the case of the interleukins, whereas many peptide growth factor receptors form tetramers. Furthermore, most inflammatory cytokine receptors are not themselves tyrosine kinases, but instead activate other tyrosine kinases, whereas peptide growth factor receptors are themselves often latent kinases. Receptors for inflammatory cytokines and most peptide growth factors eventually activate tyrosine kinase activity, but a few of the latter activate serine/threonine kinases. These and other differences allow the different members of this family of extracellular peptides to activate specific intracellular signal transduction pathways, and so to evoke different cellular responses.

The following discussion highlights the actions of two peptide growth factors that have quite different effects on the heart. These are fibroblast growth factor (FGF), which in cardiac myocytes can be viewed as a cell cycle activator, and transforming growth factor β (TGF-β), which plays an important role in healing and fibrous tissue proliferation. These generalizations, like the distinction between "inflammatory cytokines" and "growth factors," are not always valid. In the case of the FGF and TGF-β families, different peptides have different effects in different tissues—even in the same tissue under different conditions.

Fibroblast Growth Factor

The FGFs constitute a ubiquitous family of signaling peptides that plays a major role in cell-cell communication, and in communicating changes in the external environment to the cell interior (for review, see McKeehan et al., 1998). Their actions are mainly local, within tissues, so that these peptides operate quite differently than the circulating mediators of the hemodynamic defense reaction, which have effects on distant organs. The actions of FGF generally oppose those of the bHLH myogenic factors, which, as discussed earlier, inhibit proliferation and stimulate differentiation by direct effects on gene transcription and by "locking" the pocket proteins in their hypophosphorylated growth-inhibitory state. In general, FGF stimulates proliferation and inhibits differentiation (Engelmann et al., 1993; Mima et al., 1995; Corda et al., 1997), although different FGFs can evoke quite different cellular responses (Parker et al., 1990). The effects of FGF generally oppose not only those of bHLH, but also of TGF-β (Table 6-3).

The FGFs communicate their signals much as the inflammatory cytokines described in Chapter 5: both bind to receptors to form aggregates, often involving additional proteins, and both modify cell function when they activate tyrosine kinases. As shown in Table 6-4 and Fig. 6-9, three protein families participate in FGF signaling (McKeehan and Kan, 1994; Green et al., 1996; Vlodavsky et al., 1996; McKeehan et al., 1998). In ad-

---

TABLE 6-3. *General patterns of the effects of FGF and TGF-β in the heart*

FGF (fibroblast growth factor)
    Stimulates proliferation (acidic FGF)
    Inhibits differentiation and myogenesis
    Promotes expression of the fetal gene program (basic FGF)
    Promotes expression of more primitive gene programs (acidic FGF)
TGF-β (transforming growth factor-β)
    Inhibits proliferation
    Stimulates differentiation and myogenesis
    Promotes expression of the fetal gene program
    Stimulates fibrosis

TABLE 6-4. *Three components that mediate signaling by fibroblast growth factors*

Fibroblast growth factor (FGF): regulatory peptides that are members of the cytokine family. Most contain heparin-binding sites that interact with the extracellular matrix.
FGF receptor tyrosine kinase (FGFRTK): membrane proteins that bind FGF with high affinity. These receptors also contain an extracellular heparin-binding domain, intracellular tyrosine kinase sites, and tyrosine molecules that are substrates for regulatory phosphorylations.
FGF receptor heparan sulfate proteoglycan (FGFRHS): glycoproteins that contain polysaccharides which potentiate FGF effects, stabilize and protect FGFs from inactivation, help to aggregate FGF-receptor complexes, and sequester FGFs near their high affinity receptors.

dition to FGF itself, a class of receptors called *FGF receptor tyrosine kinases* (*FGFRTK*) binds this peptide growth factor with high affinity. The FGF receptors contain extracellular FGF- and heparin-binding domains; their intracellular domain includes both tyrosine kinase catalytic sites and tyrosine residues that serve as substrates for "downstream" phosphorylation reactions (see Fig. 6-9). When bound to FGF, the extracellular heparin-binding domain of the FGF receptors associates with the third component of the signal transduction complex, called *FGF receptor heparan sulfate proteoglycan* (*FGFRHS*). The latter are glycoproteins that potentiate the actions of FGF; they also stabilize FGFs, help to aggregate FGF-receptor complexes, and possibly sequester FGFs near their high affinity receptors (Vlodavsky et al., 1996). The FGF receptor heparan sulfate proteoglycans are anchored in the plasma membrane by their membrane-spanning domains, which allows the sugar moieties to interact with the FGF-FGF receptor complex in the extracellular space (see Fig. 6-9).

As is so common in biology, there are many isoforms of FGF. Members of this family of signaling proteins, which are encoded by at least ten genes, are sometimes divided into acidic and basic peptides, both of which are expressed in the heart. There are also many different FGF receptors, which are encoded by at least four genes; this diversity is increased further by alternative splicing. FGF receptors are found in many mammalian tissues, including adult cardiac myocytes (Liu et al., 1995).

A clue as to the evolutionary origin of the FGFs is provided by participation of the proteoglycan FGFRHS in the complex formed between FGFs and the FGFRTK receptors (see Table 6-4, see Fig. 6-9). This proteoglycan is a member of a family of sugar-rich proteins found in the extracellular matrix, where they make up a meshwork of proteins and complex polysaccharides that holds cells together. In addition to contributing to the connective tissue scaffolding of the extracellular matrix, proteoglycans are found in cartilage and basal laminae. The participation of proteoglycans in FGF signaling suggests that this peptide growth factor may have evolved to communicate changes in the extracellular matrix as signals that modify the growth of nearby cells. Echoes of this type of interaction are discussed later, when we examine the role of adhesion molecules and the cytoskeletal proteins in mediating signals that regulate growth and proliferation.

Members of the FGF family of peptides appear to be essential for cardiac myocyte proliferation early in embryonic development (Mima et al., 1995) and to mediate autocrine growth-promoting stimuli following a transient increase in plasma membrane permeability ("wounding") (Clarke et al., 1995; Kaye et al., 1996). Some proliferative effects of FGF are mediated by the ability of these peptides to increase the number of calcium channels (Merle et al., 1995). Although FGFs generally stimulate proliferation and inhibit myogenesis, the many members of this peptide family have divergent effects (for review, see Schneider and Parker, 1992; Cummins, 1993; Schneider et al., 1994). For example, whereas basic FGFs selectively increase the expression of fetal cardiac genes in the heart,

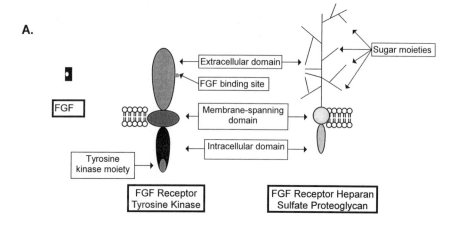

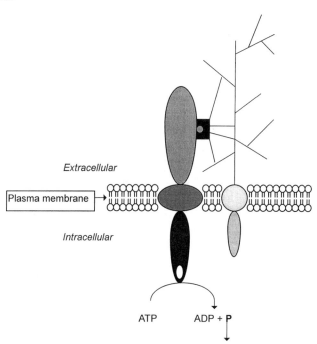

FIG. 6-9. Components of the FGF signaling system (**A**) include three proteins: FGF, its plasma membrane receptor (FGF receptor tyrosine kinase), and an FGF receptor heparan sulfate proteogylcan. Sugar moieties in the latter participate in FGF binding and link this complex to the extracellular matrix. Formation of the heterotrimeric complex (**B**) activates a latent tyrosine kinase in the intracellular domain of the FGF receptor. The resulting tyrosine phosphorylation activates steps further "downstream" in this signal transduction cascade.

acidic FGFs can exert opposing effects on some genes (Parker et al., 1992). These peptides, which play a role in the highly orchestrated growth response following injury, probably participate in the signaling mechanisms that generate the different cardiac phenotypes that appear in overloaded and failing hearts (see later discussion). Much remains to be learned of the role of the FGFs in mediating the hypertrophic response of the heart following the imposition of a chronic overload, so that the possibility that modifying the FGF signal transduction system might improve prognosis in patients with heart failure remains largely conjectural.

Transforming Growth Factor β (TGF-β)

The cellular actions of TGF-β highlight the many ways by which peptide growth factors can regulate cellular behavior. Members of the large TGF-β family influence a variety of functions, including fibrous tissue growth, cell proliferation, differentiation, embryogenesis, and programmed cell death, and like other signaling peptides, TGF-β can operate by autocrine, paracrine, and endocrine mechanisms. One of the major effects of TGF-β is to activate fibrosis, which plays a major role in the response to issue injury (Border and Noble, 1994, 1998; Grande, 1998). Members of the TGF-β family also regulate dorsal-ventral patterning (for review, see Hill, 1996) and left-right asymmetry (Meno et al., 1996; Collignon et al., 1996; Lowe et al., 1996) at the beginning of embryonic life. These major programs of gene expression complement the anterior-posterior patterning controlled by the homeobox genes discussed earlier. Many of the effects of TGF-β on the heart oppose those of FGF (see Table 6-3).

The cellular actions of TGF-β, like those of the other cytokines, are initiated when this growth factor binds to specific plasma membrane receptors (for review, see Hill, 1996; Grande, 1997; Cox and Maurer, 1997; Whitman, 1997; Heldin et al., 1997). TGF-β signaling depends on two classes of TGF-β receptors, called type I and type II, which operate together in forming aggregates that mediate the signals initiated by the arrival of TGF-β at the cell surface (Fig. 6-10). These two receptor types, which play different roles in the ligand-receptor aggregates, include extracellular, membrane-spanning, and intracellular domains; both contain serine/threonine kinase catalytic sites, but only the type II receptors actually bind TGF-β.

TGF-β signaling begins when two of the type II receptors bind to a homodimer formed by two TGF-β molecules (see Fig. 6-10). The tetrameric ligand–receptor complexes formed by the TGF-β dimer and the two type II receptors then aggregate with two type I receptors to form a heterohexamer that activates a latent protein kinase activity in the type II receptors. This stimulates the type II receptors to phosphorylate the type I receptors (see Fig. 6-10), which activates the protein kinase moieties on the type I receptors. This is key to subsequent signaling by TGF-β because the activated type I receptors then catalyze a series of serine/threonine phosphorylations that propagate the TGF-β signal into the cell interior.

A major substrate for phosphorylation by the activated type I TGF-β receptors is a family of signaling molecules, called SMADS or MADs (Niehrs 1996; Wrana and Pawson, 1997), names that illustrate the whimsy seen in molecular biology: *MAD* is an acronym for "mothers against dpp," with *dpp* being the TGF-β that controls the dorsal-ventral patterning mentioned earlier. When phosphorylated, the SMAD proteins form aggregates that enter the nucleus where they generally inhibit cell proliferation and induce fibrosis. The SMADs, which are directly phosphorylated by the TGF-β receptor aggre-

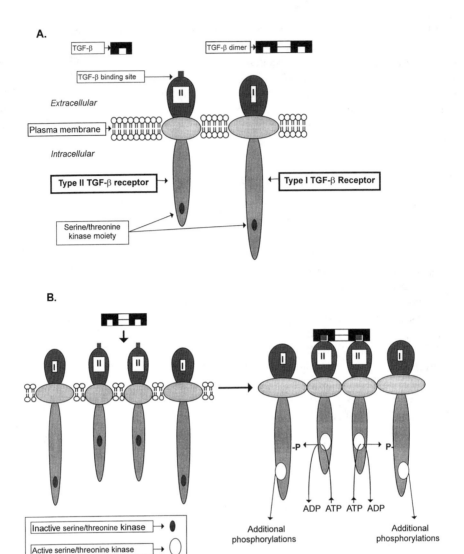

FIG. 6-10. Components of the TGF-β signaling system (**A**) include TGF-β and two types of TGF-β receptor called type I and type II. Signals are generated by a hexameric complex (**B**) made up of the TGF-β homodimer, two type II receptors, and two type I receptors. Formation of this aggregate activates the latent serine/threonine kinase activity of the type II receptor, which phosphorylates and activates the type I receptor. The activated type I receptor then mediates further signal transduction within the cell by phosphorylating additional cytosolic proteins.

gates, provide a "shortcut" that bypasses the more highly regulated MAP kinase pathways (see Chapter 7).

Other substrates for type I TGF-β receptor-catalyzed phosphorylation include the CD-KIs, which as discussed earlier, inhibit the cell cycle by inactivating cyclin-activated CDKs (see Fig. 6-5). This response allows TGF-β to slow the cell cycle by inhibiting CDK-mediated phosphorylation of pRb. These effects—activation of growth-inhibitory effects of the SMADs and inhibition of the activity of the pocket proteins—represent but two of the many ways that TGF-β can inhibit cell proliferation. Additional effects of TGF-β to slow the cell cycle reflect the ability of these peptides to modify the synthesis of various CDKs and other cell cycle regulators (for review, see Cummins, 1993; Ravitz and Wenner, 1997).

In neonatal cardiac myocytes, TGF-β generally opposes the growth-promoting effects of FGF by inhibiting DNA synthesis and cell proliferation (for reviews, see Cummins, 1993; Brand and Schneider, 1996). In the adult heart, TGF-β promotes fibrosis and, like FGF, can redirect the pattern of protein synthesis to favor expression of fetal genes (Parker and Schneider, 1990). This reprogramming of the patterns of gene expression is similar to that which accompanies hypertrophy of the overloaded heart. The early appearance of TGF-β in the overloaded heart (Villareal and Dillmann, 1992) suggests that this growth factor plays a role both in the fibrotic reaction and in redirecting the overall pattern of gene expression. At this time, however, little is known of the clinical effects that could be caused by modification of the actions of this peptide growth factor.

Other Peptide Growth Factors

The actions of the other peptide growth factors listed in Table 6-2 are not discussed in this text for several reasons. First, a role for these peptides in the pathophysiology of heart failure is not yet clear. Second, it is not likely that most readers will gain much from an elaboration of the mechanisms by which additional peptide growth factors modify cellular function; the effects of FGF and TGF-β just summarized should provide sufficient insight into the general actions of these peptides. Third, and even more compelling, their effects on cell division, growth, and differentiation are not the same in all tissues. Even in a given tissue, the response to a single peptide growth factor can vary, depending on the state of the cells. This remarkable variability is due to in part to tissue- and age-dependent changes in the receptors that bind these peptides and to variations in the signal transduction cascades that are activated by these receptors. Although posing a daunting challenge to those who seek to understand these important signaling systems, this complexity also represents an opportunity for developing new means to slow the progression of the maladaptive growth in the failing heart.

THE CYTOSKELETON AS A SIGNAL MEDIATOR

Cells are not merely bags containing a "soup" in which float such functional elements as myofilaments, membrane delimited organelles, enzymes that generate chemical energy, and regulatory systems. Instead, the cell interior is a highly organized structure, surrounded by the plasma membrane and supported by a protein framework. The latter, called the *cytoskeleton*, is made up of a number of structural proteins that, like the steel work of a modern building—or more realistically like our articulated endoskeletons—maintain the architecture of the cell. In addition to holding key cellular elements in their proper orientation, the cytoskeleton interacts with the proteins of the extracellular matrix and with adjacent cells. These interactions not only serve architectural roles but also allow cells to communicate with the surrounding environment. The proteins that make up the cytoskeleton, therefore, represent more than "beams and girders" that maintain cell shape and organization. The participation of this complex structure in cell signaling creates a situation that is analogous to a wired building, in which the steel framework serves also as the telephone system.

Among the most important regulatory roles of the cytoskeleton are its ability to modify cell growth, cell cycling, and cell proliferation (for reviews, see Davies and Tripathi, 1993; Yamazaki et al., 1995; Meredith et al., 1996; Assoian and Zhu, 1997; Giancotti, 1997, Katz and Yamada, 1997). These effects are initiated when cells adhere to the extracellular matrix or when they contact other cells. These attachments involve much more than such simple physical processes as hydrophobic or electrostatic interactions. Instead, cell attachment to surrounding structures is mediated by proteins that project from the cell surface to bind specifically to proteins in the extracellular connective tissue matrix, or on the surfaces of adjacent cells. Central to these interactions is a family of plasma membrane proteins, called *adhesion molecules*, which associate with nonreceptor tyrosine kinases similar to those that bind the inflammatory cytokines. In terms of the "wired building" analogy, the ability of adhesion molecules to modify cell function in response to mechanical perturbations at the cell surface resembles a situation in which changes in structures that contact the surface of a building generate signals that modify the behavior of the building's occupants.

Adhesion Molecules

The ability of cell adherence to adjoining structures in regulating cell growth and cell cycling was discovered many years ago, when it was noted that, in order for most mammalian cells to proliferate in tissue culture, they needed to adhere to a surface (Stoker et al., 1968). These and other observations demonstrated that interactions between normal cells and both the surrounding extracellular matrix and adjacent cells could stimulate the cell cycle. The dependence of cell cycling on interactions with surrounding structures can be lost, but like cell proliferation in the absence of growth factors, such independence is a hallmark of malignancy.

The responses evoked when a cell contacts its surroundings are mediated by membrane receptors called *adhesion molecules*. These adhesion molecules, which are members of the same family of membrane receptors that bind cytokines and peptide growth factors, fall into several classes (for review, see Hynes and Lander, 1992; Hillis and MacLeod, 1996; Schwartz et al., 1995; Thiery, 1996; Yap et al., 1997). These include the *integrins*, which link cells to the surrounding extracellular matrix, and *cadherins*, which link cells to other cells (Table 6-5).

TABLE 6-5. *Some proteins that participate in cell-matrix and cell-cell communication in the heart*

Cell-matrix communication
  Extracellular matrix proteins
    Fibronectin, laminin, vitronectin, heparans
  Adhesion molecules
    Integrins
  Intracellular cytoskeletal proteins
    Talins, paxillins, vinculins, α-actinin, actin
  Other intracellular mediators
    Focal adhesion kinases
Cell-cell communication
  Gap junction(electrical): the connexins (connexin 43)
  Desmosome (mechanical)
    Adhesion molecules
      Desmogleins
    Intracellular cytoskeletal proteins
      Intermediate (desmin) filaments, desmoplakins, desmin
  Fascia adherens (mechanical)
    Adhesion molecules
      Cadherins
    Intracellular cytoskeletal proteins
      Actin filaments, α-actinin, catenins

Adhesion molecules not only link the proteins of the cytoskeleton to the extracellular matrix and surfaces of adjacent cells, but they also can activate signal transduction systems that modify cell function. Signaling by the adhesion molecules is mediated in part by phosphorylations similar to those initiated by the cytokines discussed in Chapter 5 and the peptide growth factors described earlier in this chapter. Unlike the inflammatory cytokines and peptide growth factors, which are soluble proteins that bind to cytokine receptors, the extracellular ligands that bind to adhesion molecules are fixed in the extracellular matrix (cell-matrix adhesion) or on the surfaces of other cells (cell-cell adhesion).

Mediators of Cell-Extracellular Matrix Interactions: Integrins

The *integrins* are among the most important of the adhesion molecules that link the cytoskeleton to the extracellular matrix. These membrane proteins, which are made up of α- and β-subunits, function as heterodimers. Both subunits bind to extracellular ligands, but only the β subunits link this complex to the cytoskeleton (Fig. 6-11). The integrin family includes at least 16 different α subunits and 8 β subunits, which determine both binding specificity and the cellular effects that are initiated when different integrins bind to various proteins in the extracellular matrix (for reviews, see Meredith et al., 1996: Assoian and Zhu, 1997; Giancotti, 1997; Lafrenie and Yamada, 1997; Hsueh et al., 1998). Besides linking cells to the surrounding connective tissue, this diverse family regulates cell growth and motility, and so plays an important role in the remodeling of the overloaded heart. These effects are due in part to stimulation of the G_0-G_1 and G_1-S transitions of the cell cycle. Interactions between integrins and the extracellular matrix also generate signals that regulate apoptosis (see later discussion). The GPIIb/IIIa molecules that mediate platelet adhesion are members of the integrin family, as are many of the receptors that modify the vascular endothelium (Hillis and MacLeod, 1996).

Matrix proteins that bind to the extracellular domain of the integrins include *collagen*, *fibronectin*, *laminin*, and *vitronectin* (see Table 6-5); as noted later, the response to these binding reactions is determined by the nature of the matrix protein. Sugar-containing *heparans* also participate in the interactions of integrins with fibronectin (Mohri, 1996), which illustrates further the parallels between signal transduction by adhesion molecules and that described earlier for the TGF-βs. The role of the heparans is partly to impart specificity to these interactions (Spillmann and Burger, 1997), which reflects the structural diversity of these glycoproteins, whose elaborate carbohydrate moieties, in some ways, resemble the plumage of a tropical bird.

The responses evoked by the binding of integrins to the extracellular matrix are mediated by cytoskeletal proteins that bind to the intracellular domain of the β subunit of the adhesion molecule (see Table 6-5). These cytoskeletal proteins, which include *talins*, *paxillins*, and *vinculins*, link the integrins to *α-actinin* in the actin filaments within the cell (see Fig. 6-11A). Control of cell signaling by the integrins is mediated by up to 20 additional signal transduction molecules, many of which form aggregates along the plasma membrane that include *focal adhesion kinases* (FAKs), the G protein Ras, and tyrosine kinases of the Src family. These aggregates then activate cytosolic serine/threonine kinases, such as MAP kinase and Jun kinase (Miyamoto et al., 1995), which play a key role in regulating cell growth and proliferation (see Chapter 7).

Cell signaling by the integrins is initiated when the β subunit of integrin binds first to the extracellular matrix and then to the cytoskeleton (see Fig. 6-11B). The resulting complex generally modifies growth and proliferation by activating protein kinases that phosphorylate transcription factors within the cell; in some cases, these complexes can attract

A.

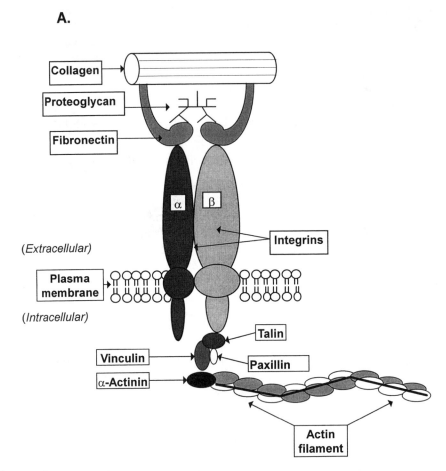

FIG. 6-11. Integrin-binding to the extracellular matrix or to other cells can initiate cell adhesion and stimulate cell signaling. Cell adhesion (**A**) occurs when the heterodimer formed by an α- and a β-subunit of the integrin becomes linked in the extracellular space to collagen (or other matrix proteins) by fibronectin and proteoglycan, and within the cell to actin through interactions with cytoskeletal proteins like talin, paxillin, and vinculin.

mRNA and ribosomes (Chicurel et al., 1998). Other signals are generated when the matrix-bound integrin activates members of a family of FAKs (see Fig. 6-11B), which catalyze the phosphorylation of many of the regulatory peptides discussed earlier. The latter include CDK, cyclins, pocket proteins, and E2F. Integrins also regulate signaling pathways that activate other protein kinases, such as protein kinase C, in reactions that allow these adhesion molecules to activate transcription factors that participate in the *immediate-early gene response* that mediates hypertrophy and remodeling in the overloaded heart (see Chapter 6). Integrins can also induce and suppress apoptosis (Sugahara et al., 1994; Schwartz et al., 1995; Malik, 1997). Together, these actions maintain cell viability, which explains why cell detachment often initiates programmed cell death (Malik, 1997). In the heart, integrin-activated signaling pathways allow cell deformation to regulate protein synthesis and cell proliferation. Along with responses triggered by neurohumoral mediators, inflammatory cytokines, and peptide growth factors, those initiated by the inte-

B.

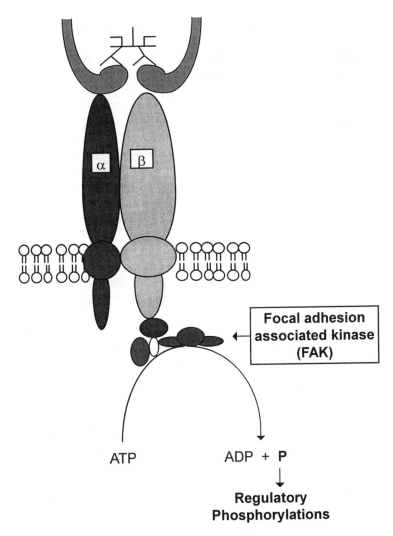

FIG. 6-11. *Continued.* Cell signaling (**B**), like cell adhesion, involves the heterodimer made up of the α- and β-subunits of integrin, the extracellular fibronectin-proteoglycan complex, and the cytoskeletal proteins talin, paxillin, and vinculin. Integrin signaling is mediated by a tyrosine kinase called focal adhesion associated kinase (FAK), which effects signal transduction by phosphorylating additional cytosolic proteins.

grins provide the heart with an array of mechanisms that regulate both cell growth and cell death.

Cell-Cell Interactions in the Heart

Cardiac muscle contains specialized cell-cell junctions, called *intercalated discs*, that provide both mechanical and electrical communication between cells. The intercalated discs include three specialized structures (Table 6-6). One is the *gap junction*, which contains a channel protein called *connexin 43* that allows the relatively free diffusion of ions between the cytosol of adjacent cells. The gap junction channels provide the low resistance intracellular electrical connections needed to conduct the wave of depolarization rapidly through the heart. The second is the *fascia adherens*, which provides mechanical connections between actin filaments in adjacent cells. The *desmosome*, the third structure of the intercalated disc, provides a strong, rivet-like, connection between the intermediate filaments of adjacent cardiac myocytes.

Mechanical connections between cells at the intercalated disc depend on a family of *cell adhesion molecules* (CAMs) that link the cytoskeleton to the extracellular matrix. The most important mediators of cell-cell communication in the heart are the *cadherins*, found in the fascia adherens, and *desmogleins* that are located in desmosomes. Other members of this family include *CAM-Igs*, and *selectins* (for review, see Hynes and Lander, 1992; Thiery, 1996, Kostin et al, 1998). The CAM-Igs, which are members of the immunoglobulin superfamily function (Ig stands for immunoglobulin), are best known for effects on the nervous system, where they play a major role in embryonic development, whereas the selectins are important for leukocyte adhesion.

Most of the cell adhesion molecules involved in cell-cell interaction form homodimers that are made up of similar receptors on the surfaces of adjacent cells (Fig. 6-12). The desmogleins, which link the intermediate ("desmin") filaments of adjacent cells to one other, interact with similar molecules on adjacent cells to form desmoglein homodimers that bind to *desmoplakins* and other cytoskeletal proteins on the intracellular side of the plasma membrane. The cadherins of adjacent cells also attach to each other to form homodimers that attach to actin filaments within the cytosol. Cadherin-binding to actin, like that of integrin, requires the participation of additional cytoskeletal proteins (see Table 6-6). These include the *catenins*, a family of actin-binding proteins that is homologous to vinculin, both contain talin-, paxillin-, and α-actinin-binding regions.

The cadherins, like the integrins, serve a dual function: they form calcium-dependent bonds that link adjacent cells to one another, and they participate in cell signaling, generally by activating tyrosine kinases (for review, see Aberle et al., 1996; Yap et al., 1997). Another link between calcium and mitogenic signaling is provided by calreticulin, a calcium-binding protein found in the subsarcolemmal cisternae of the sarcoplasmic reticulum, which participates in integrin-mediated functions (Coppolino et al., 1997). Both the cadherins and the CAM-Igs mentioned earlier share structural homologies with the FGF receptor, which accounts for the ability of these adhesion molecules to activate FGF receptor tyrosine kinase activity (Baldwin et al., 1996).

Many of the signals initiated by the interactions of cadherins with catenins, and desmogleins with desmin, are mediated by tyrosine phosphorylations within the cell. The latter include reactions that are essential for the development of the vertebrate heart (Nakagawa and Takeichi, 1997; Linask et al., 1997). In addition to regulating cell function, these phosphorylations can also modify the strength of bonds that link adjacent cells to one another.

TABLE 6-6. *Cell-cell communication across the intercalated disc*

Specialized junction	Function	Membrane-spanning protein	Cytoplasmic linkage	Intracellular filament
Gap junction	Electrical communication	Connexin 43	—	—
Fascia adherens	Mechanical linkage	Cadherins	Catenins	Actin
Desmosome	Mechnaical linkage	Desmoglyeins	Desmoplakins	Desmin

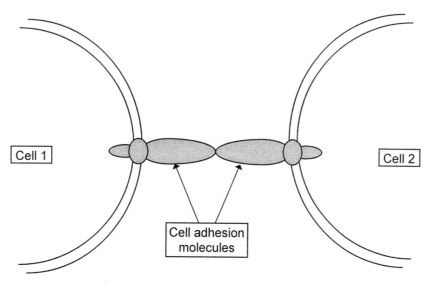

FIG. 6-12. Cell-cell adhesion occurs by formation of a homodimer between two cell adhesion molecules, such as cadherin. Not shown are the many cytoskeletal proteins that participate in these linkages.

Significance of Cytoskeletal Signal Transduction in Overloaded Hearts

Overload-induced mechanical stresses on the walls of the heart can be "sensed" by the adhesion molecules. The responses depend on several factors, including the structure of the adhesion molecule and the matrix proteins with which the adhesion molecules interact. Adherence of myoblast integrins to the matrix protein fibronectin, for example, causes myoblasts to remain in an undifferentiated state where they continue to proliferate, whereas adherence to laminin, another matrix protein, causes the same cells to differentiate and proliferation to cease. The actions of fibronectin in this setting are much like those of a growth factor, whereas laminin acts more like a myogenic determinant. One implication of the specificity of these interactions is seen later in this chapter, when the different cardiac myocyte phenotypes generated by pressure and volume overload are examined.

The ability of cytoskeletal deformation to "sense" changes in the interactions between cardiac myocytes and the surrounding extracellular matrix probably plays an important role in adapting cell size and shape to abnormal physical forces. A remarkable adaptation of form to function is seen in the normal heart, whose violent contractions propel blood through the ventricles in a manner that generates no turbulence, which explains why no murmurs are heard. In the context of the present text, the most important of these deforming forces are those generated by overload. The ability of cytoskeletal deformation to activate a variety of signal transduction cascades undoubtedly contributes to both the short-term adaptive and long-term maladaptive features of the hypertrophic response in failing hearts.

The different responses to increased afterload (pressure overload) and increased preload (volume overload) can be explained if different molecular signals are initiated by increased systolic stress and diastolic stretch, respectively (Wollert et al., 1996). Pressure overload, as in aortic stenosis, causes systolic stress, whereas diastolic stretch is a major consequence of a sustained volume overload, as occurs in aortic insufficiency. Replacement of myocardial tissue with scar after a myocardial infarction causes ventricular dilatation, which, by the operation of the Law of Laplace, increases both diastolic stretch and systolic stress. These different mechanical stimuli can explain the different types of hypertrophy that were noted in the 19th century—the active and passive aneurism described by Corvisart (Chapter 1). As described in subsequent paragraphs, the ability of pressure overload to cause wall thickening with little or no increase in cavity volume (concentric hypertrophy) and of volume overload to cause eccentric hypertrophy and cavity dilatation appear to be due in large part to different patterns of cardiac myocyte enlargement.

STRETCH-OPERATED ION CHANNELS

Mechanical signals that can regulate cellular function are generated by stretch-operated ion channels (for review, see Hu and Sachs, 1997) as well as when cytoskeletal deformation activates various adhesion molecules. These channels open in response to cell stretch; depending on their ion-selectivity, they can carry either inward or outward currents. Most known stretch-operated channels in the heart are either nonselective for sodium and calcium ions (both of which carry depolarizing inward currents) or potassium-selective (which carry repolarizing outward currents). The former play an important role in the pacemaker acceleration caused by right atrial dilatation (the "Bainbridge reflex"), whereas activation of the latter has been suggested to play a role in regulating cell proliferation (for review, see Dubois and Rouzaire-Dubois, 1993).

Stretch of heart muscle has long been known to activate protein synthesis (Peterson and Lesch, 1972), and stretch-operated calcium channels have been implicated as mediators of growth-promoting signals (Whitaker and Patel, 1990). The ability of calcium-mediated signals to stimulate cell growth (Gruver et al., 1993; McDonough et al., 1997; Molkentin et al., 1998) provides some support for the view that stretch-operated calcium channels mediate signals that cause the overloaded heart to hypertrophy. Stretch-operated sodium channels have also been proposed to regulate protein synthesis in the heart (Kent et al., 1989). However, recent studies using various blockers of stretch-operated channels do not support a major role for these channels in regulating the hypertrophic response of overloaded cardiac myocytes (for review, see Yamazaki et al., 1995).

ABNORMAL CARDIAC MYOCYTE PHENOTYPES

The architectural abnormalities seen in the failing heart are due in part to reorganization of myocardial cells and supporting structures (e.g., fiber slippage), and to changes in the size, shape, and molecular composition of individual cardiac myocytes. This cellular plasticity is apparent during normal development, as was discussed earlier in terms of the programs and subprograms that regulate myogenesis. Such structures as nodal cells and His-Purkinje fibers have long been known to represent specialized cardiac myocytes, whose morphology and ultrastructure are highly specialized. The voltage-gated ion channels that generate the action potentials in these cells differ significantly from one another, as well as from those in the atria and ventricles. More recent studies have shown that the specialized electrophysiologic properties of the epicardium, endocardium, and middle regions of the ventricular wall are caused by the expression of different ion channel isoforms (see earlier discussion) and that the myosin heavy chain isoforms expressed in atrial and ventricular myocardial cells also differ, even in adjacent myocytes. This remarkable heterogeneity is made possible by the existence of many different cardiac myocyte phenotypes (Table 6-7), which is almost certainly due partly to local regulation of gene expression by autocrine and paracrine effects of locally produced peptide growth factors and by the operation of the adhesion molecules discussed previously. There are many more cardiac myocyte phenotypes in the heart than are listed in Table 6-7. Normal cardiac development, for example, is not simply a transition from the fetal to the adult phenotype, but instead proceeds by a series of changes in both overall structure and molecular composition that differ in the many regions of the embryonic heart.

Several lines of research point to an important role for changing cardiac phenotype in the pathophysiology of heart failure (for review, see Bugaisky and Zak, 1986; Swynghedauw, 1990, 1999; Bugaisky et al., 1992). Most striking is the reexpression of fetal genes. The pattern of phenotypic changes induced by overload, however, is far more elaborate, and plastic, than a simple reversion to a fetal pattern; for example, the abnormal cardiac myocytes that appear in response to different types of hemodynamic overloading are not all the same. The myocytes generated in exercise-induced hypertrophy of the adult heart (the "athlete's heart"), which can be viewed as a physiologic growth response, are quite different from those seen in pressure overload hypertrophy. In the latter, which is an example of pathologic hypertrophy, both myosin ATPase activity and sarcoplasmic reticulum calcium transport are reduced, whereas both are increased in physiologic hypertrophy (Penpargkul et al., 1977; Scheuer and Bhan, 1979; Malhotra et al., 1981; Scheuer and Buttrick, 1987). More recently, major differences have been found in the molecular composition of pressure- and volume-overloaded hearts (Calderone et al., 1995).

Although much remains to be learned about the signaling systems that program the many phenotypic patterns listed in Table 6-7, it seems reasonable to postulate that physiologic hypertrophy is initiated during training by brief periods of intense adrenergic stimulation accompanied by increased preload and reduced afterload. In pathologic hypertrophy, where growth stimuli persist both day and night, different patterns of cardiac myocyte growth are initiated by increased systolic stress, which causes concentric hyper-

---

TABLE 6-7. *Some examples of different cardiac myocyte phenotypes*

Normal embryonic phenotypes
Normal adult phenotypes
  Working myocardial cells
    Atrial myocardium
    Ventricular myocardium
  Specialized cells
    Nodal cells
    His-Purkinje cells
    Transitional cells
Physiologic hypertrophy phenotype
  The "athlete's heart": exercise-induced hypertrophy
Pathological phenotypes
  Concentric hypertrophy
    Early or mild pressure overload (e.g., aortic stenosis, hypertension)
  Eccentric hypertrophy
    Early or mild volume overload (e.g., aortic and mitral insufficiency)
    Diffuse myocardial damage (e.g., viral or toxic myocarditis)
    Localized myocardial damage (myocardial infarction)
  Decompensated hypertrophy, remodeling: end-stage heart failure
Familial cardiomyopathies:
  Hypertrophic cardiomyopathies
  Dilated cardiomyopathies

trophy, and excessive diastolic stretch, which causes eccentric hypertrophy. These generalizations, however, fall far short of providing the detail needed to define how different types of overload activate different patterns of cell growth. Such knowledge is needed to explain the observation, made, almost 200 years ago, that eccentric hypertrophy (dilatation) is more deadly that concentric hypertrophy (see Chapter 1), and more recent reports that patients with systolic dysfunction have a poorer prognosis than those with diastolic dysfunction (see Chapter 8), observations that suggest that different phenotypes are associated with different rates of myocardial deterioration and cell death.

Shape Changes in the Cells of the Overloaded Heart

Perhaps the clearest manifestations of the operation of different signal transduction pathways in different types of overload are seen when myocardial cell length and cross-sectional area are compared in concentric and eccentric hypertrophy. It is well established that myocyte cross-sectional diameter is markedly increased in compensated concentric hypertrophy (Lowe and Bate, 1948; Linzbach, 1960). The changes that occur in eccentric hypertrophy are more complex. Early reports suggested that the number of fiber layers remains constant as the left ventricle enlarges progressively, which implies that the chamber enlargement is due mainly to rearrangement of unchanged muscle fibers ("fiber slippage") rather than fiber elongation (Linzbach, 1960). More recent studies of the failing human left ventricle, however, have demonstrated that myocyte length is increased in both end-stage ischemic cardiomyopathy and decompensated dilated cardiomyopathy (Gerdes et al., 1992; Beltrami et al., 1994; Zafeiridis et al., 1998). Whereas fiber slippage probably plays an important role in *acute* ventricular dilatation, such as occurs immediately after a large myocardial infarction (Olivetti et al., 1990), the slower dilatation (remodeling) of a damaged ventricle appears to be caused by a combination of myocyte elongation and myocyte death (Gerdes and Capasso, 1995).

Studies of myocytes isolated from normal and diseased human hearts provide elegant support for the view that different loading abnormalities generate different cardiac myocyte phenotypes. In nondilated, hypertrophied hypertensive hearts, myocyte size is increased largely by a greater cross-sectional area (Gerdes et al., 1994). Cell length has been found to be almost 50% greater than normal in myocytes isolated from the dilated, failing hearts of patients following myocardial infarction and with dilated cardiomyopathies (see earlier discussion), but appears to increase only minimally in pressure overload. These architectural differences are accompanied by molecular differences that point to the operation of specific signal transduction pathways in mediating the heart's response to various types of overload. Mitochondrial function, for example, has been reported to be abnormal in pressure overload (Cooper et al., 1973a), but normal in volume overload (Cooper et al., 1973b). Even more dramatic are the many differences in levels of the messenger RNAs that encode key proteins in pressure- and volume-overloaded hearts (Calderone et al., 1995) (Table 6-8). These molecular differences highlight the specificity of the signaling mechanisms and growth responses that lead to concentric and eccentric hypertrophy.

One explanation for the appearance of different hypertrophied myocyte phenotypes in compensated pressure and volume overload is that increased systolic wall stress initiates concentric hypertrophy by causing new sarcomeres to be added in parallel, which increases cell width, whereas in the eccentrically hypertrophied ventricle, diastolic stretch causes new sarcomeric units to be added in series, which increases cell length. This explanation implies that cardiac myocyte thickening and elongation are controlled by dif-

TABLE 6-8. *Left ventricular hypertrophy phenotypes induced by pressure and volume overload**

	Pressure overload	Volume overload
LV weight/body weight	+32%	+34%
Muscle proteins		
β-Myosin heavy chain	+500%	+20%
Skeletal α-actin	+380%	+15%
SERCA2 (calcium pump ATPase)	−28%	−8%
Growth factors		
TGF-β3		
Myocyte	+80%	+5%
Nonmyocyte	+20%	−50%
IGF-1	−	
Myocyte	+130%	+15%
Nonmyocyte	+20%	−35%
Acidic FGF		
Myocyte	−35%	No change
Nonmyocyte	−20%	−10%

*Values are changes in mRNA levels after 7 days compared to control (Calderone et al., 1995).

ferent signaling pathways. Experimental support for this view is found in a report that, in cultured cardiac myocytes, the cytokine cardiotrophin-1 induces cell elongation, whereas phenylephrine, an α-adrenergic agonist, causes these cells to become thicker (Wollert et al., 1996). This report provides evidence that, in the tissue culture model, growth stimuli that use tyrosine kinase-catalyzed phosphorylations cause cell elongation (eccentric hypertrophy), whereas G-protein-dependent growth stimuli, such as are activated by α-adrenergic agonists, increase in myocyte width (concentric hypertrophy). It is not clear, however, that these findings can be extrapolated to the adult heart, which responds differently to many growth stimuli.

The appearance of several abnormal cardiac myocyte phenotypes in the overloaded heart (see Table 6-7) raises the possibility that different drugs can be developed to activate signal transduction pathways that increase myocyte diameter (concentric hypertrophy), and to inhibit pathways that cause cell elongation (eccentric hypertrophy). The obvious value of such hypothetical agents would be to increase cell thickness without causing cells to elongate, an effect that could inhibit the progressive dilatation (remodeling) of the failing heart. Surprisingly, the findings of several experimental studies and clinical trials in patients with heart failure indicate that such drugs already exist. This is evidenced, for example, by the ability of both converting enzyme inhibitors and β-adrenergic blockers to inhibit remodeling. These clinical findings (see Chapter 9) demonstrate the importance of efforts currently underway to identify the molecular signals that initiate and maintain maladaptive growth in the failing heart. Such knowledge not only holds the key to understanding differences between adaptive and maladaptive cardiac hypertrophy, but may also allow development of drugs able to prevent the progressive, and eventually lethal, remodeling of damaged hearts. New means to regulate the signal transduction systems that generate abnormal cardiac phenotypes may therefore make it possible to prevent the transition from adaptive to maladaptive hypertrophy.

PROGRAMMED CELL DEATH (APOPTOSIS)

This text, in a many places, highlights the importance of myocardial cell death as a cause for the poor prognosis in patients with heart failure. The following discussion reviews one potentially important cause for this deterioration, a process called programmed cell death or *apoptosis*.

Before defining apoptosis, I cannot refrain from commenting on the pronunciation—and frequent mispronunciation—of this term. There are reasonable grounds for electing to pronounce or not to pronounce the second "p" in this word (*apo ptosis'* or *apo tosis'*), but there is no basis for the mispronunciation "*a pop' tosis*," which combines parts of the two syllables to create a third, nonsense, syllable. This term is derived from two Greek words, *apo* (away) and *ptosis* (falling), there is no "*pop*" in apoptosis!

The cell death caused by apoptosis is as "natural" as the falling of leaves from a deciduous tree in the autumn; in fact, apoptosis is as essential to our well-being as are cell growth and proliferation (Nagata, 1997; Hetts, 1998). The reason is that apoptosis provides for the orderly elimination of damaged cells, for example, premalignant cells that have a tendency for unchecked growth (for review, see van Noorden et al., 1998). Another important role of apoptosis is to remove cells that are no longer needed, as occurs during embryonic life. It has been estimated that up to half of the neurons that appear in the developing vertebrate nervous system die normally after they form synaptic connections with their target cells (Raff et al., 1993). This role of apoptosis is described elegantly by Savill et al. (1993), who notes that it "is beautifully demonstrated in the developing *drosophila* eye, where to achieve the adult form, thousands of unwanted interommatidal cells undergo programmed death and phagocytosis without disrupting the delicate architecture of the organ." If during early development unneeded cells were not eliminated, then humans would be born with gills, tails, and webs between fingers and toes!

An important feature of apoptosis, which distinguishes this process from necrosis (see later discussion), is that programmed cell death does not evoke a fibrotic reaction; instead, it allows cells to disappear without a trace. This is hardly counterintuitive considering the many cell types that appear and then disappear during embryogenesis; if programmed cell death led to fibrosis, the developing fetus would become a mass of scar tissue. This ability of embryos to remove unneeded tissue by apoptosis, without causing fibrosis, explains why children who have had surgery performed early in fetal life often have no scars at the site of the incision.

A final generalization regarding programmed cell death is based on the many similarities in the mechanisms that regulate apoptosis and proliferation (see later discussion). These similarities, which are so striking that apoptosis has been suggested to represent an abortive form of mitosis (Ucker, 1991), provide a key insight into the biologic role of this form of cell death.

Apoptosis versus Necrosis

It is generally stated that cells can die in two fundamentally different ways: they can be killed by extrinsic injurious factors (necrosis or accidental cell death), or they can be programmed to die by signal transduction systems that operate within the cell (apoptosis or programmed cell death) (for review, see Cohen, 1993; Buja et al., 1993; Manjo and Joris, 1995; Nagata, 1997; Raffray and Cohen, 1997; Wyllie, 1997a; Saini and Walker, 1998; Sabbah and Sharov, 1998; Haunsteter and Izumo, 1998). Certainly, these extremes differ markedly and have very different outcomes. This is evidenced by the vanishing of structures that undergo apoptosis, such as the tail of a tadpole, which is "reabsorbed" without scarring in the mature frog. This outcome is very different from that which follows a third-degree burn, where tissue necrosis leads to fibrous tissue deposition that causes extensive scarring and sometimes keloid formation.

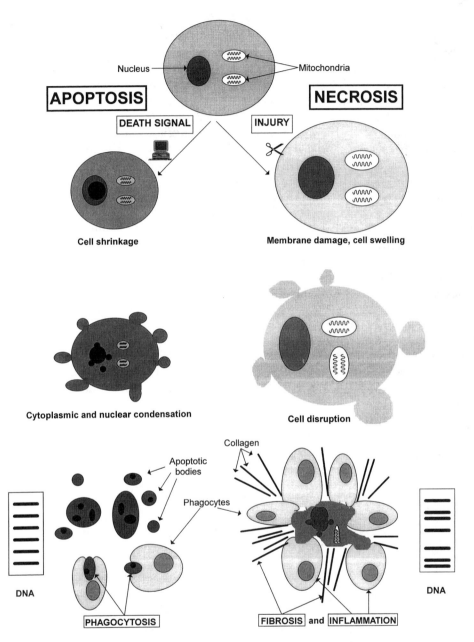

FIG. 6-13. Apoptosis and necrosis are fundamentally different mechanisms of cell death. Apoptosis (left) is a highly regulated process that induces cell shrinkage and condensation of the cytosol and nucleus. These processes yield cell fragments, called apoptotic bodies, which, because they are surrounded by plasma membrane, do not evoke an inflammatory reaction; instead, apoptotic bodies are engulfed and digested by phagocytes. The tight control exerted by the many regulators of apoptosis is seen in the orderly breakdown of DNA. which yields regularly sized fragments that, when run out on gels, resemble ladders. Necrosis (right) is generally caused by injury to the cell membrane, which, because the latter loses its ability to serve as a permeability barrier, causes cells to swell, and eventually to burst. The resulting release of the cell contents initiates an inflammatory reaction that leads to fibrosis and scarring. The breakdown of DNA into random-sized fragments prevents the appearance of the ordered laddering seen in apoptosis.

As might be expected, the processes responsible for these two processes are quite different. Whereas necrosis occurs when injury causes the plasma membrane to become leaky, apoptosis occurs when a "death signal" activates an elaborate regulatory program that requires the expenditure of energy in what can be viewed as cell suicide. The hallmark of necrosis is cell rupture, which is generally preceded by a breakdown of the plasma membrane barrier and cell swelling (Fig. 6-13). Eventually, a "catastrophic failure of cellular homeostasis" (Raffray and Cohen, 1997) causes the cell to rupture; this releases a number of reactive cellular contents, such as mitochondrial proteins, which evoke intense inflammatory and fibrotic reactions that cause scarring. These features of necrosis are especially damaging to the heart because increased membrane permeability allows calcium to leak into the cell. Exposure of the contractile proteins to this activator initiates uncontrolled interactions between the myofilaments that leads to "contraction-band necrosis," which is characterized by violent contractions that literally tear the cell to pieces.

Apoptosis, which is a highly regulated process that depends on the cell cycle (Wang and Walsh, 1996), is much less violent than necrosis. In contrast to the cell swelling seen in necrosis, during apoptosis the cell shrinks and eventually breaks up into small, membrane-surrounded fragments that often contain bits of condensed chromatin. These structures, called *apoptotic bodies*, provide an important morphologic criterion for apoptosis. Maintenance of plasma membrane integrity until late in the apoptotic process allows the dying cell to be engulfed by macrophages and prevents the release of the reactive cellular contents. Another important distinction between necrosis and apoptosis is the way that DNA is degraded. In necrosis, DNA is broken down into randomly sized fragments, whereas DNA breakdown in apoptosis gives rise to regularly sized fragments that, when run out on gels, resemble a ladder (see Fig. 6-13). According to Wyllie (1987), the four "cardinal elements" in apoptosis are (1) volume reduction, (2) chromatin condensation, (3) recognition by macrophage cells that engulf the apoptotic bodies without releasing their contents, and (4) active protein synthesis.

It is very important to recognize that the distinctions between necrosis and apoptosis described in the preceding paragraphs are not as stark as is sometimes believed. Although the extremes differ markedly, this dichotomy fails to consider gradations and variations in these two modes of death. Such gradations can occur when a population of cells becomes hypoxic or is exposed to a toxic agent (Ohno et al, 1998; for review, see Raffray and Cohen, 1997). Furthermore, similar mechanisms can operate in both types of cell death, and cell death that begins as apoptosis can end with necrosis (Kroemer et al., 1997). As discussed later, enzymes that participate in apoptosis can also be activated by ischemia, so that the extent of cell death following transient ischemia can be reduced by inhibiting some of the mediators of apoptotic damage (Kane et al., 1995; Hara et al., 1997). The many combinations and permutations of necrosis and apoptosis, which are probably best viewed as the extremes of a continuum (Kroemer et al., 1997), create an ambiguity that helps to explain widely differing estimates of the importance and frequency of apoptosis in the failing heart.

Mechanisms Causing Apoptosis

The extent to which apoptosis is a regulated process is seen in the elaborate systems that control this form of cell death. The process of programmed cell death includes at least four steps: (1) a decision by the cell to die, (2) processes that kill the cell, (3) engulfment of the dead cell by phagocytosis, and (4) degradation of the engulfed cell within phagocytes (Stellar, 1995). All have been studied extensively in the roundworm *Caenorhabditis elegans*,

TABLE 6-9. *Signaling mechanisms that induce apoptosis*

"Injury"
  DNA damage
  Membrane damage
  Mitochondrial damage
Molecular signals
  Cytokine receptors—Fas, TNF (tumor necrosis factor) receptors
  Nuclear receptors

---

known commonly as *C. elegans*. Because the appearance and fate of each cell in this organism can be followed as the adult worm develops from the fertilized egg, the genetically determined programs responsible for these changes provide a model for the study of development. Although most genes that regulate *C. elegans* development differ from those that operate in mammals, studies of this simple organism have provided clues that have identified many homologous genes that contribute to human disease.

Insofar as apoptosis plays a significant pathogenic role in heart failure (see later discussion), the most important of the four steps described in the preceding paragraph is the first: how (and why) a cardiac cell elects to die. In an organ made up of proliferating cells, the decision of a particular cell to die is really of interest only to the suicide-prone cell because other dividing cells are ready to take its place. But in the adult heart, which is made up of terminally differentiated myocytes that cannot divide, the death of any of these cells weakens the cardiac pump and initiates the vicious cycle depicted in Table 6-1. The decision of a cardiac myocyte to die, therefore, has major long-term consequences for the heart, all of them harmful.

Decision to Die: Initiating Factors

Cells do not die haphazardly by apoptosis, but instead do so in response to specific "death" signals (Table 6–9). Two types of mechanisms can initiate this process. The first is initiated by agents that injure cells, such as viruses, toxic substances, irradiation, energy starvation, and reactive oxygen species (often referred to as "free radicals"). The second class includes a variety of specialized signaling molecules that initiate apoptosis when they bind to specific plasma membrane receptors. The subsequent steps in apoptosis, which depend in part on how this process is set into motion, are not simply a series of nonspecific responses. Instead, they represent integrated and highly regulated processes that eventually kill the cell.

Cell Injury

Whereas cell damage that is so severe as to rupture the plasma membrane causes necrosis, milder forms of injury can activate signaling pathways that commit cells to apoptosis. This occurs, for example, when DNA is damaged by radiation, when a toxin injures but does not destroy the plasma membrane, or when increased mitochondrial permeability releases reactive oxygen species. Apoptosis can also be initiated by an increase in cytosolic calcium, or when free radicals are generated by mild ischemia or the inflammatory cytokines.

Increased Mitochondrial Permeability

There is substantial evidence that mitochondria can play an important role in the decision to undergo programmed cell death and that this role is mediated in part by the overproduction of reactive oxygen species (for review, see Kroemer et al., 1997; Raffray and

Cohen, 1997; Mignotte and Vayssiere, 1998) and when cytochrome c crosses a damaged mitochondrial membrane to enter the cytosol (Hengartner, 1998). Free radicals can be generated when mitochondria become damaged or when they are impaired functionally by conditions such hypoxia and calcium overload. By opening pores in the mitochondrial inner membrane, these abnormalities dissipate the normal energy-dependent proton gradient across this membrane. Further evidence supporting a causal link between mitochondrial damage and apoptosis is the ability of members of an important family of mitochondria-bound proteins to regulate apoptosis; these are Bcl-2 and related proteins (discussed in detail later) that can form pores in mitochondrial membranes. Reduction of the mitochondrial transmembrane potential by any of these mechanisms can release proteases, and possibly other substances such as cytochrome c, that serve as "pro-apoptotic factors." Mitochondria may also play the role of the "executioner" that carries out programmed cell death when the decision to die is made by other mechanisms, such as the Fas and TNF receptors.

Calcium Overload

Calcium overload has also been suggested to play an important role in a cell's decision to die by apoptosis (for review, see Dowd, 1995; McConkey and Orrenius, 1997). The many signaling functions of this cation include several that could contribute to programmed cell death; these include activation of calcium-dependent enzymes, such as proteases and endonucleases, and dissipation of the mitochondrial transmembrane potential discussed in the preceding paragraph. However, because calcium enters the cytosol when membranes are damaged by any cause, the relationship between increased cytosolic calcium and cell death could reflect one of effect-cause, rather than cause-effect.

The significance of mitochondrial damage and calcium overload in causing apoptosis in the failing heart is not yet clear. Although such abnormalities as energy starvation and membrane damage could cause myocardial cells to die by this mechanism, it must be remembered that mitochondrial rupture and calcium overload also occur in necrotic tissue, which blurs the distinction between these two forms of cell death.

Death Factors

Up to this point, the discussion has focused on apoptosis in damaged cells and how these cells can "decide" to undergo programmed cell death. A quite different way that cells can "decide" to die occurs when they respond to extracellular signals that activate cellular programs that lead to programmed cell death, or when apoptosis-preventing factors are withdrawn, which allows a preprogrammed death program to kill the cell. Signals that cause apoptosis are often referred to as *death factors*, whereas apoptosis that is initiated by removal of a survival signal can be viewed as *death by neglect* (Hetts, 1998).

The Fas/Fas Ligand System

Among the most important of the death factors is a family of a plasma membrane receptors called *Fas* (other names are Apo-1 and CD-95) that, when bound to the Fas ligand (*FasL*) initiates apoptosis (for reviews, see Nagata and Golstein, 1995; Nagata, 1997, Wallach et al., 1997). FasL is a member of the cytokine family of peptides, whose role as mediators of inflammation was discussed in Chapter 5 and as growth factors earlier in this chapter. Fas is one of the cytokine receptors. Other membrane receptors that can mediate "death-determining" signals include cytokine and growth factor receptors, as well as some glucocorticoid receptors (Saini and Walker, 1998).

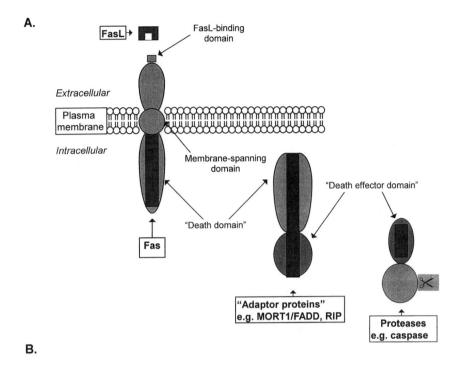

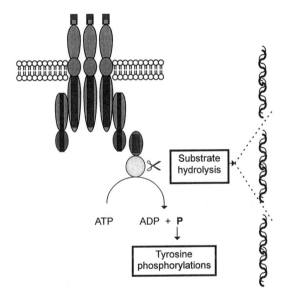

FIG. 6-14. Components of the Fas/FasL system that induces apoptosis (**A**) include the Fas ligand (FasL), which is a cytokine, its plasma membrane receptor Fas, adaptor proteins like MORT and RIP, and protease and nuclease effectors such as the caspases. Binding of the FasL to Fas (**B**) causes the latter to form a trimeric aggregate in which "death domains" in Fas interact with homologous death domains in the adaptor proteins. This interaction activates "death effector domains" in the latter, which then bind to homologous death effector domains in the ultimate effectors of the apoptotic process. The latter include not only the enzymes that break down cell constituents but also tyrosine kinases and other signaling molecules that activate additional downstream steps that regulate programmed cell death.

The FasL-Fas system is especially prominent in natural killer cells where it helps carry out the cytotoxic effects. FasL is expressed in large amounts on the surface of activated T lymphocytes and other lymphoid tissue (Suda et al., 1995; Strasser and O'Connor, 1998); smaller amounts are also found in the heart (Watanabe-Fukunaga et al., 1992). FasL can be found in two forms: one that is bound to membranes (mFasL) and a soluble form (sFasL). The membrane-bound mFasL is found on the surface of cytotoxic T cells, where this cytokine kills other cells. This occurs when the projecting FasL binds to Fas receptors on the surface of the doomed cells. Soluble sFasL, which is released when mFasL is cleaved by a metalloproteinase, can act independently of such "killer cells." Although sFasL generally induces apoptosis, in some settings, sFasL antagonizes the apoptotic effects of mFasL.

Programmed cell death that is initiated by the FasL peptides occurs when these cytokines bind to the Fas membrane receptors (Fig. 6-14), which are related to the cytokine receptors that bind TNFα. These receptors contain a 70- to 90-amino acid sequence that, because it stimulates apoptosis, represents a "death domain" (Tartaglia et al., 1993; Wallach et al., 1997). Similarities between these two types of cytokine receptor explain such findings as ability of both TNFα and FasL to induce apoptosis in T cells (Zheng et al., 1995). Binding of the Fas receptor to its ligand FasL causes the receptor to form a trimer, an aggregation that is similar to that which activates cytokine receptors (see Fig. 6-14). In this aggregate, the death domains of Fas become able to bind homologous death domains in a family of mediator proteins called "adaptors."

A role of the Fas-FasL system in the pathophysiology of heart failure has not yet been established (for review, see Wallach, 1997; Kidd, 1998), but several recent reports indicate that this system is activated in patients with this syndrome (Nishigaki et al., 1997; Okuyama et al., 1997; Schumann et al., 1997; Toyozaki et al., 1998). These findings, along with those described in Chapter 5, suggest that cytokine-induced apoptosis may contribute to the poor prognosis in this syndrome. However, additional data are needed to establish a role for this mechanism in causing progressive cell death in the failing heart.

Adaptor Proteins and Other Intracellular Mediators of Apoptosis

The adaptor proteins that participate in Fas signaling have been given names like MORT1/FADD, and RIP, terms that illustrate the wry humor of the experts in this field. For the reader who is unfamiliar with the tombstones in New England cemeteries, the commonly found letters "R.I.P." stand for "Rest in Peace." MORT recalls the Latin term for death, and the alternative name FADD is an acronym for "Fas-associated death domain protein." The latter term reflects the fact that the MORT1/FADD adaptor contains not only the death domain also found in the cytokine receptors but also a "death effector domain" (sometimes abbreviated DED) that is also found in the proteins further "downstream" in the signaling cascades that regulate subsequent steps in apoptosis (see Fig. 6-14). One way that the complex formed by the aggregated Fas receptors and the adaptors initiates apoptosis is by causing the death effector domains in the latter to bind to and activate the death effector domains in cytolytic enzymes that do the actual killing.

Other mediators of programmed cell death initiated by FasL binding to its receptors include a group of tyrosine kinases that associate with and are activated by Fas (Atkinson et al., 1996). A role of tyrosine phosphorylation as a mediator of apoptosis is not unexpected in view of the similarities between the Fas receptor and other cytokine receptors, which also activate this class of enzymes. One example of the intricate control of the systems that regulate apoptosis is seen in the ability of a tyrosine phosphatase, which has the opposite effect of reducing tyrosine phosphorylation, also to mediate the apoptotic sig-

nal. In different ways, therefore, both tyrosine phosphorylation and tyrosine dephosphorylation can initiate apoptosis.

Other regulators besides the Fas/FasL system are able to initiate apoptosis. These include stretch (Cheng et al., 1995), some integrins (Malik, 1997), nitric oxide (Iwashima et al., 1998), norepinephrine (Communal et al., 1998), and downstream signals carried by GTP-binding proteins (Troppmair and Rapp, 1997; Downard, 1998), the pocket proteins (Morgenbesser et al., 1994; Hertwig and Strauss, 1997), protein kinase C, inositol phosphate kinase, and NF-κB (for review, see Saini and Walker, 1997; Sonenshein, 1997, Chiarugi et al., 1997). Most of these signals not only initiate apoptosis but also activate cell cycling, which illustrates further the important parallels between programmed cell death and proliferation. In addition to reinforcing the fact that the world is a very dangerous place, this ability of so many different signaling systems to cause programmed cell death may provide opportunities for the development of agents to overcome a potential role of apoptosis in the progressive deterioration of the failing heart.

Executioners and Their Helpers

The final steps in apoptosis, those which actually kill the cell, occur when shrinkage and gentle disruption of the doomed cell yields small, digestible fragments that are readily engulfed by phagocytes (see Fig. 6-13). As noted earlier, the ability of phagocytes to ingest the particles formed during apoptosis represents the most important difference from necrosis, where plasma membrane disruption spills "raw," indigestible cell contents into the tissue spaces, thereby evoking an inflammatory response. One can therefore view apoptosis as resembling the preparation of a fine dinner; the shells are removed from the shrimp and clams, the meat is tenderized and cut into bite-sized pieces, and the fruits and vegetables are peeled and cooked thoroughly. The result is an easily digested meal. In necrosis, following this culinary analogy, the same ingredients are presented in raw form, often still alive, which causes the diner to experience a "stomach ache" that is analogous to the inflammatory reaction and subsequent scarring that distinguish necrosis from apoptosis. The following paragraphs deal briefly with the executioners (chefs) of programmed cell death, who in preparing cells that are damaged or no longer needed for apoptosis, make it possible for these cells to be destroyed in an orderly and tidy manner.

Caspases

The most important effectors of cell death in apoptosis are a family of cysteine proteases called *caspases,* or *ICE* (for review, see Thornberry 1997; Kidd, 1998). These enzymes, which include a previously discovered *interleukin-1β-converting enzyme* (hence the acronym ICE), are related to a key regulator of apoptosis that was first characterized in *C. elegans.* The latter, called CED-3, is a member of the caspase family that is encoded by a gene called *ced-3.* At least ten different members of this family have been isolated from human tissue (Wyllie, 1997a; Nagata, 1997; Thornberry, 1997; Hetts, 1998).

Members of the caspase family not only break down the cell contents during apoptosis but also regulate this process by activating proenzyme forms of other caspases; the result is an elaborate regulatory cascade typical of those seen in signal transduction (Liu et al., 1996; Nagata, 1997). Some caspases contain a death-effector domain similar to that found in MORT1/FADD; this domain regulates apoptosis when it binds a similar death-effector domain of the caspases to the adaptor proteins (see Fig. 6-14). Substrates for these enzymes, in addition to other caspases, include the cytoskeletal proteins fodrin and actin, proteins that maintain nuclear structure, and the pocket protein pRb (Raffray and Cohen, 1997; Nagata, 1997; Thornberry, 1997; Kidd, 1998). Caspases also hydrolyze proteins that participate in RNA splicing, cell division, and DNA repair and replication, the latter include a key enzyme called *poly (ADP) ribose polymerase* that maintains DNA integrity (Alnemri et al., 1996; Nagata, 1997). The highly regulated actions of the caspases that cause nuclear fragmentation generate an orderly complement of DNA breakdown products that, when separated on gels, give the pattern of DNA "laddering" described previously (see Fig. 6-13). As noted earlier, other enzymes, for example calcium-activated proteases, can also participate in apoptosis (McConkey and Orrenius, 1997).

Regulators of Apoptosis

The elaborate systems responsible for programmed cell death are, as might be expected, subject to many "layers" of control—death, after all, is irreversible. In many ways, apoptosis is like the death penalty in the American legal system, in which conviction, sentencing, and the many appeals that precede the actual execution allow a careful review of the death decision. The following discussion, which is limited to four of the many systems that regulate apoptosis, is not comprehensive, but instead it is intended to provide the reader with an appreciation of processes that may contribute to myocyte death in the failing heart. Hopefully, manipulation of the systems that control apoptosis may some day yield useful means by which to improve prognosis in heart failure.

The Bcl-2 Family

Considerable attention has been given to a family of proteins that can either promote or inhibit apoptosis. These are *Bcl-2* and related proteins, which first came to attention because they play a role in carcinogenesis. This feature explains the name Bcl-2, which is an acronym for *B-cell lymphoma/leukemia 2 gene* (for review, see Reed, 1994; Brown, 1997). The Bcl-2 family includes peptides that suppress apoptosis (e.g., *Bcl-2* and *Bcl-x_L*), and peptides that, by interfering with the apoptosis-suppressing proteins, promote cell death (e.g., *Bak, Bax*, and *Bad*). Bcl-2, the prototype of this family, is a "pro-apoptotic" membrane protein that is found in the outer mitochondrial membrane, nuclear envelope, and endoplasmic reticulum; this location provides some clues as to its mechanism of action. The proteins of the Bcl-2 family are highly regulated, in part by each other (for review, see Francke and Cantley, 1997).

Several proteins of the Bcl-2 family have a fascinating structure, which, like diphtheria toxin, can form pores in membranes. This structure suggests that pro-apoptotic members of the Bcl-2 family, like Bax, may induce apoptosis by increasing mitochondrial permeability (see earlier discussion; for review, see Kroemer et al., 1997). Some of these proteins also appear to have functions that are similar to those of adaptor proteins such as MORT1/FADD. In addition, to prevent mitochondrial disruption, the anti-apoptotic members of the Bcl-2 family act by inhibiting caspase and various protein kinases, or by death-inhibiting interactions with GTP-binding proteins, calcineurin, and other intracellular signal transduction molecules that initiate apoptosis (for review, see Reed, 1994, 1997; Kroemer, 1997; Hetts, 1998).

The ability of Bcl-2 to inhibit apoptosis, which prevents destruction of abnormal cells, explains why reducing the actions of Bcl-2 renders animals susceptible to malignancy, and why abnormalities in this system are emerging as a major cause of breast cancer in

women. Because overexpression of Bcl-2 can prevent cell death caused by a variety of stimuli (see Reed, 1994), there might be some value in activating Bcl-2 or related inhibitors of apoptosis in patients with heart failure, in whom the overloaded myocytes are subject to maladaptive growth signals. This line of reasoning, however, is not only highly conjectural but also simplistic. The reason is that Bcl-2 prevents the elimination of potentially malignant cells and so could increase the likelihood of malignancy in tissues other than the heart. Yet, growing evidence that apoptosis plays a role not only in heart failure but also in the genesis of such common arrhythmias as the "sick sinus syndrome," makes selective inhibition of programmed cell death in the heart a promising goal for future therapy in cardiac patients.

The Tumor Suppressor Proteins

The pocket proteins, in addition to inhibiting cell cycling and preventing the uncontrolled proliferation that leads to malignancy, can prevent apoptosis (for review, see Herwig and Strauss, 1997). The latter effect is seen, for example, when inactivation of pRb sensitizes cells to apoptosis, and overexpression of this tumor suppressor protein prolongs cell survival by inhibiting apoptosis. As discussed earlier, the growth-suppressing effects of pRb are due partly to its binding of the transcription factor E2F, which suggests that, in addition to activating the cell cycle, E2F stimulates apoptosis.

Heat Shock Proteins

The responses that help cells survive stress are mediated in part by a family of proteins that protect key cellular constituents from denaturation. These are the *heat shock proteins*, so named because they were first observed in cells that had been exposed to high temperature. These proteins are also called *chaperones* because, like the elderly aunt who accompanies a youngster who is virtuous but easily led astray, they protect innocent proteins from loss of virtue. The role of these proteins is discussed further in Chapter 8, but at this point it is important to note that at least some of the smaller members of this family of stress-activated proteins, notably hsp27, can inhibit apoptosis (Mehlen et al., 1996, 1997). This effect, which is accompanied by slowing of cell proliferation, may be due in part to the ability of these heat shock proteins to prevent accumulation of reactive oxygen species.

Interventions that decrease expression of hsp27 not only increase apoptosis but also promote cell proliferation and inhibit differentiation, responses that provide another example of the parallels between cell growth and programmed cell death. This link between growth and death is seen in the ability of growth factors such as E2F to stimulate both cell cycling and apoptosis. Other growth-stimulating factors that share these actions include some of the cyclins, the GTP-binding coupling protein *ras*, and the protooncogene c-*fos* (Hertwig and Strauss, 1997; Thompson, 1998). The effects of the protooncogene c-*myc*, whose actions parallel those of c-*fos*, also illustrate this link.

*The Protooncogene c-*myc *and Its Protein Product c-Myc*

Initiators and regulators of apoptosis include the protooncogene c-*myc* and its product c-Myc (by convention, a gene and its product are distinguished in that the name of the gene is italicized but not capitalized, whereas that of the protein is capitalized but not italicized). These transcription factors, which activate cell growth and participate in the immediate-early gene response discussed in Chapter 7, also promote apoptosis (Evan et al., 1992; Smeyne et al., 1993; Collins and Lopez Rivas, 1993; for reviews, see Henriksson and Lüscher, 1996; Thompson, 1998). As already noted, this is consistent with the view that apoptosis represents a modified form of mitosis (Ucker, 1991).

c-Myc, the protein encoded by c-*myc*, is a transcription factor that, when expressed in proliferating cells, plays a major role in regulating cell growth by increasing the expression of genes that encode cyclins and other participants in cell cycle regulation. Although Myc also induces apoptosis, the converse is not true because apoptosis does not require the participation of c-Myc. Although the pro-apoptotic actions of c-Myc cannot be separated from its ability to stimulate cell growth (Evan et al., 1992), elevated c-*myc* levels and increased c-Myc function do not always correlate with the extent of programmed cell death.

The ability of c-Myc to initiate programmed cell death is due in large part to increased expression of p53 (Henrikkson and Lüscher 1996), a transcription factor that has been called the "master watchman" of the genome during cell cycling (Saini and Walker, 1997). In growing cells, p53 regulates gene expression by an interplay with the pocket proteins (Chiarugi et al., 1997), whereas in damaged cells, p53 inhibits proliferation and causes cell death by increasing expression of genes that encode several pro-apoptotic factors (Hetts, 1998).

The transcription factor p53 can be viewed as providing a "fast-track" connection by which DNA damage inhibits both the cell cycle and programmed cell death (Wyllie, 1997b; Mowat, 1998). If DNA damage is mild, the ability of p53 to shut down cell cycling allows time for DNA repair. If the cell heals, then all is well; but if the injury is severe and the DNA damage cannot be repaired, the pro-apoptotic effects of p53 kill the irreversibly damaged cell. In this way, p53 provides a vital protective action in rapidly growing cells in that its pro-apoptotic actions prevent multiplication of malignantly transformed cells. In terminally differentiated cells such as cardiac myocytes, in which malignant transformation is rare, activation of p53 serves mainly to eliminate severely damaged cells. These considerations suggest that blocking the effects of p53 could prevent apoptotic cell death in the failing heart, although such efforts, while possibly reducing cell death in the heart, might also inhibit the removal of potentially malignant cells in other, proliferating tissues. Manipulation of these systems, therefore, could lead to unanticipated consequences, some quite dangerous.

Role of Apoptotic Cell Death in Heart Disease

There is growing evidence that apoptosis represents an important cause of cell death in the failing heart (Bing, 1993; Brömme and Holtz, 1996; Sharov et al., 1996; Teiger et al., 1996; Yao et al., 1996; Narula et al., 1996; Li et al., 1997; Olivetti et al., 1997; Sabbah and Sharov, 1998), due possibly to activation of the Fas-FasL system. Some descriptions of the frequency of apoptosis in the failing heart, however, do not seem plausible; for example, values for the fraction of "apoptotic" nuclei have been reported to be as high as 0.2% (Olivetti et al., 1997), 1% to 12% (Olivetti et al., 1994), and even 35% (Narula et al., 1996). Such high rates of cell death would destroy the heart so rapidly as to be incompatible even with the poor prognosis in heart failure. The reason is that, as noted by Savill (1997),

a little apoptosis equates to a lot of cell loss. The significance for tissue kinetics of apparently low frequencies of apoptosis is easy to appreciate if one considers a hypothetical tissue in which there is no cell birth by mitosis. Should only 1% of cells appear apoptotic in the "snapshot" of a histological section, and the clearance time is 1 h, a quarter of the cells in the tissue will have disappeared in 1 day.

This estimate of the rate of cell loss is based on a time of 1 to 2 hours between the onset of apoptosis and the point where the dying cells are no longer histologically detectable (Savill, 1997). This is, in fact, a solid estimate because it is based on studies in *C. elegans*, in which the time course of apoptosis can be followed with precision, the rate at which cells are lost in developing organs, the time required for phagocytosis of apoptotic cells *in vitro*, and the effects of inhibition of apoptosis *in vivo*. Thus, some published estimates of the frequency of cells undergoing apoptosis in sections obtained from failing human hearts are implausible because, if these values are correct, the entire heart would disappear in a few days, rather than the average survival of several years seen in the natural history of this syndrome. Explanations for high published values include counting of nonmyocyte cells undergoing programmed cell death and misidentifying necrosis as apoptosis. The latter is not unlikely in that many of the patients whose hearts were studied had end-stage disease, and so, during the period immediately before the hearts were obtained for analysis, may have been receiving drugs such as β-adrenergic agonists, which can both accelerate apoptosis and cause myocyte necrosis. As noted earlier, because the criteria used to identify apoptotic cells are subject to technical artifacts that can misidentify cells that are undergoing necrosis, some published reports are likely to have overestimated the importance of programmed cell death in these terminally ill patients (Buja and Entman, 1998).

Although a role for apoptosis in clinical heart failure remains to be established, there is solid evidence that apoptosis occurs in the heart in other settings (Umansky and Tomei, 1997). These include normal embryonic development (Takeda et al., 1996), ischemic syndromes (Tanaka et al., 1994; Olivetti et al., 1994; Gottlieb et al., 1994, 1996), arrhythmogenic right ventricular dysplasia (Mallat et al., 1996), and the sinoatrial and atrioventricular block commonly seen in the elderly as the "sick sinus syndrome" (James, 1994, 1998).

The value of pursuing an understanding of the role of apoptosis in the failing heart is underscored by evidence that caspase inhibitors can reduce the extent of the tissue injury caused by transient ischemia in the brain (Kane et al., 1995; Hara et al., 1997). This protective effect raises the possibility that inhibitors of apoptosis could also delay or prevent cell death in the energy-starved, failing heart. The clinical relevance of these speculations is suggested by the possibility that angiotensin-converting enzyme inhibitors and β-adrenergic blockers prolong survival in patients with heart failure, in part by inhibiting apoptosis-promoting effects of angiotensin II (Yamada et al., 1996; Kajstura et al., 1997) and norepinephrine (Communal et al., 1998). Hopefully, work that is currently underway in many laboratories will soon clarify the role of programmed cell death in patients with heart failure.

CONCLUSION

This rather complex chapter has wended its way through several aspects of cell growth and cell death that appear to play an important role in the progressive deterioration of the failing heart. The emergence of maladaptive cell growth as one of the most important, if not *the* most important, problem in patients with heart failure highlights the relevance of these processes to the management of these patients. The rapid advances in our understanding of the control of cell proliferation and cell differentiation, the cell cycle, growth factors, and apoptosis may therefore provide a key to new approaches to prolonging survival and alleviating symptoms in these patients. As noted in Chapter 9, several recent clinical trials have yielded findings that indicate that we are already moving toward these goals. Thus, the new and remarkably complex fields of science summarized in this chapter may also represent promising areas in which to search for new therapeutic approaches. As was true of the new science of bacteriology almost 150 years ago, the current fast-moving fields of molecular biology can be expected to provide important tools for alleviating suffering and prolonging survival in patients. It is virtually certain, however, that in the case of heart failure, we will not have to wait a century for the discovery of new and effective therapeutic agents.

BIBLIOGRAPHY

Alberty B, Bray D, Lewis J, Raff M, Roberts K, Watson JD (1994). *Molecular Biology of the Cell,* 3rd ed. Garland, New York.

Bugaisky L, Zak R (1986). Biological mechanisms of hypertrophy. In Fozzard H, Haber E, Katz A, Jennings R, Morgan HE, eds. *The Heart and Cardiovascular System.* Raven Press, New York, pp 1491–1506.

Bugaisky L, Gupta M, Gupta MG, Zak R (1992). Cellular and molecular mechanisms of hypertrophy. In Fozzard H, Haber E, Katz A, Jennings R, Morgan HE, eds. *The Heart and Cardiovascular System,* 2nd ed. Raven Press, New York, pp 1621–1640.

Cummins P, ed (1993). *Growth Factors and the Cardiovascular System.* Kluwer, Boston.

Darnell J, Lodish H, Baltimore D (1990). *Molecular Cell Biology,* 2nd ed. Scientific American, New York.

Keating MT, Sanguinetti MC (1996). Molecular insights into cardiovascular disease. *Science* 272:681–688.

Roberts R, ed (1993). *Molecular Basis of Cardiology,* Blackwell, Oxford.

Swynghedauw B, ed (1990). *Cardiac Hypertrophy and Failure.* INSERM, Paris.

Swynghedauw B (1997). Molecular mechanisms of myocardial remodeling. *Physiol Rev* 79:215–262.

REFERENCES

Aberle H, Schwartz H, Kemler R (1996). Cadherin-catenin complex: protein interactions and their implications for cadherin function. *J Cell Biochem* 61:514–523.

Alnemri ES, Livingston DJ, Nicholson DW, et al (1996). Human ICE/CED-3 protease nomenclature. *Cell* 87:171.

Antzelevitch C, Sicouri S, Litovsky SH, Lukas A, Krishnan SC, Di Diego JM, Gintant GA, Liu DW (1991). Heterogeneity within the ventricular wall. Electrophysiology and pharmacology of epicardial, endocardial, and M cells. *Circ Res* 69:1427–1449.

Anversa P, Kajstura J (1998). Ventricular myocytes are not terminally differentiated in the adult mammalian heart. *Circ Res* 83:1–14.

Anyukhovsky EP, Sosunov EA, Rosen MR (1996). Regional differences in electrophysiological properties of epicardium, midmyocardium, and endocardium. *In vitro* and *in vivo* correlations. *Circulation* 94:1981–1988.

Arber S, Halder G, Caroni P (1994). Muscle LIM protein, a novel essential regulator of myogenesis, promotes myogenic differentiation. *Cell* 79:221–231.

Arber S, Hunter JJ, Ross J Jr, Hongo M, Sansig G, Borg J, Perriard J-C, Chien KR, Caroni P (1997). MLP-deficient mice exhibit a disruption of cardiac cytoarchitectural organization, dilated cardiomyopathy, and heart failure. *Cell* 88:393–403.

Assoian RK, Zhu X, Giancotti FG (1997). Cell anchorage and the cytoskeleton as partners in growth factor dependent cell cycle progression. *Curr Opin Cell Biol* 9:93–98.

Atkinson EA, Ostergaard H, Kane K, Pinkowski MJ, Caputo A, Olszowy MW, Bleackley RC (1996). A physical interaction between the cell death protein fas and tyrosine kinase p59^{fynT}. *J Biol Chem* 271:5968–5971.

Baig MK, Goldman JH, Caforio ALP, Coonar AS, Keeling PJ, McKenna WJ (1988). Familial dilated cardiomyopathy: cardiac abnormalities are common in asymptomatic relatives and may represent early disease. *J Am Coll Cardiol* 31:195–201.

Baldwin TJ, Fazeli MS, Doherty P, Wlash FS (1996). Elucidation of the molecular actions of NCAM and structurally related cell adhesion molecules. *J Cell Biochem* 61:502–513.

Bartek J, Bartkova J, Lukas J (1997). The retinoblastoma protein pathway in cell cycle control and cancer. *Exp Cell Res* 237:1–6.

Beltrami CA, Finato N, Rocco M, Feruglio GA, Puricelli C, Cigola E, Quaini F, Sonnenblick EH, Olivetti G, Anversa P (1994). Structural basis for end-stage failure in ischemic cardiomyopathy in humans. *Circulation* 89:151–163.

Bernards R (1997). E2F: a nodal point in cell cycle regulation. *Biochim Biophys Acta* 1333:M33–M40.

Bing OHL (1993). Hypothesis: apoptosis may be a mechanism for the transition to heart failure with chronic pressure overload. (Editorial). *J Mol Cell Cardiol* 26:943–948.

Bloom S, Lockard VG, Bloom M (1996). Intermediate filament-mediated stretch-induced changes in chromatin: a hypothesis for growth initiation in cardiac myocytes. *J Mol Cell Cardiol* 28:2123–2127.

Border WA, Noble NA (1994). Transforming Growth Factor β in tissue fibrosis. *N Engl J Med* 331:1286–1292.

Border WA, Noble NA (1998). Interactions of transforming growth factor-β and angiotensin II in renal fibrosis. *Hypertension* 31:181–188.

Bouvagnet P, Leger J, Dechesne C, Pons F, Leger JJ (1984). Fiber types and myosin types in human atrial and ventricular myosin. An anatomical description. *Circ Res* 55:794–804.

Brand T, Schneider MD (1996). Transforming growth factor-β signal transduction. *Circ Res* 78:173–179.

Brodsky VY, Chernyaev AL, Vasilieva IA (1991). Variability of the cardiomyocyte ploidy in normal human hearts; range of values. *Virchow's Archiv [B]* 61:289–294.

Brodsky VY, Sarkisov DS, Arefyeva AM, Panova NW, Gvasava IG (1994). Polyploidy in cardiac myocytes of normal and hypertrophic human hearts; range of values. *Virchow's Archiv* 424:429–435.

Brömme HJ, Holtz J (1996). Apoptosis in the heart: when and why? *Mol Cell Biochem* 163–164:261–275.

Brown R (1997). The Bcl-2 family of proteins. *Br Med Bull* 53:466–477.

Buja LM, Eigenbrodt ML, Eigenbrodt EH (1993). Apoptosis and necrosis. Basic types of cell death. *Arch Pathol Lab Med* 117:1208–1214.

Buja LM, Entman ML (1998). Models of myocardial cell injury and cell death in ischemic heart disease. *Circulation* 98:1355–1357.

Calderone A, Takahashi N, Izzo NJ Jr, Thaik CM, Colucci WS (1995). Pressure- and volume-induced left ventricular hypertrophies are associated with distinct myocyte phenotypes and differential induction of peptide growth factor mRNAs. *Circulation* 92:2385–2390.

Chiarugi V, Magnelli L, Cinelli M (1997). Complex interplay among apoptosis factors: RB, P53, E2F, TGF-β, cell cycle inhibitors and the Bcl-2 gene family. *Pharmacol Res* 35:257–261.

Cheng W, Li B, Kajstura J, Li P, Wolin MS, Sonnenblick EH, Hintze TH, Olivetti G, Anversa P (1995). Stretch-induced programmed myocyte cell death. *J Clin Invest* 96:2247–2259.

Chicurel ME, Singer RH, Meyer CJ, Ingber DE (1998). Integrin binding and mechanical tension induce movement of mRNA and ribosomes to focal adhesions. *Nature* 392:730–733.

Chien KR, Zhu H, Knowlton KU, Miller-Hance W, van-Bilsen M, O'Brien TX, Evans SM (1994). Transcriptional regulation during cardiac growth and development. *Annu Rev Physiol* 55:77–95.

Clarke MS, Caldwell RW, Chiao H, Miyake K, McNeil PL (1995). Contraction-induced cell wounding and release of fibroblast growth factor in heart. *Circ Res* 76:927–934.

Cohen J, Shah PM, eds (1974). Cardiac hypertrophy and cardiomyopathy. *Circ Res* 34-35(Suppl):II-3–II-11.

Cohen JJ (1993). Apoptosis. *Immunol Today* 14:126–130.

Collignon J, Varlet I, Robertson EJ (1996). Relationship between asymmetric nodal expression and the direction of embryonic turning. *Nature* 381:155–158.

Collins MKL, Lopez Rivas A (1993). The control of apoptosis in mammalian cells. *TIBS* 18:307–309.

Communal C, Singh K, Pimentel DR, Colucci WS (1998). Norepinephrine stimulates apoptosis in adult rat ventricular myocytes by activation of the β-adrenergic pathway. *Circulation* 98:1329–1334.

Cooper G IV, Satava RM Jr, Harrison CE, Coleman HN III (1973a). Mechanism for the abnormal energetics of pressure-induced hypertrophy of cat myocardium. *Circ Res* 33:213–223.

Cooper G IV, Puga F, Zujko KJ, Harrison CE, Coleman HN III (1973b). Normal myocardial function and energetics in volume-overload hypertrophy in the cat. *Circ Res* 32:140–148.

Coppolino MG, Woodside MJ, Demaurex N, Grinstein S, St-Arnaud R, Dedhar S (1997). Calreticulin is essential for integrin-mediated calcium signalling and cell adhesion. *Nature* 386:843–847.

Corda S, Mebazaa A, Gandolfini MP, Fitting C, Marotte F, Peynet J, Charlemagne D, Cavaillon JM, Payen D, Rappaport L, Samuel JL (1997). Trophic effect of human pericardial fluid on adult cardiac myocytes. Differential role of fibroblast growth factor-2 and factors related to ventricular hypertrophy. *Circ Res* 81:679–687.

Cox DA, Maurer T (1997). Transforming growth factor-β. *Clin Immunol Immunopathol* 83:25–30.

Cummins P (1993). Fibroblast and transforming growth factor expression in the cardiac myocyte. *Cardiovasc Res* 27:1150–1154.

Davis PF, Tripathi SC (1993). Mechanical stress mechanisms and the cell. An endothelial paradigm. *Circ Res* 72:3239–3245.

Di Diego JM, Sun ZQ, Antzelevitch C (1996). I(to) and action potential notch are smaller in left vs. right canine ventricular epicardium. *Am J Physiol* 271:H548–H561.

Doevendans PA, van Bilsen M (1996). Transcription factors and the cardiac gene programme. *Int J Biochem Cell Biol* 28:387–403.

Dowd DR (1995). Calcium regulation of apoptosis. *Adv Second Messenger Phosphoprotein Res* 30:255–280.

Downard J (1998). Ras signaling and apoptosis. *Curr Opin Genet Dev* 8:49–54.

Dubois JM, Rouzaire-Dubois B (1993). Role of potassium channels in mitogenesis. *Prog Biophys Mol Biol* 59:1–21.

Dynlacht BD (1997). Regulation of transcription by proteins that control the cell cycle. *Nature* 389:149–152.

Edmondson DG, Olson EN (1993). Helix-loop-helix proteins as regulators of muscle-specific transcription. *J Biol Chem* 268:755–758.

Engelmann GL, Dionne CA, Jaye MC (1993). Acidic fibroblast growth factor and heart development. Role in myocyte proliferation and capillary angiogenesis. *Circ Res* 72:7–19.

Evan GI, Wyllie AH, Gilbert CS, Littlewood TD, Land H, Brooks M, Waters CM, Penn LZ, Hancock DC (1992). Induction of apoptosis in fibroblasts by c-myc protein. *Cell* 69:119–128.

Ewen ME, Sluss HK, Sherr CJ, Matsushime H, Kato J-y, Livingston DM (1993). Functional interactions of the retinoblastoma protein with mammalian D-type proteins. *Cell* 73:487–497.

Firulli AB, Olson EN (1997). Modular regulation of muscle gene transcription: a mechanism for muscle cell diversity. *Trends Genet* 13:364–369.

Fishman MC, Olson EN. Parsing the heart: genetic modules for organ assembly. *Cell* 91:153–156, 1997.

Francke TF, Vantley LC (1997). A bad kinase makes good. *Nature* 390:116–117.

Gerdes AM, Kellerman SE, Moore JA, Muffy KE, Clark LC, Reeves PY, Malec KB, McKeown PP, Schocken DD (1992). Structural remodeling of cardiac myocytes in patients with ischemic cardiomyopathy. *Circulation* 85: 426–430.

Gerdes AM, Kellerman SE, Malec KB, Schocken DD (1994). Transverse shape characteristics of cardiac myocytes from rats and humans. *Cardioscience* 5:31–36.

Gerdes AM, Capasso JM (1995). Editorial review: structural remodeling and mechanical dysfunction of cardiac myocytes in heart failure. *J Mol Cell Cardiol* 27:849–856.

Giancotti FG (1997). Integrin signaling: specificity and control of cell survival and cell cycle progression. *Curr Opin Cell Biol* 9:691–700.

Goss RJ (1966). Hypertrophy versus hyperplasia. *Science* 153:1615–1620.

Gottlieb RA, Burleson KO, Kloner RA, Babior BM, Engler RL (1994). Reperfusion injury induces apoptosis in rabbit cardiomyocytes. *J Clin Invest* 94:1621–1628.

Gottlieb RA, Gruol DL, Zhu JY, Engler RL (1996). Preconditioning in rabbit cardiomyocytes. Role of pH, proton ATPase and apoptosis. *J Clin Invest* 97:2391–2398.

Grande JP (1997). Role of transforming growth factor-β in tissue injury and repair. *Proc Soc Exp Biol Med* 214: 27–40.

Green PJ, Walsh FS, Doherty P (1996). Promiscuity of fibroblast growth factor receptors. *Bioessays* 18:639–646.

Grove D, Nair KG, Zak R (1969). Biochemical correlates of cardiac hypertrophy. III. Changes in DNA content; the relative contributions of polyploidy and mitotic activity. *Circ Res* 25:463–471.

Grünig E, Tasman JA, Kücherer H, Franz W, Kübler W, Katus HA (1998). Frequency and pehnotypes of familial dilated cardiomyopathy. *J Am Coll Cardiol* 31:186–194.

Gruver CL, DeMayo F, Goldstein MA, Means AR (1993). Targeted developmental overexpression of calmodulin induces proliferative and hypertrophic growth of cardiomyocytes in transgenic mice. *Endocrinology* 133:376–388.

Gu W, Schneider JW, Condorelli G, Kaushal S, Mahdavi V, Nadal-Ginard B (1993). Interaction of myogenic factors and the retinoblastoma protein mediates muscle cell commitment and differentiation. *Cell* 72:309–324.

Hara H, Friedlander RM, Gagliardini V, Ayata C, Fink K, Huang Z, Shimizu-Sasamata M, Yuan J, Moskowitz MA (1997). Inhibition of interleukin 1β converting enzyme family proteases reduces ischemic and excitotoxic neuronal damage. *Proc Nat Acad Sci U S A* 94:2007–2012.

Haunstetter A, Izumo S (1998). Apoptosis. Basic mechanisms and implications for cardiovascular disease. *Circ Res* 82:1111–1129.

Heldin C-H, Miyazono K, ten Dijke P (1997). TNF-β signaling from cell membrane to nucleus through SMAD proteins. *Nature* 390:465–471.

Hengartner MO (1998). Death cycle and Swiss army knives. *Nature* 391:441–442.

Henriksson M, Lüscher B (1996). Proteins of the Myc network: essential regulator of cell growth and differentiation. *Adv Cancer Res* 68:109–182.

Herwig S, Strauss M (1997). The retinoblastoma protein: a master regulator of cell cycle, differentiation, and apoptosis. *Eur J Biochem* 246:581–601.

Hetts SW (1998). To die or not to die: an overview of apoptosis and its role in disease. *JAMA* 279:300–307.

Hill CS (1996). Signaling to the nucleus by members of the transforming growth factor-β (TGF-β) superfamily. *Cell Signal* 8:533–544.

Hillis GS, MacLeod AM (1996). Integrins and disease. *Clin Sci* 91:639–650.

Hsueh WA, Law RE, Do YS (1997). Integrins, adhesion, and cardiac remodeling. *Hypertension* 31:176–180.

Hu H, Sachs F (1997). Stretch-activated ion channels in the heart. *J Mol Cell Cardiol* 29:1511–1523.

Hynes RO, Lander AD (1992). Contact and adhesive specificities in the associations, migrations, and targeting of cells and axons. *Cell* 68:303–322.

Iwashima M, Shichiri M, Marumo F, Hirata Y (1998). Transfection of inducible nitric oxide synthase gene causes apoptosis in vascular smooth muscle cells. *Circulation* 98:1212–1218.

James TN (1994). Normal and abnormal consequences of apoptosis in the human heart. From postnatal morphogenesis to paroxysmal arrhythmias. *Circulation* 90:556–573.

James TN (1998). Normal and abnormal consequences of apoptosis in the human heart. *Annu Rev Physiol* 60:309–325.

Jeffrey PD, Russo AA, Polyak K, Gibbs E, Hurwitz J, Massagué J, Pavletich NP (1995). Mechanism of CDK activation revealed by the structure of a cyclin A-CDK2 complex. *Nature* 376:313–320.

Kajstura J, Cigola E, Malhotra A, Li P, Cheng W, Meggs LG, Anversa P (1997). Angiotensin II induces apoptosis of adult ventricular myocytes in vitro. *J Mol Cell Cardiol* 29:859–870.

Kane DJ, Örd T, Anton R, Bredesan DE (1995). Expression of Bcl-2 inhibits necrotic neural cell death. *J Neurosci Res* 40:269–275.

Katz AM (1990). Cardiomyopathy of overload. A major determinant of prognosis in congestive heart failure. *N Engl J Med* 322:100–110.

Katz AM (1994). The cardiomyopathy of overload: An unnatural growth response in the hypertrophied heart. *Ann Intern Med* 121:363–371.

Katz AM (1997). Evolving concepts of heart failure: cooling furnace, malfunctioning pump, enlarging muscle. Part I. Heart failure as a disorder of the cardiac pump. *J Cardiac Failure* 3:319–334.

Katz AM (1998). Evolving concepts of heart failure: cooling furnace, malfunctioning pump, enlarging muscle. Part II. Hypertrophy and dilatation of the failing heart. *J Cardiac Failure* 4:67–81.

Katz AM, Katz PB (1989). Homogeneity out of heterogeneity. *Circulation* 79:712–717.

Katz BZ, Yamada KM (1997). Integrins in morphogenesis and signaling. *Biochimie* 79:467–476.

Katz LN, Shaffer AB (1966). Hemodynamic aspects of congestive heart failure. In Blumgart HL, ed. *Symposium on Congestive Heart Failure.* Am Heart Assn Monograph No. 1:12–31.

Kaye D, Pimental D, Presad S, Mäki T, Berger H-J. McNeil PL, Smith TW (1996). Role of transiently altered sarcolemmal membrane permeability and basic fibroblast growth factor release in the hypertrophic response of adult rat ventricular myocytes to increased mechanical activity in vitro. *J Clin Invest* 97:281–291.

Keeling PJ, Gang Y, Smith G, et al (1995). Familial dilated cardiomyopathy in the United Kingdom. *Br Heart J* 73: 417–421.

Kent R, Hoober K, Cooper G IV (1989). Load responsiveness of protein synthesis in adult mammalian myocardium: role of cardiac deformation linked to sodium influx. *Circ Res* 64:L74–L85.

Kidd VJ (1998). Proteolytic activities that mediate apoptosis. *Annu Rev Physiol* 60:533–573.

Kirshenbaum LA, Abdellatif M, Chakraborty S, Schneider MD (1996). Human E2F-1 reactivates cell cycle progression in ventricular myocytes and represses cardiac gene expression. *Dev Biol* 179:402–411.

Kompmann M, Paddags I, Sandritter W (1966). Feulgen cytophotometric DNA determinations on human hearts. *Arch Pathol* 82:303–308.

Kostin S, Heling A, Hein S, Scholz D, Klövekorn W-P, Schaper J (1998). The protein composition of the normal and diseased cardiac myocyte. *Heart Failure Rev* 2:245–260.

Kroemer G (1997). The proto-oncogene Bcl-2 and its role in regulating apoptosis. *Nature Med* 3:614–620.

Kroemer G, Zamzami N, Susin SA (1997). Mitochondrial control of apoptosis. *Immunol Today* 18:44–51.

Kuisk IR, Tran D, Capetanaki Y (1996). A single MEF2 site governs desmin transcription in both heart and skeletal muscle during mouse embryogenesis. *Dev Biol* 174:1–13.

Lafrenie RM, Yamada, KM (1997). Integrin-dependent signal transduction. *J Cell Devel Biol* 61:543–553.

Li Z, Bing OHL, Long X, Robinson KG, Lakatta EG (1997). Increased cardiomyocyte apoptosis during the transition to heart failure in the spontaneously hypertensive rat. *Am J Physiol* 272:H2313–H2319.

Lin Q, Schwarz J, Bucana C, Olson EN (1997). Control of mouse cardiac morphogenesis and myogenesis by transcription factor MEF2C. *Science* 276:1404–1407.

Linask KK, Knudsen KA, Gui YH (1997). N-cadherin-catenin interaction: necessary component of cardiac cell compartmentalization during early vertebrate heart development. *Dev Biol* 185:148–164.

Linzbach AJ (1960). Heart failure from the point of view of quantitative anatomy. *Am J Cardiol* 5:370–382.

Litovsky SH, Antzelevitch C (1988). Transient outward current prominent in canine ventricular epicardium but not endocardium. *Circ Res* 62:116–126.

Liu L, Pasumarthi KBS, Paua R, Massaeli H, Fandrich R, Pierce GN, Cattini PA, Katdami E (1995). Adult cardiomyocytes express functional high affinity receptors for basic fibroblast growth factor. *Am J Physiol* 37: H1927–H1938.

Liu X, Kim CN, Yang J, et al (1996). Induction of apoptotic program in cell free extracts: requirements for DATP and cytochrome c. *Cell* 86:147–157.

Lowe LA, Supp DM, Sampath K, Yokoyama T, Wright CVE, Potter SS, Overbeek P, Kuehn MR (1996). Conserved left-right asymmetry of notal expression and alterations in murine situs inversus. *Nature* 381:159–161.

Lowe TE, Bate EW (1948). The diameter of cardiac muscle fibres: a study of the diameter of muscle fibres in the left ventricle in normal hearts and in the left ventricular enlargement of simple hypertension. *Med J Aust* i:467–469.

Mably JD, Liew C-C (1996). Factors involved in cardiogenesis and the regulation of cardiac-specific gene expression. *Circ Res* 79:4–13.

Maione R, Amati P (1997). Interdependence between muscle differentiation and cell-cycle control. *Biochim Biophys Acta* 1332:M19–M30.

Malhotra A, Penpargkul S, Schaible T, Scheuer J (1981). Contractile proteins and sarcoplasmic reticulum in physiologic cardiac hypertrophy. *Am J Physiol* 241:H263–H267.

Malik RK (1998). Regulation of apoptosis by integrin receptors. *J Pediatr Hematol Oncol* 19:541–545.

Mallat Z, Tedgui A, Fontaliran F, Frank R, Durigon M, Fontaine G (1996). Evidence of apoptosis in arrhythmogenic right ventricular dysplasia. *N Engl J Med* 335:1190–1196.

Manjo G, Joris I (1995). Apoptosis, oncosis, and necrosis. An overview of cell death. *Am J Pathol* 146:3–15.

Martelli F, Cenciarelli C, Santarelli G, Polikar B, Felsini A, Caruso M (1994). MyoD induces retinoblastoma gene expression during myogenic differentiation. *Oncogene* 9:3579–3590.

McConkey DJ, Orrenius S (1997). The role of calcium in the regulation of apoptosis. *Biochem Biophys Res Comm* 239:357–366.

McDonough PM, Hanford DS, Sprenkle AB, Mellon NR, Glembotski CC (1997). Collaborative roles for c-Jun N-terminal kinase, c-Jun, serum response factor, and Sp 1 in calcium-regulated myocardial gene expression. *J Biol Chem* 272:24046–24053.

McKeehan WL, Kan M (1994). Heparan sulfate fibroblast growth factor receptor complex: structure-function relationships. *Mol Reprod Dev* 39:69–81.

McKeehan WL, Wang F, Kan M (1998). The heparan sulfate-fibroblast growth factor family: diversity of structure and function. *Prog Nucleic Acid Res Mol Biol* 59:135–176.

Meerson FZ (1961). On the mechanism of compensatory hyperfunction and insufficiency of the heart. *Cor et Vasa* 3:161–177.

Mehlen P, Kretz-Remy C, Préville X, Arrigo A-P (1996). Human hsp27 and human αβ-crystallin expression-mediated increase in glutathione is essential for the protective activity of these proteins against TNFα-induced death. *EMBO J* 15:2695–2706.

Mehlen P, Mehlen A, Godet J, Arrigo A-P (1997). hsp27 as a switch between differentiation and apoptosis in murine embryonic stem cells. *J Biol Chem* 272:31657–31665.

Meno C, Saijoh Y, Fujii H, Ikeda M, Yokoyama T, Yokoyama M, Toyoda Y, Hamada H (1996). Left-right asymmetric expression of the TGFβ-family member *lefty* in mouse embryos. *Nature* 381:151–155.

Meredith JE Jr, Winitz S, Lewis JM, Hess S, Ren X-D, Renshaw MW, Schwartz MA (1996). The regulation of growth and intracellular signaling by integrins. *Endocrinol Rev* 17:207–220.

Merle PL, Feige JJ, Verdetti J (1995). Basic fibroblast growth factor activates calcium channels in neonatal rat cardiomyocytes. *J Biol Chem* 270:17361–17367.

Mignotte B, Vayssiere J-L (1998). Mitochondria and apoptosis. *Eur J Biochem* 252:1–15.

Mima T, Ueno H, Fischman DA, Williams LT, Mikawa T (1995). Fibroblast growth factor receptor is required for in vivo cardiac myocyte proliferation at early embryonic stages of heart development. *Proc Nat Acad Sci U S A* 92: 467–471.

Miyamoto S, Termoto H, Coso OA, Gutkind JS, Burbelo PD, Akiyama SK, Yamada KM (1995). Integrin function: molecular hierarchies of cytoskeletal and signaling molecules. *J Cell Biol* 131:791–805.

Mohri H (1996). Fibronectin and integrins interactions. *J Invest Med* 44:428–441.

Molkentin JD, Lu J-R, Antos CL, Markham B, Richardson J, Robbins J, Grant SR, Olson EN. A calcineurin-dependent transcriptional pathway for cardiac hypertrophy. *Cell* 1998;93:215–228.

Morgan DO (1995). Principles of CDK regulation. *Nature* 374:131–134.

Morgenbesser Sd, Williams BO, Jacks T, DePinho RA (1994). p53-dependent apoptosis produced by *Rb*-deficiency in the developing mouse lens. *Nature* 371:72–74.

Mowat MRA (1998). p53 in tumor progression: life, death and everything. *Adv Cancer Res* 74:25–48.

Nagata S (1997). Apoptosis by death factor. *Cell* 88:355–365.

Nagata S, Golstein P (1994). The Fas death factor. *Science* 267:1449–1456.

Nakagawa S, Takeichi M (1997). N-cadherin is crucial for heart formation in the chick embryo. *Dev Growth Differentiation* 39:451–455.

Narula J, Haider N, Virmani R, DiSalvo TG, Kolodgie FD, Hajjar RJ, Schmidt U, Semigran MJ, Dec WG, Khaw B-A (1996). Apoptosis in myocytes in end-stage heart failure. *N Engl J Med* 335:1182–1189.

Nasmyth K, Hunt T (1993). Cell cycle: dams and sluices. *Nature* 366:634–635.

Niehrs C (1996). Mad connection to the nucleus. *Nature* 381:561–562.

Nishigaki K, Minatoguchi S, Seishima M, Asano K, Noda T, Yasuda N, Sano H, Kumada H, Takemura M, Noma A, Tanaka T, Watanabe S, Fujiwara H (1997). Plasma Fas ligand, an inducer of apoptosis, and plasma soluble Fas, an inhibitor of apoptosis, in patients with chronic congestive heart failure. *J Am Coll Cardiol* 29:1214–1220.

Okuyama M, Yamaguchi S, Nozaki N, Yamaoka M, Shirakabe M, Tomoike H (1997). Serum levels of soluble form of Fas molecule in patients with congestive heart failure. *Am J Cardiol* 79:1698–1701.

Olivetti G, Capasso JM, Sonnenblick EH, Anversa P (1990). Side-to-side slippage of myocytes participates in ventricular wall remodeling acutely after myocardial infarction in rats. *Circ Res* 67:23–34.

Olivetti G, Quaini E, Sala R, Lagrasta C, Corradi D, Bonacina E, Gambert S, Cigola E, Anversa P (1994). Acute myocardial infarction in humans is associated with activation of programmed myocyte cell death in the surviving portion of the heart. *J Mol Cell Cardiol* 28:2005–2016.

Olivetti G, Abbi R, Quaini F, Kajstura J, Cheng W, Nitihara JA, Quaini E, DiLoreto CD, Beltrami CA, Krajewski S, Reed JC, Anversa P (1997). Apoptosis in the failing human heart. *N Engl J Med* 336:1131–1141.

Olson EN (1993). Regulation of muscle transcription by the MyoD family. The heart of the matter. *Circ Res* 72:1–6.

Pardee AB (1989). G₁ events and regulation of cell proliferation. *Science* 246:603–608.

Parker TG, Chow K-L, Schwartz RJ, Schneider MD (1990). Differential control of the skeletal α-actin transcription in cardiac muscle by two fibroblast growth factors. *Proc Nat Acad Sci U S A* 87:7066–7070.

Parker TG, Chow K-L, Schwartz RJ, Schneider MD (1992). Positive and negative control of skeletal α-actin promoter in cardiac muscle. *J Biol Chem* 267:3343–3350.

Parker TG, Schneider MD (1990). Peptide growth factors can provoke "fetal" contractile protein gene expression in rat cardiac myocytes. *J Clin Invest* 85:507–514.

Peeper DS, Bernards R (1997). Communication between the extracellular environment, cytoplasmic signaling cascades and the nuclear cell-cycle machinery. *FEBS Lett* 410:11–16.

Penpargkul S, Repke DI, Katz AM, Scheuer J (1977). Effect of physical training on calcium transport by rat cardiac sarcoplasmic reticulum. *Circ Res* 40:134–138.

Peters G (1994). Cell cycle: stifled by inhibitions. *Nature* 371:204–205.

Peterson MB, Lesch M (1972). Protein synthesis and amino acid transport in isolated rabbit right ventricular muscle. *Circ Res* 31:317–327.

Qin X-Q, Livingston D, Kaelin WG, Adams PD (1994). Deregulated transcription factor E2F-1 expression leads to S-phase entry and p53-mediated apoptosis. *Proc Nat Acad Sci U S A* 91:10918–10922.

Rabinowitz M (1974). Overview on pathogenesis of cardiac hypertrophy. *Circ Res* 34-35(Suppl):II-3–II-11.

Raff MC, Barres BA, Burne JF, Coles HS, Ishizaki Y, Jacobson MD (1993). Programmed cell death and the control of cell survival: lessons from the nervous system. *Science* 262:695–700.

Raffray M, Cohen GM (1997). Apoptosis and necrosis in toxicology: a continuum or distinct modes of cell death? *Pharmacol Ther* 75:153–177.

Ravitz MJ, Wenner CE (1997). Cyclin-dependent kinase regulation during G1 phase and cell cycle regulation by TGF-β. *Adv Cancer Res* 71:165–207.

Reed JC (1994). Bcl-2 and the regulation of programmed cell death. *J Cell Biol* 124:1–6.

Reed JC (1997). Double identity for proteins of the Bcl-2 family. *Nature* 387:773–776.

Rumyantsev PP (1977). Interrelations of the proliferation and differentiation of processes during cardiac myogenesis and regeneration. *Int Rev Cytol* 51:187–273.

Sabbah HN, Sharov VG (1998). Apoptosis in heart failure. *Prog CV Dis* 40:549–562.

Sadoshima J, Aoki H, Izumo S (1997). Angiotensin II and serum differentially regulate expression of cyclins, activity of cyclin-dependent kinases, and phosphorylation of retinoblastoma gene product in neonatal cardiac myocytes. *Circ Res* 80:228–241.

Saini KS, Walker NI (1998). Biochemical and molecular mechanisms regulating apoptosis. *Mol Cell Bioochem* 178:9–25.

Sandritter W, Scomazzoni G (1964). Deoxyribonucleic acid content (Feulgen photometry) and dry weight (interference microscopy) of normal and hypertrophic heart muscle fibres. *Nature* 202:100–101

Sartore S, Gorza L, Pierobon Bormioli S, Dalla Liber L, Schiaffino S (1981). Myosin types and fiber types in cardiac muscle. I: Ventricular myocardium. *J Cell Biol* 88:226–233.

Sartorelli V, Kurabayashi M, Kedes L (1993). Muscle-specific gene expression. A comparison of cardiac and skeletal muscle transcription strategies. *Circ Res* 72:925–931.

Savill J (1997). Recognition and phagocytosis of cells undergoing apoptosis. *BMJ* 53:491–508.

Savill J, Fadok V, Henson P, Haslett C (1993). Phagocyte recognition of cells undergoing apoptosis. *Immunol Today* 14:131–136.

Scheuer J, Bhan AK (1979). Cardiac contractile proteins. Adenosine triphosphatase activity and physiological function. *Circ Res* 45:1–12.

Scheuer J, Buttrick P (1987). The cardiac hypertrophic responses to pathologic and physiologic loads. *Circulation.* 75(1 Pt 2):163–168.

Schmeichel KL, Beckerle MC (1994). The LIM domain is a modular protein-binding interface. *Cell* 79:211–219.

Schneider MD, Parker TG (1992). Cardiac myocytes as targets for the action of peptide growth factors. *Circulation* 81:1443–1456.

Schneider MD, Kirshenbaum LA, Brand T, MacLellan WR (1994). Control of cardiac gene transcription by fibroblast growth factors. *Molec Reprod Dev* 39:112–117.

Schumann H, Morawietz H, Hakim K, Zerkowski HR, Eschenhagen T, Holtz J, Darmer D (1997). Alternative splicing of the primary Fas transcript generating soluble Fas antagonists is suppressed in the failing human ventricular myocardium. *Biochem Biophys Res Comm* 239:794–798.

Schwartz MA, Schaller MD, Ginsberg MH (1995). Integrins: emerging paradigms of signal transduction. *Ann Rev Cell Dev Biol* 11:549–599.

Sharov VG, Sabbah HN, Shimoyama H, Goussev AV, Lesch M, Goldstein S (1996). Evidence for cardiocyte apoptosis in myocardium of dogs with chronic heart failure. *Am J Pathol* 148:141–149.

Smeyne RJ, Vendrell M, Hayward M Baker SJ, Miao GG, Schilling K, Robertson LM, Curran T, Morgan JI (1993). Continuous c-fos expression precedes programmed cell death in vivo. *Nature* 363:166–169.

Sonenshein GE (1997). Rel/NK-κB transcription factors and the control of apoptosis. *Cancer Biol* 8:113–119.

Spillman D, Burger MM (1997). Carbohydrate-carbohydrate interactions in adhesion. *J Cell Biochem* 61:562–568.

Stellar H (1995). Mechanisms and genes of cellular suicide. *Science* 267:1445–1449.

Stoker M, O'Neill C, Berryman S, Waxman V (1968). Anchorage and growth regulation in normal and virus transformed cells. *Int J Cancer* 3:683–693.

Strasser A, O'Connor L (1998). Fas ligand—caught between Scylla and Charibdis. *Nature Med* 4:21–22.

Suda T, Okazaki T, Naito Y, Yokota T, Arai N, Ozaki S, Nakao K, Nagata S (1995). Expression of the Fas ligand in cells of T lineage. *J Immunol* 154:3806–3813.

Sugahara H, Kanakura Y, Furitsu T, Ishihara K, Oritani K, Ikeda H, Kitayama H, Ishikawa J, Hashimoto K, Kanayama Y (1994). Induction of programmed cell death in human hematopoietic cell lines by fibronectin via its interaction with very late antigen 5. *J Exp Med* 170:1757–1766.

Suzuki ST (1996). Structural and functional diversity of cadherin superfamily: Are new members of cadherin superfamily involved in signal transduction pathway? *J Cell Biochem* 6:531–542.

Takeda K, Yu ZX, Nishikawa T, Tanaka M, Hosoda S, Ferrans VJ, Kasajima T (1996). Apoptosis and DNA fragmentation in the bulbus cordis of the developing rat heart. *J Mol Cell Cardiol* 28:209–215.

Tanaka M, Ito H, Adachi S, Akimoto H, Nishikawa T, Kasajima T, Marumo F, Hiroe M (1994). Hypoxia induced apoptosis with enhanced expression of Fas antigen messenger RNA in cultured neonatal rat cardiomyocytes. *Circ Res* 75:426–433.

Tartaglia LA, Ayres TM, Wong GHW, Goeddel DV (1993). A novel domain within the 55 kd TNF receptor signals cell death. *Cell* 74:845–853.

Teiger E, Than VD, Richard L, Wisnewsky C, Tea BS, Gaboury L, Tremblay J, Schwartz K, Hamet P (1996). Apoptosis in pressure overload-induced heart hypertrophy in the rat. *J Clin Invest* 97:2891–2897.

Thiery JP (1996). The saga of adhesion molecules. *J Cell Biochem* 61:489–492.

Thompson EB (1998). The many roles of c-Myc in apoptosis. *Annu Rev Physiol* 60:575–600.

Thornberry NA (1997). The caspase family of cysteine proteases. *Br Med Bull* 53:478–490.

Toyozaki T, Hiroe M, Saito T, Iijima Y, Takano H, Hiroshima K, Kohno H, Ishiyama S, Marumo F, Masuda Y, Ohwada H (1998). Levels of soluble Fas in patients with myocarditis, heart failure of unknown origin, and in healthy volunteers. *Am J Cardiol* 81:798–800.

Troppmair J, Rapp UR (1997). Apoptosis regulation by Raf, Bcl-2, and R-ras. *Rec Res Cancer Res* 143:245–249.

Ucker DS (1991). Death by suicide: one way to go in mammalian development? *New Biologist* 3:103–109.

Umansky SR, Tomei LD (1997). Apoptosis in the heart. *Adv Pharmacol* 41:383–407.

van Noorden CFJ, Meade-Tollin LC, Bosman FT (1998). Metastasis. *Am Scientist* 86:130–141.

Villareal FJ, Dillmann WH (1992). Cardiac hypertrophy-induced changes in mRNA levels for TGF-β1, fibronectin and collagen. *Am J Physiol* 262:H1861–H1866.

Vliegen HW, Eulderink E, Bruschke AV, van der Laarse A, Cornelisse CJ (1995). Polyploidy of myocyte nuclei in pressure overloaded human hearts: a flow cytometric study in left and right ventricular myocardium. *Am J Cardiovasc Pathol* 5:27–31.

Vlodavsky I, Miao H-Q, Medalion B, Danagher P, Ron D (1996). Involvement of heparan sulfate and related molecules in sequestration and growth promoting activity of fibroblast growth factor. *Cancer Metastasis Rev* 15:177–186.

Wallach D (1997). Placing death under control. *Nature* 388:123–126.

Wallach D, Boldin M, Varfolomeev E, Beyaert R, Vandenabeele P, Fiers (1997). Cell death induction by receptors of the TNF family: towards a molecular understanding. *FEBS Lett* 410:96–106.

Walsh K, Perlman H (1997). Cell cycle exit upon myogenic differentiation. *Curr Opin Genet Dev* 7:597–602.

Waltenberger J (1997). Modulation of growth factor activation. Implications for the treatment of cardiovascular diseases. *Circulation* 96:4083–4094.

Wang J, Walsh K (1996). Resistance to apoptosis conferred by Cdk inhibitors during myocyte differentiation. *Science* 273:359–361.

Wang J, Guo K, Walsh K (1997). Rb functions to inhibit apoptosis during myocyte differentiation. *Cancer Res* 57:351–354.

Watanabe-Fukunaga R, Brannan CI, Itoh N, Yonehara S, Copeland NG, Jenkins NA, Nagata S (1992). The cDNA structure, expression, and chromosomal assignment of the mouse Fas antigen. *J Immunol* 148:1274–1279.

Weber K (1992). Cardiac interstitium: extracellular space of the myocardium. In Fozzard H, Haber E, Katz A, Jennings R, Morgan HE, eds. *The Heart and Cardiovascular System,* 2nd ed. Raven Press, New York, pp 1465–1480.

Weng W, Li B, Kajstura J, Li P, Wolin MS, Sonnenblick EH, Hintze TH, Olivetti G, Anversa P (1995). Stretch-induced programmed cell death. *J Clin Invest* 96:2247–2259.

Whitaker M, Partel R (1990). Calcium and cell cycle control. *Development* 108:525–542.

Whitman M (1997). Feedback from inhibitory SMADs. *Nature* 389:549–551.

Wollert KC, Taga T, Saito M, Narazaki M, Kishimoto T, Glembotski CC, Vernallis AB, Heath JK, Pennica D, Wood WI, Chien KR (1996). Corticotrophin-1 activates a distinct form of cardiac muscle cell hypertrophy. Assembly of sarcomeric units in series via gp130/leukemia inhibitory factor receptor-dependent pathways. *J Biol Chem* 271:9535–9545.

Wrana J, Pawson T (1997). Mad about SMADS. *Nature* 388:28–29.

Wyllie AH (1987). Apoptosis: cell death in tissue regulation. *J Pathol* 153:313–316.

Wyllie AH (1997a). Apoptosis: an overview. Br Med Bull 53:451–465.

Wyllie AH (1997b). Clues in the p53 murder mystery. *Nature* 389:237–238.

Yamada T, Horiuchi M, Dzau VJ (1996). Angiotensin II type 2 receptor mediates programmed cell death. *Proc Nat Acad Sci U S A* 93:156–160.

Yamazaki T, Komuro I, Yazaki Y (1995). Molecular mechanism of cardiac hypertrophy by mechanical stress. *J Mol Cell Cardiol* 27:133–140.

Yao M, Keogh A, Spratt P, dos Remedios CG, Keissling PC (1996). Elevated DNase I levels in human idiopathic dilated cardiomyopathy: an indicator of apoptosis? *J Mol Cell Cardiol* 28:95–101.

Yap AS, Brieher WM, Gumbiner BM (1997). Molecular and functional analysis of cadherin-based adherens junction. *Ann Rev Cell Dev Biol* 13:119–146.

Yoshizumi M, Lee W-S, Hsieh C-M, Tsai J-C, Li J, Perrella MA, Patterson, Endege WO, Schlegel R, Lee M-E (1995). Disappearance of cyclin A correlates with permanent withdrawal of cardiomyocytes from the cell cycle in human and rat hearts. *Cell* 95:2275–2280.

Zafeiridis A, Jeevanandam V, Houser SR, Margulies KB. Regression of left ventricular hypertrophy following left ventricular assist device support. *Circulation* 1998;98:656–662.

Zheng L, Fisher G, Miller RE, Peschon J, Lynch DH, Lenardo MJ (1995). Induction of apoptosis in mature T cells by tumour necrosis factor. *Nature* 377:348–351.

7

Signal Transduction Within Cells of the Failing Heart

The farther researches we make into this admirable scene of things [the flow of fluids in plants], the more beauty and harmony we see in them: And the stronger and clearer convictions they give us, of the being, power and wisdom of the divine Architect, who has made all things to concur with a wonderful conformity, in carrying on, by various and innumerable combinations of matter, such a circulation of causes, and effects, as was necessary to the great ends of nature.

Stephen Hales, *Vegetable Staticks,* 1727, The Introduction

And how vastly more numerous are the many Branchings, Windings and Turnings of the Arteries and Veins, how innumerable the lymphatic Vessels, and secretory Ducts? And these all adjusted and ranged, in the most exact Symmetry and Order, to serve the several Purposes of the animal Oeconomy; So curiously are we wrought, so fearfully and wonderfully are we made!

Stephen Hales, *Statickal Essays: Containing Hæmastaticks,* 1733, p. 72

Among the most eloquent comments on the complexity of biological regulation are those of Stephen Hales (1677–1761), who made the first accurate determinations of blood pressure in living animals. Hales, who was educated as a minister, saw a "beauty and harmony" in the control of integrated biological systems. But unlike the normal circulation studied by Hales, where the end result of homeostasis is "Symmetry and Order," the compensatory responses in heart failure are not only adaptive but also initiate and perpetuate degenerative processes that can destroy the heart.

In virtually every patient who suffers with heart failure, the body's "attempts" to compensate for the reduced cardiac function are made possible by responses that, while initially adaptive, eventually harm both the heart and the patient. In other words, the hemodynamic abnormalities that initiate these compensatory responses are made worse by the body's efforts to "put the circulation right." As described in Chapters 4 through 6, misdirected efforts at compensation include the neurohumoral response, hemodynamic and inflammatory defense reactions, and stimulation of myocardial growth.

The earlier discussions of the maladaptive responses in heart failure focused on extracellular messengers and the membrane receptors that bind these signaling molecules. This chapter carries the description of these responses across the plasma membrane, into the cell, highlighting signal transduction cascades that are activated by the extracellular messengers. These intracellular cascades lead to such "downstream" responses as protein phosphorylation by an activated protein kinase, and DNA binding by an activated transcription factor. The final result is a molecular change that modifies both biochemical properties, notably contractile performance, and gene expression. These responses hold the key to understanding both the pathophysiology and practical management of heart failure.

AN OVERVIEW OF CELL SIGNALING

The homeostatic mechanisms that adjust cardiac myocyte function to meet the needs of the body require effective, ongoing communication with the environment outside the cell. The heart's ability to interpret changing circulatory demands, therefore, depends on signal transduction pathways that "notify" cardiac myocytes of a change in hemodynamics or the inadequate perfusion of a vital organ, and then evoke an appropriate response. In exercise, the most important of the physiologic stimuli, the heart must be made aware of the body's need for a large increase in cardiac output. This is brought about by responses that not only augment pump function, but when called upon repeatedly during training, also cause a growth response called physiologic hypertrophy (the "athlete's heart"). The pathologic response to a sustained overload initiates quite different growth patterns that, depending on the nature of the hemodynamic stress, favor the appearance of one or another abnormal cardiac myocyte phenotypes. Different pathologic stimuli, such as systolic stress and diastolic stretch (pressure and volume overload), cause concentric and eccentric hypertrophy, which at the cellular level are due in part to increased myocyte diameter and length, respectively (see Chapter 6). This ability to generate different myocyte phenotypes in response to different mechanical stimuli requires intracellular signaling systems that, with both sensitivity and selectivity, evoke appropriate molecular responses. The intracellular signal transduction systems that control contractile performance and myocyte phenotype are the focus of this chapter.

The Response to Exercise: A Model for Intracellular Signal Transduction

The neurohumoral response to exercise is among the best understood of the mechanisms that adjust the heart's output to a change in circulatory dynamics. Key to this re-

FIG. 7-1. Depiction of the signal cascade by which exercise leads to an increase in myocardial contractility. This cartoon shows 11 of these steps as a series of buckets where, in each step, the incoming signal causes the bucket to overflow its contents, thereby transmitting the signal to the next bucket in the cascade. In cellular signal transduction, different substances pass from one "bucket" to the next. The first, sympathetic stimulation (Step 1) activates an elaborate system that releases norepinephrine into the space outside cardiac myocytes (Step 2). Step 3, binding of norepinephrine to the β receptor, occurs in the extracellular space at the outer surface of the plasma membrane. The remaining steps, which all take place within the myocardial cell, include activation of a "coupling protein" (Step 4), increased adenylyl cyclase activity (Step 5), generation of the second messenger cyclic AMP (Step 6), activation of a cyclic-AMP dependent protein kinase (Step 7), phosphorylation of several substrates, including plasma membrane L-type calcium channels (Step 8), and increased open probability of the channel that allows more calcium to enter the cell (Step 9). The resulting increase in intracellular calcium stores makes more of this activator cation available for release during excitation-contraction coupling (Step 10), which allows calcium to bind to a greater number of troponin molecules. This activates a greater number of actin-myosin interactions (Step 11), which increases contractility.

sponse are mechanisms that operate together to increase cardiac output. One is an increase in venous return, brought about when vasodilatation in the exercising muscles increases blood flow into the veins from the arteries. The resulting increase in diastolic volume stretches the cardiac myocytes, thus increasing their ability to do work through the operation of Starling's Law of the Heart. The response to exercise is also aided by the he-

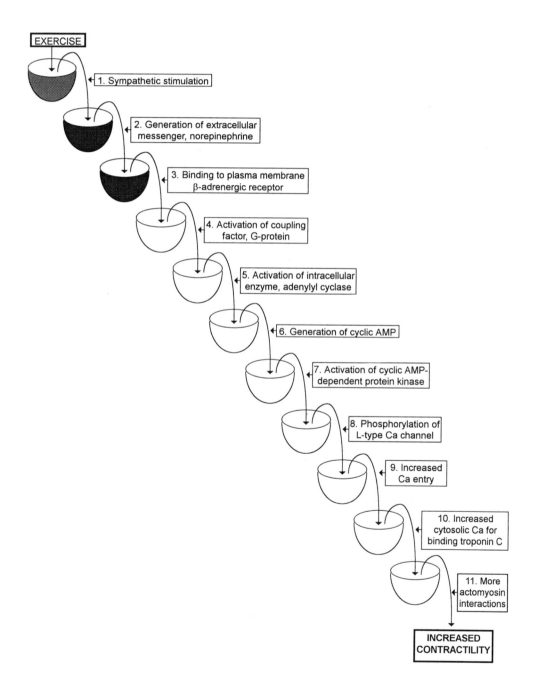

modynamic defense reaction discussed in Chapter 4. The most important elements of this response are increases in heart rate, myocardial contractility, and relaxation, all of which are initiated when norepinephrine binds to β-adrenergic receptors on cardiac myocytes. The following brief overview highlights the inotropic response in illustrating the operation of one of the best known of the heart's signal transduction systems.

The Inotropic Response to Exercise

The major stimulus for the increased contractility during exercise is norepinephrine release from sympathetic nerve endings in the heart. Norepinephrine does not act directly on the heart's contractile machinery, rather it initiates its inotropic effects when it binds to β-adrenergic receptors on the surface of working myocardial cells. Because β-adrenergic receptors also cannot interact directly with the contractile proteins, additional means of communication are required to initiate the positive inotropic response. These are provided by the multistep signaling system, in which each step is controlled by a messenger or chemical reaction generated in the preceding step. Like a series of waterfalls along a river, these steps are linked one to another in a "signal transduction cascade."

The signal transduction cascade shown schematically in Fig. 7-1 depicts 11 of the steps by which exercise increases myocardial contractility as a series of "buckets." In each step of this "bucket brigade," an incoming signal causes one bucket to transmit its signal to the next bucket. Unlike a bucket brigade, in which a single substance (water) is passed from firefighter to firefighter, a different substance transmits the signal from each step to the next in a cellular signaling cascade.

The first two steps in Fig. 7-1 (sympathetic stimulation and norepinephrine release) take place outside of the heart, between cells in the autonomic nervous system and at sympathetic nerve endings, respectively. The third step, activation of the β receptor by its binding to norepinephrine, occurs in the extracellular space immediately outside the myocardial cell. All of the remaining steps take place within the myocardial cell, where each uses a different signaling mechanism. These include activation of a "coupling protein" (step 4), which increases the catalytic activity of adenylyl cyclase (step 5), which generates cyclic adenosine monophosphate (cyclic AMP) (step 6), which activates a protein kinase (step 7), which phosphorylates a calcium channel (step 8), which admits more calcium into the cell (step 9), which increases the cell's store of calcium (step 10), which allows more of this cation to be released to activate a greater number of troponin molecules, thereby increasing the number of active actin-myosin interactions (step 11). It is not until the last step in this sequence that contractility is actually increased. As discussed later in this chapter, signaling cascades similar in complexity to that shown in Fig. 7-1, yet quite different in detail, mediate virtually every signal that modifies cardiac function.

Detailed accounts of the intracellular signal transduction cascades that operate in the patient with heart failure are available elsewhere. The following discussion highlights a conceptual approach that should be useful to those who deal with heart failure. Important principles of signal transduction are reviewed, using examples that seem to be of greatest importance for understanding and managing this syndrome.

WHY ARE THERE SO MANY STEPS IN A SIGNAL TRANSDUCTION CASCADE?

One might reasonably ask why, as shown in Fig. 7-1, so many steps intervene between a change in hemodynamic function and the molecular response that increases myocardial contractility. (In fact, the "real" response is even more elaborate than is shown in Fig. 7-1, which has simplified this signal transduction cascade by omitting or combining several steps.) The answer lies in the ability of these multistep sequences to enhance the control of cell signaling. Thus, the many steps that link sympathetic stimulation to increased myocardial contractility, which at first glance might seem almost perverse, actually provide the cell with important options.

The linear sequence of reactions depicted in Fig. 7-1 is, in fact, not an accurate representation of how most cellular signal transduction systems actually work. Instead of a simple linear cascade, in which one step couples to a single downstream reaction, these pathways generally branch, loop both forward and backward, and interconnect with other pathways. These patterns illustrate several important principles in biological regulation. In the first place, these many steps provide rich opportunities for control in terms of grading the response ("fine tuning"), amplifying the signal, and providing feedback loops to prevent the response from going out of control ("runaway signaling"). For example, each of the eight steps in Fig. 7-1 that take place within the cell (steps 4 through 11) can be regulated by other steps in this cascade, as well as by entirely separate signaling systems. The result is "intrapathway" and "extrapathway" cross-talk that allows the increased contractility to be graded to match the rapidly changing needs of the circulation, yet remain within the limitations of the myocardial cell. This cross-talk also provides for amplifications that allow myocardial contractility to increase rapidly, as well as a flexibility of response that maintains contractility within a range that is appropriate for the circulation at any moment. None of this would be possible if the increase in contractility were simply an "all-or-none" inotropic response.

Two of many mechanisms that can fine tune this cascade are shown in Fig. 7-2. One sensitizes the increased calcium entry caused by phosphorylation of L-type calcium channels (step 9) to allosteric control by adenosine triphosphate (ATP). This cross-talk can allow a decrease in ATP concentration to inhibit L-type calcium channel opening and thus blunt the inotropic response in an energy-starved heart. The second example illustrates one way that the norepinephrine-induced increase in contractility is integrated with changes in other systems to prevent "runaway signaling." This is the ability of increased cytosolic calcium (step 10) to inhibit the rate at which adenylyl cyclase generates cyclic AMP (Tada et al., 1975), an effect that slows the cascade at step 5.

The many steps in most signal transduction cascades also allow a single extracellular messenger to evoke an integrated response. For example, the large number of isoforms found for most enzymes and substrates that participate in these signal transduction cascades allows a single messenger to cause distinct responses both in different tissues and in a single tissue that contains several cell types. Chapter 4 noted how different receptor subtypes (step 3 in Fig. 7-1) make it possible for norepinephrine to evoke different responses in different tissues. Later in this chapter, another example is discussed, the generation of two intracellular signaling molecules when a ligand-bound receptor interacts

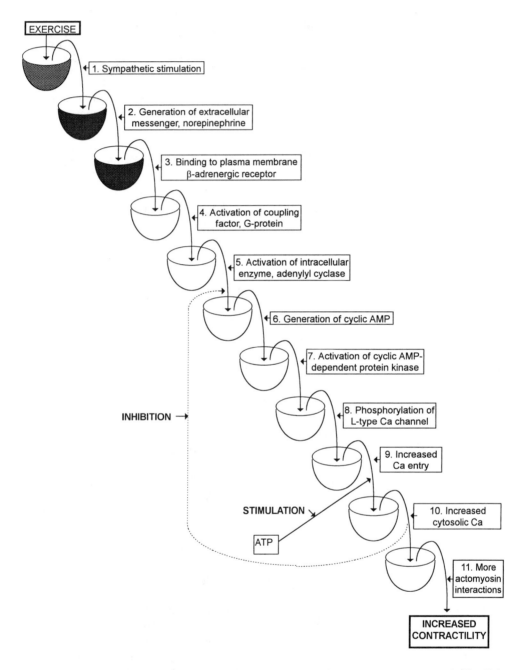

FIG. 7-2. Two mechanisms that "fine tune" the signal transduction cascade shown in Fig. 7-1. The first is seen when cytosolic calcium, elevated by increased opening of L-type calcium channels (Step 9), inhibits adenylyl cyclase activity so as to slow the cascade at Step 5. The second reflects an allosteric control exerted by ATP, which allows a decrease in ATP concentration to inhibit L-type calcium channel opening (Step 10), a feedback that attenuates this cascade in an energy-starved heart.

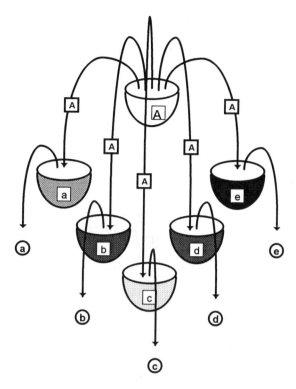

FIG. 7-3. Cartoon showing showing how a single class of signaling molecule (labeled "A") can interact with five targets to generate five different "products" (labeled "a" through "e").

with the heterotrimeric G proteins. This signal diversification is depicted schematically in Fig. 7-3, in which a single signaling molecule (labeled "A") interacts with five different targets (buckets "a" through "e") to generate five different "products," each of which can produce a different effect. Yet another level of control is shown in Fig. 7-4, in which interactions between the five products can amplify and inhibit both "upstream" and "downstream" reactions.

With some imagination, the reader can expand on the cartoons in Figs. 7-1 through 7-4 to grasp the precision of control made possible by cross-talk within a given signaling cascade, and the integration and fine tuning of signals by interactions between different cascades. Several examples of these principles are encountered later in this chapter, wherein a single extracellular messenger evokes a multifaceted response that is integrated with other cellular responses. These principles illustrate Hales' remarkable insight that biological control exhibits a

> symmetry and Order... a wonderful conformity, in carrying on, by various and innumerable combinations of matter, such a circulation of causes, and effects, as [is] necessary to the great ends of nature.

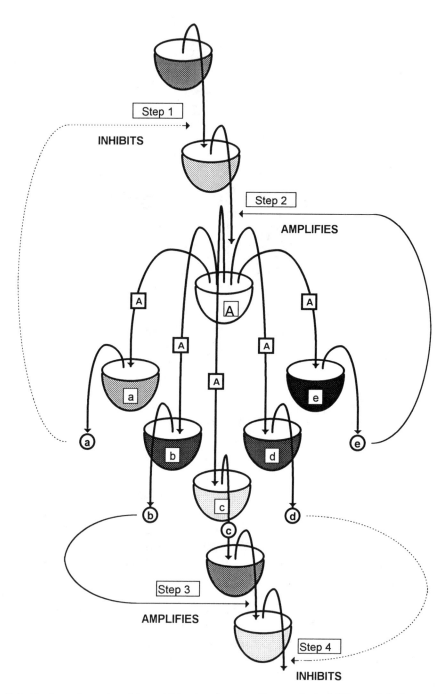

FIG. 7-4. Cartoon, based on Figure 7-3, showing how the products "a" through "e," generated in response to a single messenger ("A"), can modify other reactions in the signal cascade. Product "a" inhibits upstream Step 1 and product "e" amplifies upstream Step 2. The downstream reactions, which are mediated by product "c," are amplified by product "b" at Step 3 and inhibited by product "d" at Step 4.

RECEPTORS

Most signal transduction cascades are initiated when a small molecule, referred to throughout this text as an *extracellular messenger*, arrives at the surface of the cell. Because these messengers initiate their cellular effects when they bind to membrane receptors, they are also called *ligands* or *agonists*. Extracellular messengers can reach their targets by way of the bloodstream (endocrine signaling), from adjacent nerve endings (neurohumoral signaling), from nearby cells (paracrine signaling), or from the cell whose function is modified (autocrine signaling) (Table 7-1).

The affinity with which various ligands bind to membrane receptors varies considerably (Table 7-2). Some toxins saturate their receptors at concentrations around 10^{-12} M, whereas most neurohumoral transmitters and drugs occupy their receptors at concentrations between 10^{-8} and 10^{-6} M. Some compounds, such as ethanol, interact with membranes only at higher concentrations, around 10^{-3} M. These affinities are important determinants of the specificity of the effects of a ligand. As might be expected, the responses to ligands that bind their receptors at low concentrations (high binding affinities) are very specific and accompanied by few side effects. The reason is that a high binding affinity allows the ligand to occupy a specific receptor at very low concentrations, which minimizes nonspecific interactions with other components of the membrane. Ligands that bind to their receptors at high concentrations tend to have more extraneous, nonspecific actions.

The receptors that recognize and bind extracellular messengers can be divided into two broad classes: *plasma membrane receptors* located on the cell surface, which interact with ligands in the extracellular space, and *intracellular receptors*, which bind to ligands that have entered the cytosol (Table 7-3). Hydrophilic molecules, because they are unable to cross the lipid barrier of a phospholipid bilayer and so cannot enter the cytosol, bind to sites on the extracellular surface of the plasma membrane. Because most mediators of the neurohumoral response discussed in Chapter 4, as well as the cytokines and related peptide growth factors discussed in Chapters 5 and 6, are water-soluble molecules, their effects depend on interactions with plasma membrane receptors. Major exceptions are steroid and thyroid hormones, which, because they are lipophilic molecules, can cross the plasma membrane to enter the cytosol, where they bind to intracellular receptors.

TABLE 7-1. *Major routes of signal transduction by extracellular messengers*

Endocrine signaling: extracellular messenger arrives via the bloodstream
Neurohumoral signaling: extracellular messenger arrives from an adjacent nerve ending
Paracrine signaling: extracellular messenger arrives from a nearby cell
Autocrine signaling: extracellular messenger is secreted by the cell whose function is modified

TABLE 7-2. *Binding affinities of cardiac plasma membrane receptors to various ligands*

Ligand	Receptor	Approximate K_d*
Tetrodotoxin	Sodium channel	10^{-12} M
Nitrendipine	Calcium channel	10^{-10} M
Epinephrine	β-adrenergic receptor	10^{-8} M
Ouabain	Sodium pump	10^{-6} M
Ethanol	Unknown	10^{-3} M

*K_d, the dissociation constant, is the ligand concentration at which half of the receptors are occupied. The lower the K_d, the tighter is the binding. The reciprocal of K_d is the binding constant K_b, so that a higher K_b means the ligand binds more tightly to its receptor.

TABLE 7-3. *Major receptor classes*

Plasma membrane receptors
    Ion channel receptors: L-type calcium channels, acetylcholine receptors
    Enzyme-linked receptors: cytokine receptors, cell adhesion molecules
    Heptahelical, G protein-coupled receptors: See Table 7-4
        α- and β-Adrenergic receptors
        Muscarinic receptors
        Angiotensin II receptors
        Endothelin receptors
Intracellular receptors
    Steroid, thyroxin, vitamin D, and retinoic acid receptors

Intracellular Receptors

Signaling molecules that enter the cell generally bind to receptors located within the nucleus (for review, see Evans, 1988). The resulting ligand-receptor complexes often function as transcription factors that directly modify gene expression when they recognize and bind to a specific DNA sequence. One example of this mechanism is seen in the ability of thyroxin to form a complex with nuclear thyroxin receptors that modifies the expression of genes that encode myosin heavy chains (for review, see Izumo et al., 1990). This effect of thyroxin, which favors synthesis of the fast α-myosin heavy chain (Everett et al., 1983), is the opposite of the isoform shift seen in the overloaded failing heart, where the slower, β-myosin heavy chain gene is expressed preferentially (Izumo et al., 1987). Actions of steroid hormones on the heart (Beznak, 1964; Rannels et al., 1977; Lengsfeld et al; 1988; March et al., 1998) appear to be clinically significant in light of recent evidence, discussed in Chapter 9, that aldosterone receptor blockade improves prognosis in patients with moderately severe heart failure.

Plasma Membrane Receptors

There are three major types of plasma membrane receptors (see Table 7-3). The first are channel molecules that contain ligand-binding sites, which, when occupied by an agonist, directly modify transitions from one channel state to another, for example, between open and closed channels. Ion channel receptors include the acetylcholine receptor of the neuromuscular junction, which opens when bound to this agonist.

The two other major types of plasma membrane receptor are the *enzyme-linked receptors*, so-named because, when bound to their ligand, these receptors directly activate an intracellular enzyme, usually a protein kinase, and the *heptahelical receptors*, so named because they share a common structure that includes seven membrane-spanning α helices. The signals initiated by the latter are coupled to a family of GTP-binding (guanosine triphosphate) proteins, called *G proteins*, which couple the activated receptor to a variety of downstream reactions. For this reason, heptahelical receptors are also called *G protein-coupled* receptors.

Several enzyme-linked receptors were discussed in the review of cytokines, peptide growth factors, and adhesion molecules. When bound to their ligands, or in the case of the adhesion molecules to the extracellular matrix or to other cells, these receptors activate an intracellular enzyme, generally a latent tyrosine kinase that is part of the receptor molecule. In most cases, the ligand-bound receptor forms an aggregate that activates tyrosine kinase sites on another receptor-bound protein. In other signal transduction systems, enzyme-linked receptors activate serine/threonine kinases or enzymes other than protein kinases; the latter include a tyrosine phosphatase, which by catalyzing tyrosine dephosphorylation, mediates a proapoptotic signal, and guanylyl cyclase, which is part of a receptor that, when bound to atrial natriuretic peptide, synthesizes the intracellular second messenger cyclic GMP (Maack, 1992). Chapters 5 and 6 have already discussed the enzyme-linked receptors that mediate cytokine and peptide growth factor actions, so that the following discussion highlights the actions of the heptahelical G protein-coupled receptors.

HEPTAHELICAL (7 MEMBRANE-SPANNING), G PROTEIN-COUPLED RECEPTORS

The most important mediators of the hemodynamic defense reaction are members of the family of heptahelical receptors depicted schematically in Fig. 7-5. This extensive family of plasma membrane receptors is among the largest in biology and includes as many as 1,000 different proteins (Wess, 1997); about 1 in 80 of the human genes have been estimated to encode members of this class of receptors (Clapham and Neer, 1997), a few of which are listed in Table 7-4.

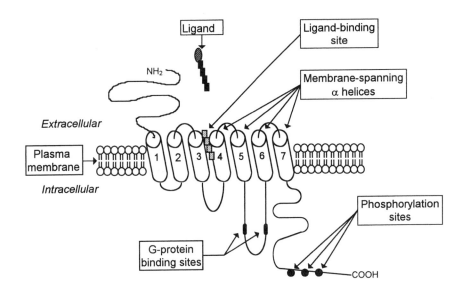

**HEPTAHELICAL (7 MEMBRANE-SPANNING)
G PROTEIN-COUPLED RECEPTOR**

FIG. 7-5. Heptahelical membrane receptor showing the seven membrane spanning α helices (tilted "cans") and both intracellular and extracellular peptide loops. Portions of several transmembrane helices (shaded) bind to the ligand. The intracellular peptide loop linking the fifth and sixth membrane spanning helices contains sites that bind the coupling G protein. Phosphorylation sites on the C-terminal intracellular peptide loop participate in receptor downregulation.

TABLE 7-4. *Some of the major signal transduction systems activated by heptahelical G-protein-coupled receptors*

Receptor	Ligand	"Target"	Second messenger or effector
α-adrenergic	α-Agonists	Phospholipase C	↑ Diacylglycerol, InsP₃
β-adrenergic	β-Agonists	↑ Adenylyl cyclase	↑ cyclic AMP
Muscarinic	Acetylcholine	K channel	↑ Outward K current
Muscarinic	Acetylcholine	↓ Adenylyl cyclase	↓ Cyclic AMP
Purinergic (P₁)	Adenosine	K channel	↑ Outward K current
Purinergic (P₁)	Adenosine	↓ Adenylyl cyclase	↓ Cyclic AMP
Angiotensin (AT₁)	Angiotensin II	Phospholipase C	↑ Diacylglycerol, InsP₃
Endothelin	Endothelin	Phospholipase C	↑ Diacylglycerol, InsP₃

InsP₃, inositol 1,4,5-trisphosphate; AMP, adenosine monophosphate

The seven membrane-spanning α-helices that give these receptors their name contain hydrophobic amino acids that anchor these proteins in the plasma membrane bilayer (see Fig. 7-5). The ligand-binding site of most, if not all, members of this class of receptors faces the extracellular surface and includes parts of the hydrophobic regions of the membrane-spanning α-helices numbers 4 through 7 and, in the case of receptors that bind cationic agonists such as norepinephrine, acetylcholine, dopamine, and serotonin, an aspartate residue in the middle of helix-number 3. (For review, see Herbette and Mason, 1992; Trumpp-Kallmeyer et al., 1992). The G-protein binding sites that are in contact with the cytosol also include portions of some membrane-spanning α-helices and one of the intracellular loops (Wess, 1997). Phosphorylation sites located on the C-terminal intracellular loop desensitize the receptors in a process that is discussed further later, when mechanisms that blunt the response of the failing heart to β-adrenergic agonists are discussed. The immediate targets of ligand-bound heptahelical receptors are members of the large family of heterotrimeric G proteins.

Regulation of Receptor Sensitivity and Number

The number of receptors available to respond to their extracellular messengers is not fixed but can increase or decrease. One important change in receptor number occurs when the heart is chronically stimulated by β-adrenergic agonists, which reduces the response to these neurohumoral mediators. This phenomenon, once referred to as "tachyphylaxis," is generally called *desensitization* or *downregulation* (for review, see Lefkowitz et al., 1997).

Desensitization

There are three steps in desensitization: uncoupling, internalization, and digestion, which occur in the sequence shown in Fig. 7-6. Although the following description highlights β-adrenergic receptor desensitization, similar mechanisms reduce the responsiveness of other members of this family of receptors.

Uncoupling (Phosphorylation)

The first step in β-adrenergic receptor desensitization occurs when a ligand-bound receptor is phosphorylated by a protein kinase, commonly referred to as *βARK (β-adrenergic receptor kinase)*. βARK is one of a family of protein kinases, called *G protein re-*

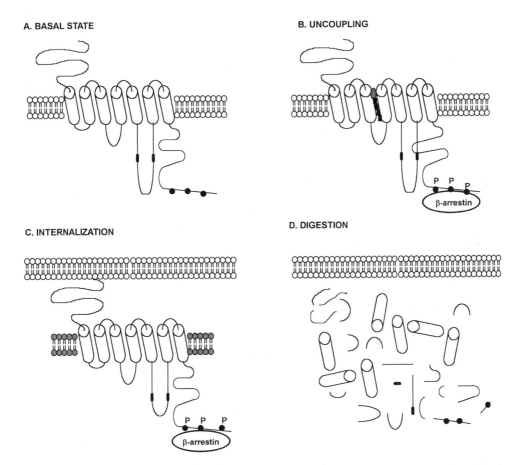

FIG. 7-6. β-Adrenergic receptor desensitization. **A:** Basal state of the receptor. **B:** Prolonged binding of the receptor to its ligand stimulates a G protein receptor kinase called βARK (β-adrenergic receptor kinase) to catalyze the phosphorylation of the C-terminal intracellular peptide chain. This phosphorylated peptide chain then binds a cofactor called arrestin, which prevents the receptor from interacting with its G protein. **C:** Internalization occurs by transfer of the phosphorylated receptors from the plasma membrane to other membrane systems within the cell, where the internalized receptors, although structurally intact, can no longer interact with either their agonists or their G protein. Dephosphorylation (not shown), by allowing the internalized receptors to return to the plasma membrane, can resensitize the receptors. **D:** If the receptors remain internalized for a long period, they are digested by intracellular proteolytic enzymes. This mechanism, unlike uncoupling and internalization, is irreversible.

ceptor kinases (GRK), that catalyze phosphorylation reactions that are targeted to ligand-bound receptors so as to prevent the activated receptor from interacting with its G protein (see Fig. 7-6B). By uncoupling the receptor from its downstream signal transduction pathway, these phosphorylations provide a negative feedback that inactivates the cascade. Receptor desensitization by βARK is mediated by a cofactor called *β-arrestin*, which binds to the phosphorylated C-terminal intracellular peptide chain so as to block the receptor's interactions with its G protein. This step in receptor desensitization is fully reversible where receptor activity is restored by a process called *resensitization,* in which the receptor is dephosphorylated by a *G protein-coupled receptor phosphatase.*

The G protein receptor kinases that phosphorylate and desensitize G protein-coupled receptors can be activated by other signal transduction systems, for example, by phospholipid-activated protein kinases (DebBurman et al., 1996). The ability of one signal transduction system to stimulate a protein kinase that inactivates another signal transduction system represents a "cross-phosphorylation" by which one signal transduction cascade shuts down another system.

Internalization (Sequestration)

The second step in desensitization, called "internalization," occurs when the phosphorylated receptors that have been uncoupled from their G proteins are removed from the plasma membrane. The internalized, β-arrestin-bound receptors, which are transferred to clathrin-coated pits within the cell (Luttrell et al., 1999), initially remain structurally intact, although they cannot interact with either their agonists or their G proteins. As discussed later in this chapter, the internalized complex between the β receptor and β-arrestin can participate in mitogenic signaling, which provides an example of how inactivation of one signal transduction system (the β receptor cascade) can activate another system (mitogenic signaling).

Internalization, like phosphorylation, is reversible as long as the phosphorylated receptors remain intact. The internalized receptors can return to the plasma membrane if they are dephosphorylated by a phosphoprotein phosphatase. However, if the receptors remain internalized for long periods, they become susceptible to proteolytic digestion, a final and irreversible step in desensitization.

Digestion (Degradation)

After prolonged exposure of the cell to an agonist, the internalized receptors are digested by proteolytic enzymes within the cell. Unlike uncoupling and internalization, this mechanism is irreversible, so that full return of function after prolonged exposure to high concentrations of an agonist requires that new receptors be synthesized.

Enhanced Sensitivity

The sensitivity of the heart's β receptors to β-adrenergic agonists can also be increased. This is seen in laboratory animals after the heart is denervated, a phenomenon that is sometimes called "denervation sensitivity." Clinically, a similar phenomenon can occur after prolonged administration of β-adrenergic blockers. The heightened sensitivity of these receptors makes it dangerous to stop β-blocker therapy abruptly, so that when therapy with these drugs must be stopped, the dose should be "tapered," (i.e., lowered gradually) when possible. This enhanced sensitivity of receptors to β agonists following prolonged administration of β blockers appears to result from an increase in β receptor number (Heilbrunn et al., 1989), an effect that may be due to externalization of receptors that, under normal conditions, are held in reserve within the cell.

ROLE OF GTP-BINDING PROTEINS IN THE RESPONSE TO HEPTAHELICAL RECEPTORS

Guanyl nucleotide-binding proteins (G proteins), which provide a critical link between ligand-bound heptahelical receptors (step 3 in Fig. 7-1) and downstream signal transduction (step 4 in Fig. 7-1), interact with heptahelical receptors as heterotrimers made up of G_α, G_β, and G_γ subunits. Because binding of the ligand to its receptor generates two G protein-mediated signals, the actions of these heterotrimers exemplify the principle of diversification shown schematically in Fig. 7-3. One signal is mediated by G_α, the guanyl nucleotide-binding component that, when bound to GTP, functions on its own; the other is mediated by G_β and G_γ, which operate together as a dimer that is referred to as $G_{\beta\gamma}$.

Reactions Between the Heptahelical Receptors and GTP-Binding Coupling Proteins

An elaborate minuet allows activation of a heterotrimeric G protein by its ligand-bound heptahelical receptor to generate two different signals. This process can be viewed as the five-step sequence that is depicted schematically in Fig. 7-7 and described below.

Step 1: Binding of the ligand to its receptor and activation of G_α. In the "basal state" (see Fig. 7-7A), in which the ligand-binding site on the receptor is unoccupied, the free receptors are bound to the G protein trimer ($G_{\alpha\beta\gamma}$). In this state, the inactive G protein increases the binding affinity of the unoccupied receptor (R) for its ligand (L), which favors ligand-receptor binding, the first step in the activation sequence (see Fig. 7-7B):

$$R-G_\alpha-GDP-G_{\beta\gamma} + L \rightarrow R-L-G_\alpha-GDP-G_{\beta\gamma}$$

Step 2: Formation of G_α–GTP and dissociation of $G_{\beta\gamma}$. Binding of the ligand to the receptor complex stimulates G_α to bind GTP. This forms the activated G_α–GTP complex, which initially remains bound to $G_{\beta\gamma}$:

$$R-L-G_\alpha-GDP-G_{\beta\gamma} + GTP \rightarrow R-L-G_\alpha-GTP-G_{\beta\gamma} + GDP$$

The activated G_α-GTP then becomes dissociated from $G_{\beta\gamma}$, but remains bound to the ligand-receptor complex. Release of $G_{\beta\gamma}$ allows the latter to interact with its targets ($T_{\beta\gamma}$) (see Fig. 7-7C):

$$R-L-G_\alpha-GTP-G_{\beta\gamma} \rightarrow R-L-G_\alpha-GTP + G_{\beta\gamma} \rightarrow T_{\beta\gamma}.$$

Step 3: Dissociation of G_α–GTP from the receptor: Dissociation of $G_{\beta\gamma}$ from the R–L–G_α–GTP complex causes G_α–GTP to separate from the ligand-receptor complex (R–L). This has two consequences (see Fig. 7-7D). The first is to reduce the ligand-binding affinity of the receptor, which releases the ligand. The second is to allow the free G_α–GTP to participate in additional signaling cascades by interacting with its own targets (T_α).

$$R-L-G_\alpha-GTP \rightarrow R + L + G_\alpha-GTP \rightarrow T_\alpha$$

Step 4: Dissociation of the ligand-receptor complex from G_α-GTP and dephosphorylation of bound GTP. Dissociation of the G_α-GTP complex from the receptor stimulates the intrinsic GTPase activity of G_α, which dephosphorylates its bound GTP (see Fig. 7-7E). Dephosphorylation of GTP regenerates G_α-GDP, which returns G_α to its basal state. The G_α-GDP then rebinds and inactivates the $G_{\beta\gamma}$ released in step 2. As a result, signaling by both G_α and $G_{\beta\gamma}$ is ended:

$$G_\alpha-GTP + G_{\beta\gamma} \rightarrow G_\alpha-GDP-G_{\beta\gamma} + P_i.$$

The rate of GTP hydrolysis, which is key to turning off the signal, is a major determinant of the duration of the response. As discussed below, this key reaction is controlled by several additional regulatory proteins.

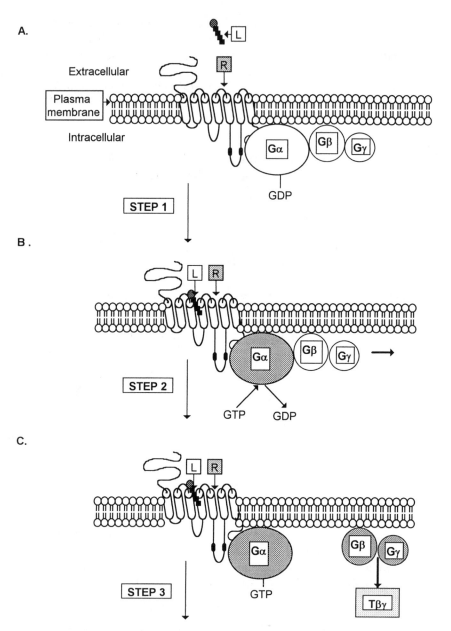

FIG. 7-7. Simplified scheme showing five steps in the interactions between a heptahelical receptor, its ligand, and the heterotrimeric G proteins. **A:** Basal state, where the ligand (L), is not bound to its receptor (R) and G_α is bound to GDP. In this state, binding of the complex formed by G_α and the $G_{\beta\gamma}$ dimer activates the receptor, increasing its ligand-binding affinity. In this and subsequent drawings, inactive forms of these proteins are unshaded, whereas the active forms are shaded. **B:** Binding of the ligand to the receptor stimulates G_α to bind GTP, which forms the active G_α-GTP complex. At the same time, $G_{\beta\gamma}$ becomes dissociated from G_α. **C:** Dissociation activates $G_{\beta\gamma}$, allowing it to modify its targets ($T_{\beta\gamma}$).

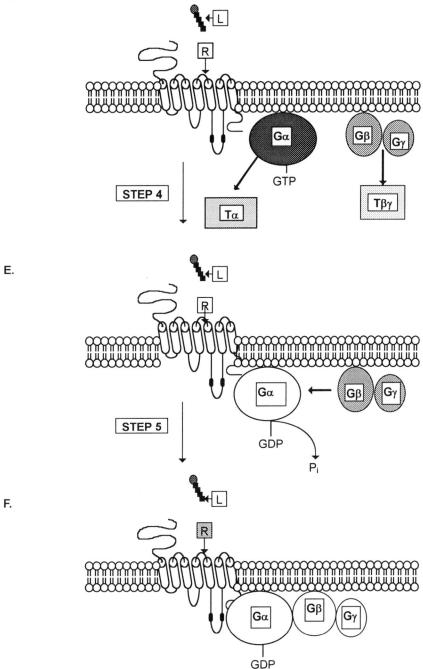

FIG. 7-7. D: The activated G_α-GTP complex becomes dissociated from the receptor, which by reducing its ligand-binding affinity, releases the ligand. The free G_α-GTP complex released in this step becomes further activated (increased shading), which allows G_α to interact with its targets (T_α). **E:** Dissociation of activated G_α from the receptor causes the former to become a GTPase enzyme, which by dephosphorylating its bound GTP, forms the inactive G_α-GDP complex. The latter then rebinds $G_{\beta\gamma}$. **F:** The inactivated $G\alpha$ subunit rebinds and activates the receptor, and rebinds and inactivates the $G_{\beta\gamma}$ subunit. The transitions in E and F turn off both G protein-mediated signals and bring these signaling elements back to the situation in F, which is identical to A.

Step 5: Rebinding of G_α to $G_{\beta\gamma}$ and rebinding of the receptor to the $G_{\alpha\beta\gamma}$ complex: Formation of the complex between G_α-GDP and $G_{\beta\gamma}$ allows the $G_{\alpha\beta\gamma}$ complex to rebind the free receptor, increasing its affinity for the ligand (see Fig. 7-7F).

$$R + G_\alpha\text{–}GDP\text{–}G_{\beta\gamma} \rightarrow R\text{–}G_\alpha\text{–}GDP\text{–}G_{\beta\gamma}$$

This step returns the system to its original state.

Regulators of the G Protein Cycle

At least three protein families regulate GTP hydrolysis, which is the major rate-limiting reaction in G protein-coupled signaling. These are *GTPase-activating proteins (GAPs)*, which accelerate GTPase activity, *guanine nucleotide exchange factors (GEFs)*, which accelerate the release of G_α-bound GDP, and *guanine nucleotide dissociation inhibitors (GDIFs)*, which counteract GEFs by inhibiting GDP release. The control of these regulators, which involves several additional reactions, is not discussed further.

Overview of the G Protein Cycle

The elaborate reactions of the heterotrimeric G proteins allow the binding of a single ligand to its heptahelical receptor to release two messengers: activated G_α-GTP and free $G_{\beta\gamma}$, each of which activates many downstream messengers (shown schematically in Fig. 7-3). This control also amplifies some of these signals ("positive" feedback) and, by turning off many steps more or less "automatically" ("negative" feedback), avoids runaway signaling. This "negative" feedback occurs because the G_α-GTP complex is unstable, spontaneously hydrolyzing its bound nucleotide to form the inactive G_α-GDP. In addition, when the latter rebinds $G_{\beta\gamma}$, the other messenger is also inactivated. Runaway signaling is also avoided because dissociation of activated G_α-GTP from the ligand-bound receptor reduces the affinity of the bound receptor for its ligand, which helps turn off the G protein-mediated signal by favoring dissociation of the ligand from the receptor. A quite different effect is seen in the dependence of this signaling system on a continuing supply of GTP, which slows G protein-coupled systems in energy-starved cells, when the GTP: GDP ratio decreases.

SIGNAL TRANSDUCTION BY HEPTAHELICAL
G PROTEIN-COUPLED RECEPTORS

The richness of signaling made possible by the hundreds of known heptahelical receptors is increased still further by at least 20 G_α subunits, 6 G_β subunits, and 12 G_γ subunits (for reviews, see Neer, 1995; Clapham and Neer, 1997; Gudermann et al., 1997). This diversity provides for both precision and variety in cell signaling. The G_α subunits are often divided into four families: $G_{\alpha s}$, $G_{\alpha i}$, $G_{\alpha q}$, and $G_{\alpha 12}$. $G_{\alpha s}$ is involved in stimulatory responses, such as adenylyl cyclase activation by norepinephrine, whereas $G_{\alpha i}$ mediates inhibition of cyclic AMP production by muscarinic and purinergic agonists (see Table 7-4).

Coupling of different ligand-bound receptors with their G_α subunits follows several patterns. A few ligand-bound receptors interact with a single G_α subtype to generate a tightly focused signal. However, most extracellular messengers activate several G_α subtypes to transmit signals down many cascades so as to generate integrated, multifaceted responses. In some cases, a single receptor can activate as many as ten different G_α subunits, including members of all four families (Laugwitz et al., 1996). Not all responses initiated by ligand binding to G protein-coupled receptors involve activation; many are inhibitory. As noted earlier, different G proteins can exert opposite effects on cellular function, for example, $G_{\alpha s}$ stimulates cyclic AMP production, whereas $G_{\alpha i}$ inhibits formation of this second messenger.

G Protein Alterations in the Failing Heart

Desensitization of the failing heart to the stimulatory effects of β-adrenergic agonists blunts some of the maladaptive features of the hemodynamic defense reaction. As discussed in Chapter 4, mechanisms for this desensitization include a reduced number of β adrenergic receptors caused by inhibition of β-receptor synthesis and β receptor downregulation. A third mechanism that inhibits the response of the failing heart to sympathetic stimulation is brought about by changes in the levels of the G proteins that couple activated β receptors to adenylyl cyclase. Levels of $G_{\alpha s}$, which stimulates cyclic AMP formation, although reported in early studies to be unchanged in the failing heart (Feldman et al., 1988; Insel and Ransnäs, 1988; Schnabel et al., 1990), are probably decreased when this stimulatory protein is inactivated and internalized in a manner similar to that described for the β receptors (Roth et al., 1993; Ping and Hammond, 1994; Nash et al., 1996). Conversely, levels of $G_{\alpha i}$, which inhibits adenylyl cyclase, are increased in the failing heart (Feldman et al., 1988; Neumann et al., 1988; Böhm et al., 1994), so that the ratio $G_{\alpha i}:G_{\alpha s}$ is increased in this syndrome. These changes, along with reduced β receptor synthesis and β receptor downregulation explain a decrease in cyclic AMP content in failing hearts (Danielsen et al., 1989).

Direct (Membrane-Delimited) and Indirect (Second Messenger-Mediated) Coupling

Activated G proteins can transmit signals by two general mechanisms (Table 7-5). In the first, which is referred to as direct or *membrane-delimited coupling*, the activated G protein itself interacts with the target that alters cell function. One example is the ability of muscarinic receptor-activated G proteins to modify membrane potential by interacting directly with plasma membrane potassium channels. The other way that G proteins modify cell function is by indirect, or *second messenger-mediated coupling*, which takes place when the target of an activated G protein is an enzyme that modifies the concentration of one or more intracellular signaling molecules, called second messengers (Table 7-6).

Intracellular Second Messengers

Intracellular second messengers are substances that carry signals from one place to another when they diffuse along the cytosolic surface of the plasma membrane or through the cytoplasm. These intracellular signaling molecules include nucleotides, lipids, and phosphosugars whose synthesis is controlled by signals that are generated by heptaheli-

TABLE 7-5. *Two mechanisms for signaling by heptahelical receptor-GTP-binding coupling protein*

Direct signaling: direct actions of the coupling proteins on effector systems
Indirect (second messenger) signaling: second messengers mediate the effects of the coupling proteins on effector systems

TABLE 7-6. *Major intracellular messengers*

Second messenger	Initiation of signal	Termination of signal
Cyclic AMP	Synthesized from ATP by adenylyl cyclase	Degraded to AMP by phosphodisterases
Cyclic GMP	Synthesized from GTP by guanylyl cyclase	Degraded to GMP phosphodiesterases
InsP$_3$	Synthesized from PIP$_2$ by phospholipase C	Dephosphorylated by phosphatases
Diacylglycerol	Synthesized from PIP$_2$ by phospholipase C	Phosphorylated to form phosphatide or hydrolyzed to form monogylceride
Calcium	Diffuses into the cytosol from a region of high concentration	Pumped out of cytosol

PIP$_2$, Phosphatidylinositol 4,5-bisphosphate; InsP$_3$, inositol 1,4,5-trisphosphate

cal G protein-coupled receptors (see Table 7-6). Examples include cyclic AMP and cyclic GMP, which are synthesized by activated *adenylyl cyclase* and *guanylyl cyclase*, respectively. Adenylyl cyclase is generally stimulated or inhibited by different G proteins, whereas regulators of guanylyl cyclase often act directly on this enzyme, as occurs when cyclic GMP synthesis is stimulated by the binding of nitric oxide (EDRF) to an intracellular guanylyl cyclase, or when atrial natriuretic peptide (ANP) binds to receptors that contain a latent guanylyl cyclase. Other second messengers provide additional signal diversification, as is seen in the actions of *phospholipase C* (*PLC*), a family of G protein-activated lipolytic enzymes made up of three major groups (PLCβ, PLCγ, and PLCδ), each of which includes several isoforms (Nishizuka, 1995; Schnabel et al., 1996). When activated, this lipolytic enzyme hydrolyzes the membrane phospholipid *phosphatidyl-inositol 4,5-bisphosphate* (*PIP$_2$*) to release two intracellular messengers: *diacyl glycerol* (*DAG*) and *inositol trisphosphate* (*InsP$_3$*). *Phospholipase D*, another lipolytic enzyme that can be activated when mitogens bind to their plasma membrane receptors, hydrolyzes *phosphatidylcholine* to release *phosphatidic acid*, another second messenger that generates DAG. *Ceramide*, a recently discovered second messenger derived from yet another family of membrane phospholipids, the *sphingomyelins*, is discussed later, when the stress-activated MAP kinases are considered.

Calcium, another important intracellular messenger listed in Table 7-6, is not synthesized within cells. Instead, this cation enters the cytosol from regions of high concentration, either the extracellular space or an internal membrane-delimited structure called the sarco(endo)plasmic reticulum. Many calcium fluxes into and out of the cytosol are controlled by G protein-coupled receptors and their second messengers.

Signal Transduction Cascades Regulated by Ras and other Monomeric G Proteins

The signal transduction cascades that modify growth and proliferation are generally coupled by GTP-binding proteins that function as monomers. These monomeric G proteins, which resemble G$_\alpha$, generally do not interact with plasma membrane receptors but instead are activated by other intracellular signal transduction cascades, such as those initiated by ligand-binding to enzyme-linked receptors. The monomeric G protein *Ras* transmits proliferative signals that modify gene expression, whereas other members of this family, such as *Rho* and *Rac*, participate in signal transduction cascades that impinge on the cytoskeleton.

Ras targets are usually serine/threonine kinases that, when activated, initiate mitogenic signals that are transmitted to the nucleus where they stimulate protein synthesis, cell

growth, and proliferation. Among the most important of the Ras-coupled signal transduction cascades are those that activate a family of enzymes, discussed later, called *mitogen-activated protein kinases (MAP kinases)* (Vojtek and Cooper, 1995). Ras, like G_α,
binds guanyl nucleotides, is active when bound to GTP, contains an intrinsic GTPase, and
is inactivated when the bound GTP is dephosphorylated to form GDP. Hydrolysis of GTP
by Ras is slower than that by G_α, which means that Ras-mediated signals are generally
long lasting. The duration of the Ras signal, like that of the G protein heterotrimers described earlier, can be modified by proteins that stimulate and inhibit GTPase activity and
GDP release.

PATHWAYS ACTIVATED BY ENZYME-LINKED AND
G PROTEIN-COUPLED RECEPTORS

There are several parallels between the signals generated by enzyme-linked receptors,
such as those that bind cytokines and peptide hormones, and the signals initiated by G
protein-coupled heptahelical receptors. Some of these parallels are shown schematically
in Fig. 7-8 and, for a few major signaling pathways, are listed in Table 7-7. Furthermore,
both receptor classes generally use G proteins to link receptor activation at the "top" of
the cascade to the downstream phosphorylations within the cell by activating protein kinases.

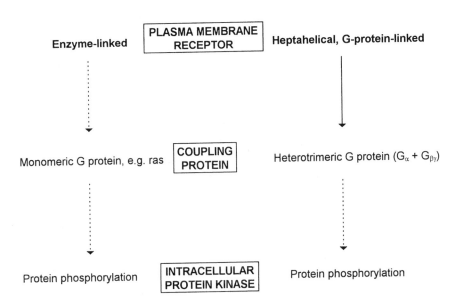

FIG. 7-8. Parallels between signals generated by enzyme-linked plasma membrane receptors,
such as those that bind cytokines and peptide hormones (left), and the signals initiated by G
protein-coupled heptahelical receptors (right). Both classes of receptor generally utilize GTP-
binding proteins to link receptor activation at the "top" of the cascade to the downstream phosphorylations that are catalyzed by protein kinases. Whereas heptahelical receptors interact directly with the heterotrimeric G proteins (solid arrow), activation of the monomeric G proteins
by enzyme-linked receptors is indirect and involves several coupling steps (dashed arrows), as
do the downstream phosphorylations in both signaling cascades.

TABLE 7-7. *Key signal transduction systems that operate in the mammalian cardiovascular system*

Extracellular signal	Receptor	Coupling proteins	Second messenger or mediator system	Intracellular target
β-Adrenergic agonists	β-adrenergic receptor	G protein*	adenylyl cyclase, cyclic AMP	protein kinase A
α-Adrenergic agonists	α-adrenergic receptor	G protein*, ras	phospholipase C, DAG, InsP₃	protein kinase C
Angiotensin II	AT₁ receptor	G protein*, ras	phospholipase C, DAG, InsP₃	protein kinase C
Endothelin	ET_A receptor			
Inflammatory cytokines	cytokine receptors	ras		SAPKs
Peptide growth factors	tyrosine kinase receptors	ras		MAP kinases
Extracellular matrix contact, cell/cell contact kinases	integrins cadherins	ras ras		tyrosine kinases tyrosine

*Heterotrimeric G protein. Other abbreviations: SAPK; stress-activated protein kinase, MAP kinase: mitogen activated protein kinases

Most enzyme-linked receptors either form aggregates with proteins that contain latent tyrosine kinase activity or are themselves latent tyrosine kinases, so that the initial signal generated by these receptors is tyrosine phosphorylation. A major exception is the TGF-β receptor, which is a serine/threonine kinase (see Chapter 6). G protein-coupled receptors, on the other hand, generally activate serine/threonine kinases, usually in signaling cascades that require the participation of intracellular second messengers. Unlike G protein-coupled receptors, which interact directly with heterotrimeric G proteins, activation of monomeric G proteins (e.g., Ras) by tyrosine kinase receptors occurs further downstream (see Fig. 7-8). As the signals generated by these two classes of receptor are transmitted down the signaling cascades, both tyrosine and serine/threonine protein kinases become activated.

Protein Kinases and Phosphatases

At this point it is useful to define explicitly the actions of two classes of enzyme that mediate the phosphorylations that have been mentioned at many points in this text. The first are the *protein kinases*, which catalyze the transfer of the terminal phosphate of ATP to hydroxyl groups found on three amino acids: tyrosine, serine, and threonine (Table 7-8). The result is the formation of a stable *phosphoester* bond that is quite different from the more labile, high-energy, *acyl-phosphate* reaction intermediates formed by such ATP-utilizing structures as ion pumps and the contractile proteins (Fig. 7-9).

A second class of enzyme mentioned frequently in this text are the *phosphoprotein phosphatases*, often called simply *phosphatases*, which dephosphorylate the phosphoesters described in the preceding paragraph (for review, see van Hoof et al., 1993). Phosphotyrosine phosphatases are found both in soluble form and bound to membranes; the

TABLE 7-8. *Major intracellular protein kinases*

Protein kinase	Activated by (second messenger)
Cyclic AMP-dependent (*protein kinase A, PK-A*)	Cyclic AMP
Cyclic GMP-dependent	Cyclic GMP
Phospholipid-dependent (*protein kinase C, PK-C*)	Diacyl glycerol
Calcium, calmodulin-dependent (*CAM kinase*)	Calcium

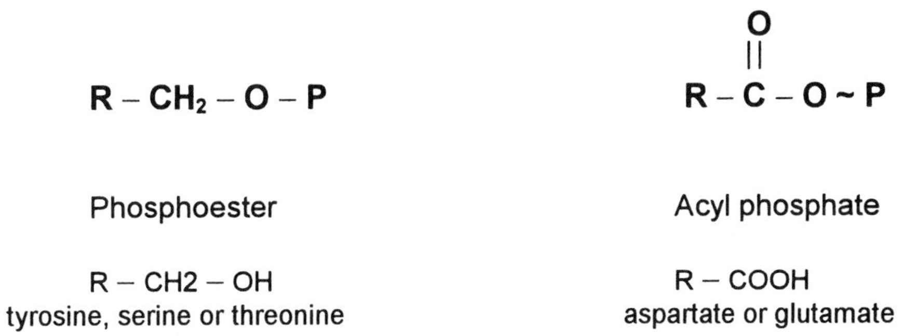

$$R - CH_2 - O - P$$

$$R - \overset{\overset{\displaystyle O}{\displaystyle \|}}{C} - O \sim P$$

Phosphoester

Acyl phosphate

R − CH2 − OH
tyrosine, serine or threonine

R − COOH
aspartate or glutamate

FIG. 7-9. Differences between a phosphoester (left) and an acyl-phosphate (right) bond. A stable phosphoester is formed when phosphate binds to a hydroxyl moiety on tyrosine, serine, or threonine, whereas in the more labile, high-energy acyl-phosphate reaction intermediates are formed by bonds linking phosphate to the carboxyl moiety of aspartic or glutamic acid.

latter, by responding to the arrival of an extracellular messenger at the cell surface, can participate directly in signal transduction. Nonreceptor and receptor phosphotyrosine phosphatases are closely related to one another and include many isoforms whose substrate specificity allows these enzymes to participate in the tight control of cellular function. Some soluble phosphotyrosine phosphatases are related to *src* family of "adaptor proteins" that participate in the MAP kinase pathways discussed below. Together, protein kinase-catalyzed phosphorylations and phosphatase-catalyzed dephosphorylations participate in many of the reactions that regulate cell function, growth, and proliferation.

"Proliferative" versus "Functional" Signaling

The rapid progress in our understanding of signal transduction is described in an elegant editorial by H. R. Bourne (1995) as advancing from "a few discrete clans" of signaling molecules, organized in two discrete pathways of functional and proliferative signaling, to a series of "wheels within wheels!...bustling communication networks within and between clans of signaling proteins within the average cell." Cell function and cell proliferation, once thought to be controlled by two independently regulated, nonoverlapping signal transduction pathways (Fig. 7-10), can no longer be viewed as a simple dichotomy between distinct systems, one regulating cell function and the other growth and proliferation. The G protein-linked heptahelical receptors, initially identified as regulating cell function, are currently known to modify growth responses once thought to be under the "exclusive" control of the enzyme-linked tyrosine kinase receptors. The latter include cell proliferation, gene expression, and protein synthesis. Similarly, the tyrosine kinase receptors that were initially viewed as mediating only growth responses are known to have effects on such cellular functions as myocardial contractility and membrane potential (Cachero et al., 1998). It is clear, therefore, that there is a great deal of cross-talk between the two pathways depicted in Fig. 7-10.

The clinical importance of this cross-talk is enormous. Signals once thought to be highly specific are now known to modify a number of cellular functions, often with surprising clinical consequences. This cross-talk can explain why, in a number of clinical trials, agents designed to modify "functional" signaling in a manner that improves symptoms over the short term, were found to worsen long-term outcome by effects on proliferative signaling. It also can account for the beneficial effects of some drugs, like the converting enzyme inhibitors, which block proliferative as well as functional pathways. One reason that drugs such as vaso-

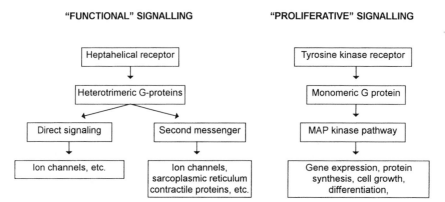

FIG. 7-10. Early view of cell signaling as involving two independent systems for "functional" and "proliferative" signaling. The former, which is mediated by heptahelical receptors that are linked to heterotrimeric G proteins, was viewed as regulating such functions as contraction, whereas the latter, thought to regulate only growth and proliferation, was thought to be mediated by tyrosine kinase receptors coupled to a monomeric GTP-binding protein such as Ras. These two pathways were thought to use different signaling mechanisms: functional signaling by either membrane-delimited or second messenger mediated mechanisms, and proliferative signaling by mitogen-activated protein kinase (MAP kinase) pathways.

dilators and inotropes, which by reducing afterload and increasing contractility have obvious short-term beneficial effects on function, worsen long-term survival is that they also have effects, both direct and indirect, that appear to exacerbate maladaptive growth in the failing heart. It is becoming increasingly clear that "secondary" effects of many drugs on cell growth are often of greater clinical significance than their more obvious hemodynamic effects, in accord with the principle that what is obvious is not always important, whereas what is important is not always obvious. These topics are discussed in Chapter 9, where possible foundations for new therapeutic approaches for the management of heart failure are discussed.

ADRENERGIC SIGNALING BY HEPTAHELICAL G PROTEIN-LINKED RECEPTORS

The two major adrenergic pathways by which norepinephrine modifies cell function are illustrated in Fig. 7-11. Both are mediated by heptahelical receptors that are coupled

FIG. 7-11. Two major adrenergic pathways that are activated when norepinephrine binds to its heptahelical receptors. **A:** Binding of the catecholamine to a β-receptor modifies cell function by indirect (upper) and direct (lower) mechanisms. In the former, the ligand-bound receptor activates G_α, which stimulates adenylyl cyclase to form cyclic AMP (cAMP). This intracellular second messenger then activates protein kinase A (PK-A), which modifies cellular function by phosphorylating one or more proteins, such as the calcium channel depicted in this example. In direct coupling, the activated G protein, in this case $G_{\beta\gamma}$, interacts directly with its target, such as a plasma membrane potassium channel. **B:** Binding of norepinephrine to an α_1-receptor modifies cell function by activating $G_{\beta\gamma}$. (Signaling molecules in their basal state are unshaded and in their activated state are shaded.) The latter then stimulates phospholipase C. This lipolytic enzyme hydrolyzes phosphatidylinositol, a membrane phospholipid, to generate two second messengers: diacylglycerol (DAG) and inositol trisphosphate ($InsP_3$). Angiotensin II, endothelin, and other extracellular messengers also use this pathway to modify cell function.

β-RECEPTOR ACTIVATION

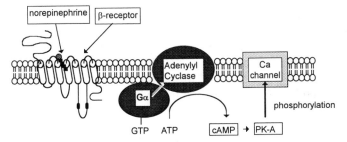

INDIRECT (SECOND MESSENGER-MEDIATED) COUPLING

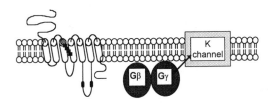

DIRECT (MEMBRANE-DELIMITED) COUPLING

A

α₁-RECEPTOR ACTIVATION

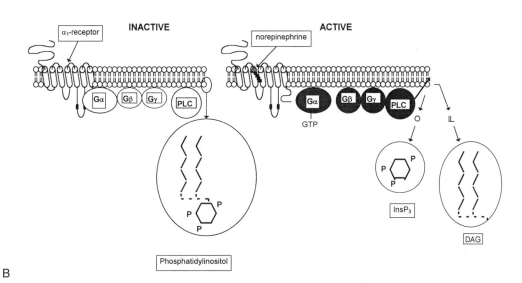

B

to the heterotrimeric G proteins, although they allow the catecholamine to generate quite different cardiovascular responses. One pathway is mediated by β-receptor activation, which generally modifies cell function by cyclic AMP-mediated mechanisms, but occasionally operates by indirect signaling (see Fig. 7-11A). The other, which is activated when norepinephrine binds to α_1-receptors, generates two quite different second messengers (see Fig. 7-11B). The following description of these signal transduction cascades, although not an exhaustive review of these cellular mechanisms, should provide an overview of adrenergic signaling and an introduction to key "players" in these communication pathways.

β-Adrenergic Receptors, Adenylyl Cyclase, and Cyclic AMP

The signals initiated by ligand-binding to adrenergic receptors vary among different tissues. In the heart, norepinephrine binding to β receptors leads to the formation of the active G_α-GTP complex and the liberation of $G_{\beta\gamma}$, each of which transmits its own signals within the cell (see Fig. 7-7). Activated G proteins can act directly to modify the function of a target protein, such as an ion channel, or they can activate adenylyl cyclase, which synthesizes cyclic AMP (see Fig. 7-11A). This intracellular second messenger generally stimulates cyclic AMP-dependent protein kinases (PK-A), which catalyze serine/threonine phosphorylations that both modify cell function and regulate cell growth and proliferation. Recognizing the close relationship between cell growth and programmed cell death, it is not surprising that norepinephrine can also induce apoptosis.

α-Adrenergic Receptors, Phospholipase C, Inositol Trisphosphate, Diacylglycerol, and Protein Kinase C

Norepinephrine binding to α_1-adrenergic receptors, which in the human cardiovascular system are found mainly on vascular smooth muscle, initiates very different cellular responses than does the binding of this neurotransmitter to β receptors. This is true even in the heart, where norepinephrine-binding to the small number of α_1 receptors exerts a weak inotropic effect. Activation of β receptors, on the other hand, evokes a much more powerful inotropic response. Although norepinephrine-binding to α_1 receptors and β receptors activates both G_α and $G_{\beta\gamma}$, different isoforms of these G proteins transmit the α_1 and β adrenergic signals to different downstream signaling cascades. Among the most important of these differences is that α_1 agonists activate $G_{\alpha q}$, which does not stimulate adenylyl cyclase but instead activates phospholipase C. As discussed earlier, this lipolytic enzyme hydrolyzes phosphatidylinositol 4,5-bisphosphate (PIP$_2$) to release inositol trisphosphate (InsP$_3$), a phosphosugar, and the lipid diacylglycerol (DAG) (see Fig. 7-11B). The family of phospholipases C, which can be activated by both G_α-GTP and free $G_{\beta\gamma}$, appears to be the most important mediator of the signaling molecules that are activated by α_1 agonists, and by other mediators of the hemodynamic defense reaction, including angiotensin II, endothelin, and vasopressin (for review, see van Biesen et al., 1996; Hefti et al., 1997).

The cellular actions of InsP$_3$ and DAG not only differ from those of cyclic AMP but also from each other (Fig. 7-12). The major effect of InsP$_3$ is to increase cytosolic calcium concentration by opening intracellular calcium release channels that differ from the "ryanodine receptors" discussed in Chapter 3. DAG, on the other hand, activates lipid-dependent protein kinases called protein kinase C (PK-C). Although PK-C, like PK-A, alters cellular function by catalyzing serine/threonine phosphorylations, the substrates for

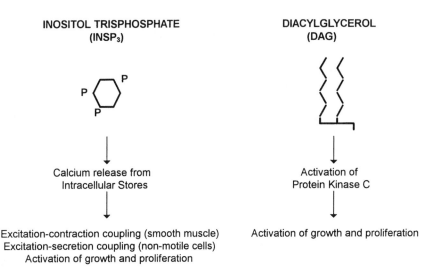

FIG. 7-12. The two products released by phospholipase C cleavage of inositol phospholipids, inositol trisphosphate (InsP₃), and diacylglycerol (DAG), have different effects on cellular function. InsP₃ binds to receptors that release calcium from intracellular membrane stores into the cytosol. In smooth muscle, this calcium participates excitation-contraction coupling, whereas in nonmotile cells, InsP₃-induced calcium release mediates excitation-secretion coupling. InsP₃-induced calcium release also activates gene expression, cell proliferation, and protein synthesis. DAG activates protein kinase C (PK-C), a family of lipid-activated serine/threonine kinases that phosphorylate a variety of targets. Many of the latter participate in signal transduction cascades that regulate gene expression, cell growth and proliferation, and protein synthesis.

these two enzymes are different, so that α_1 and β adrenergic signaling evoke quite different responses.

The protein kinase C family, like so many of the signaling molecules discussed in this chapter, is very diverse (for review, see Nishizuka, 1995; Simpson, 1999). These enzymes can be activated by DAG and calcium (*cPKCs*; c = conventional), by DAG but not calcium (*nPKCs*; n = novel), or by phospholipids other than DAG (*nPKCs*; a = atypical). Each of these groups includes several subspecies, and as many as ten isoforms of this enzyme can be found in the mammalian heart. Major substrates for the PK-Cs include the monomeric G protein Ras, and Raf-1, a key enzyme in the mitogenic MAP kinase pathway discussed later. Members of the PK-C family also regulate cell growth and proliferation by activating nuclear transcription factors. Elevated levels of calcium-activated isoforms of this family of key enzymes in the failing heart (Bowling et al., 1999) are consistent with a central tenet of this text, that activation of mitogenic pathways plays a major role in causing the poor prognosis in this syndrome.

Other Activators of Phospholipase C, Inositol Trisphosphate, and Diacylglycerol

Signaling cascades mediated by phospholipase C, PK-C, DAG, and InsP₃ are central to signaling systems activated by α_1-adrenergic agonists, angiotensin II, endothelin, and vasopressin. In addition to modifying such cellular functions as vasomotor tone, these neurohumoral mediators regulate gene expression, although in different ways. The ability of a cell to "direct" a phospholipase C- or PK-C-mediated signal so as to target an appropriate response is made possible by the existence of a number of different phospholipase C and PK-C isoforms, which are activated by different G proteins (the many isoforms of G_α, G_β, and G_γ) in response to the binding of different ligands to their specific plasma membrane receptors (Fig. 7-13). This targeting implies a spatial "compartmentation" within the cell, as can occur when a given set of isoforms is inserted into a specialized segment of an internal membrane, such as a unique lipid "domain" formed by a cluster of distinct membrane phospholipids (Klausner et al., 1980; Katz et al., 1982). A more important mechanism of compartmentation is the association of proteins kinases and their targets through anchoring proteins, such as the *AKAPs* (*A kinase anchoring proteins*), which direct cyclic AMP-dependent protein kinases to specific sites on the cytosolic face of a membrane (for review, see Gray et al., 1998).

Functional and Proliferative Signaling and Calcium

The control of tension developed by the heart and blood vessels in response to α- and β-adrenergic signaling is due largely to effects on calcium fluxes into and out of the cytosol.

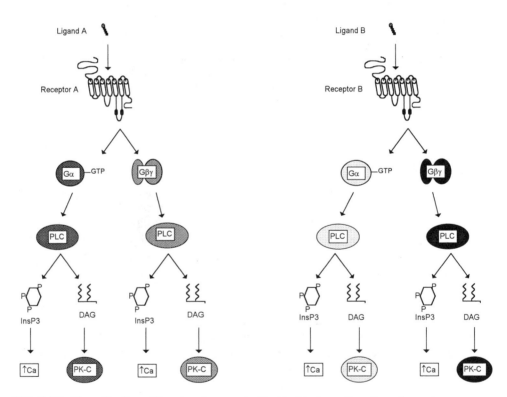

FIG. 7-13. Diversification of the signal generated by the binding of two ligands, such as an norepinephrine and angiotensin II, to different heptahelical receptors. Each ligand-bound receptor generates both activated G_α-GTP and free $G_{\beta\gamma}$, each of which can stimulate the lipolytic activity of a different isoform of phospholipase C (PLC). These, in turn, can hydrolyze phosphatidylinositols located in different regions of the cell, where by activating different isoforms of protein kinase C, can generate different responses. The inositol trisphosphate generated by PLC in these reactions can also elevate calcium concentration in different regions of the cell.

In the heart, cyclic AMP generated by β-adrenergic signaling stimulates the ion channels and pumps that control calcium fluxes across both the plasma membrane and sarcoplasmic reticulum. Cyclic AMP accelerates heart rate by increasing the pacemaker current, i_f, and calcium currents that control pacemaker activity in the sinoatrial node. This second messenger also increases contractility and facilitates relaxation by accelerating calcium fluxes across the plasma membrane and sarcoplasmic reticulum in the working cells of the atria and ventricles.

In vascular smooth muscle, the InsP$_3$ generated by $α_1$-adrenergic signaling opens InsP$_3$-gated channels that, by releasing calcium from intracellular stores, play a critical role in vasoconstriction. Other mediators of the neurohumoral response, notably angiotensin II, endothelin, and arginine vasopressin, also activate signal transduction cascades that constrict vascular smooth muscle. These effects, like those of $α_1$-adrenergic stimulation, are mediated by G protein-coupled activation of phospholipase C, and by the second messengers InsP$_3$ and DAG. The importance of the cross-talk between "functional" and "proliferative" signaling is seen in the ability of the calcium released by these signal transduction cascades also to regulate cell growth and proliferation.

The role of InsP$_3$-induced calcium release in cardiac myocytes is not yet fully understood. Because the calcium flux through InsP$_3$-gated calcium channels is quite slow, much less than that through the ryanodine receptors (Ehrlich and Watras, 1988), the former is unlikely to play an important role in beat-to-beat excitation-contraction coupling. The increased cytosolic calcium mediated by InsP$_3$-gated receptors can cause a weak, slowly developing inotropic response, and may increase diastolic tension. The slow increase in cytosolic calcium may also participate in controlling gene expression.

Elevated cytosolic calcium can stimulate proliferative responses by several mechanisms. In addition to the cPKCs described above, these include a family of protein kinases called *calcium, calmodulin kinases* (*CAM*) kinases (for review, see Lewis et al., 1998). The role of the CAM kinases in regulating gene expression has been studied extensively in neurons, which like cardiac myocytes are terminally differentiated cells. Calcium entry through neuronal L-type channels, by activating CAM kinase, initiates signals that are transmitted to the nucleus (Bading et al., 1993), possibly by the MAP kinase pathways. These proliferative effects are mediated in part by interactions with the GTP-binding protein Ras (Rosen et al., 1994; Farnsworth et al., 1995; Zwick et al., 1997) and in part by direct effects of calcium to stimulate transcription factors such as *cyclic AMP response element binding protein* (*CREB*).

One fascinating example of the signaling cross-talk encountered so often in biology is the presence of a high-affinity EF hand calcium-binding site on some phospholipase C (PLC) isoforms (Irvine, 1996). Because InsP$_3$, one of the products of PLC lipolysis, releases calcium from intracellular stores, this positive feedback can amplify signals generated by these PLCs.

Calcium also regulates gene expression by activating a phosphatase called *calcineurin*, which activates gene transcription by dephosphorylating the inactive form of a transcription factor called NF-AT3. The latter, which was initially discovered as a regulator of gene expression in the immune response (hence the family name *NF-AT*, for *nuclear factor of activated T cells*), is found in many cell types, where it participates in cytokine receptor-mediated responses and mediates the immunosuppressive actions of drugs such as cyclosporin (for review, see Rao et al., 1997). One of the more interesting properties of the NF-AT transcription factor is its ability to distinguish between short-term calcium pulses, such as those which activate contraction, and the more prolonged elevations of cytosolic calcium that stimulate cell growth and proliferation. This occurs because NF-AT is translocated to the nucleus only after cytosolic calcium has remained elevated for several minutes; a transient decrease in cytosolic calcium ends this signal by causing the rapid export of NF-AT from the nucleus (Timmerman et al., 1996). Like a high-frequency electronic filter, therefore, this transcription factor responds only to a sustained, relatively small elevation of cytosolic calcium, whereas excitation-contraction coupling depends on a brief but very large increase. These different effects are examples of a fascinating property of calcium signaling called "the AM and FM of calcium signaling" (Berridge, 1997), in which the response to an increase in cytosolic calcium depends on its frequency and amplitude.

The proliferative effects of sustained elevations of cytosolic calcium allow this cation to mediate a hypertrophic response in overloaded and failing hearts (Thompson et al., 1997; McDonough et al., 1997; Molkentin et al., 1998). These and other growth-promoting actions of calcium explain recent findings that overexpression of calcium-regulatory elements in transgenic mice can cause the heart to hypertrophy (Gruver et al., 1993; Molkentin et al., 1998).

PROLIFERATIVE SIGNALING: "MAP KINASE" PATHWAYS

As the focus of this discussion proceeds downstream along the signal transduction systems that regulate gene expression, we move further from the plasma membrane and its receptors and closer to the nucleus and its DNA. The messengers that actually diffuse from the cytosol into the nucleus include members of a family of serine/threonine kinases called *MAP kinases*. This term, which stands for *mitogen-activated protein kinases*, reflects the fact that these enzymes, when phosphorylated in response to growth-promoting stimuli that initiate a cascade of upstream cytosolic kinases, cross through large pores in the nuclear membrane. Once in the nucleus, the MAP kinases phosphorylate, and so activate, nuclear transcription factors that modify gene expression. The overlap between functional and proliferative signaling is again seen in the systems that activate the MAP kinase pathways. These activators include well recognized mitogenic signals, such as growth factors and cell adhesion molecules, and mediators of the neurohumoral response and inflammatory cytokines (Table 7-9).

Several different MAP kinase pathways can be activated by a variety of signaling systems. The result is stimulation of phosphorylation cascades that allow different MAP kinases to mediate different mitogenic signals. The nomenclature in this subject is especially maddening because key enzymes frequently have two, and sometimes more, different names. And with few exceptions, these names are abbreviated as nonsense words, generally containing guttural sounds not unlike the language of the orcs in J. R. R. Tolkien's

TABLE 7-9. *Some signals that regulate MAP kinases (mitogen-activated protein kinases) in the heart*

Peptide growth factors
   e.g., fibroblast growth factor
Cell adhesion molecules
   e.g., integrins, cadherins
Circulating mediators of the neurohumoral response
   e.g., norepinephrine, angiotensin II, endothelin
Paracrine and autocrine effects of locally released neurohumoral mediators
   e.g., angiotensin II
Inflammatory cytokines
   e.g., TNF-α

Ring Trilogy. To provide a basis for understanding the pathophysiology and management of heart failure, the following description of the MAP kinase pathways highlights signaling systems that seem most likely to cause maladaptive growth and cell death in the failing heart.

MAP kinase pathways, as shown in Fig. 7-14, carry out a "generic" sequence of regulated serine/threonine phosphorylations (for reviews, see Gotoh and Nishida, 1995; Whitmarsh et al., 1995; Krontiris, 1995; Pelech and Charest, 1995; Moriguchi et al., 1996; Sadoshima and Izumo, 1997; Lewis et al., 1998; and for elegant historical discussions, Egan

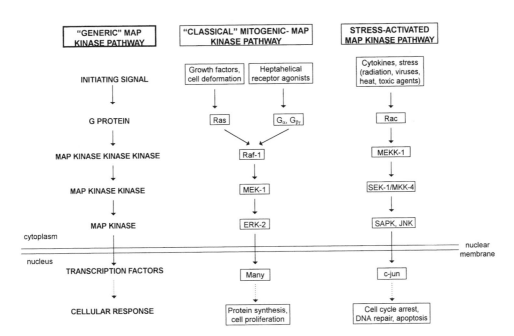

FIG. 7-14. MAP kinase pathways. A "generic" pathway (left) lists several key steps shared by these pathways, which allow an initiating signal at the "top" of the pathway to evoke a cellular response at the bottom. These pathways use a GTP-binding coupling protein to activate a series of three serine/threonine kinases; the first two (MAP kinase kinase kinase and MAP kinase kinase) phosphorylate the next enzyme "down" the pathway. When MAP kinase, the third in this series of kinases, is phosphorylated, the activated enzyme enters the nucleus, where it activates nuclear transcription factors that evoke the cellular response. Two specific pathways are also outlined. In the middle is the "classical" mitogenic pathway, and on the right is a more recently described "stress-activated" pathway. The mitogenic MAP kinase pathway (middle) is generally coupled by Ras when this pathway is activated by tyrosine kinase receptors, and by the heterotrimeric G proteins when activation is by heptahelical receptors. The latter signal can be coupled by both G_α and $G_{\beta\gamma}$. The MAP kinase kinase kinases in the mitogenic pathway include Raf-1, the MAP kinase kinases include MEK-1, and one important MAP kinase is ERK-2. Translocation of the latter to the nucleus allows this kinase to phosphorylate a large number of transcription factors. Stress-activated MAP kinase pathways (right) include the MAP kinase kinase kinase MEKK-1, whose function is analogous to that of Raf-1, the MAP kinase kinase SEK-1 (also called MKK-4), whose function is analogous to that of MEK-1, and the stress-activated protein kinase SAPK (also called JNK). As in the case of ERK-2, a SAPK-like JNK crosses into the nucleus, where it activates transcription factors like c-jun, which differ from those activated by ERK-2. Whereas the mitogenic pathways usually stimulate cell growth and cell division, stress-activated pathways act to inhibit cell proliferation and promote apoptosis.

and Weinberg, 1993; Graves et al., 1997). MAP kinase pathways were initially recognized as regulators of cell growth and proliferation that were activated when peptide growth factors bound their tyrosine kinase receptors. More recently, mitogenic MAP kinase pathways have been found to be activated when adhesion molecules are stimulated by cell deformation and by heptahelical G protein-coupled receptors. A second major group of pathways are the more recently described "stress-activated" MAP kinases (for review, see Force et al., 1996; Sugden and Clerk, 1998), which can be activated by inflammatory cytokines and a variety of toxic agents. In addition to these two MAP kinase pathways, which are outlined in Fig. 7-14, other, often overlapping, MAP kinase pathways have been described.

Both mitogenic and stress-activated MAP kinase pathways are coupled by a GTP-binding protein; the former can be activated by G_α, $G_{\beta\gamma}$ and Ras, whereas stress-activated pathways appear to utilize only monomeric G proteins such as Rac (for reviews, see Bourne, 1995; van Biesen et al., 1996; Force et al., 1996; Clapham and Neer, 1997). Mediators of the hemodynamic defense reaction that bind to G protein-coupled receptors, like norepinephrine, angiotensin II, and endothelin, activate MAP kinase pathways in reaction sequences that are coupled by both G_α (Taylor et al., 1991; Sadoshima et al., 1995; Dostal et al., 1997; Sakata et al., 1998) and the $G_{\beta\gamma}$ complex (Crespo et al., 1994; Cook and McCormick, 1994; Daaka et al., 1997). The most important G_α isoform that stimulates MAP kinase pathways in the heart appears to be $G_{\alpha q}$, which when activated by α-adrenergic agonists, angiotensin II and endothelin, causes phospholipase C to catalyze the formation of DAG and $InsP_3$. The former stimulates PK-C, a family of lipid-dependent serine/threonine kinases that, along with $G_{\beta\gamma}$, can activate MAP kinase pathways (for review, see Pelech and Charest, 1995; Steinberg et al., 1995; Luttrell et al., 1997; Hefti et al., 1997). $InsP_3$, the other second messenger generated by phospholipase C-catalyzed lipolysis, releases calcium that can activate MAP kinase pathways via both Ras-dependent (Farnsworth et al., 1995) and Ras-independent (Komoro and Yazaki, 1994) mechanisms.

Cyclic AMP, the second messenger produced by β adrenergic agonists, not only regulates cardiac function but also mediates effects on cell growth. By activating PK-A, this second messenger phosphorylates several transcriptional regulators, including both phospholipase C (Liu and Simon, 1996) and enzymes in MAP kinase pathways. In some cell types, the major effect of cyclic AMP is to inhibit MAP kinase pathways (Svetson et al., 1993; Cook and McCormick, 1993), but in mammalian cardiomyocytes the predominant effect of PK-A appears to be stimulation of protein synthesis and cell growth (Yamazaki et al., 1997). Some of the growth-promoting effects of cyclic AMP stimulate phosphorylation of the nuclear transcription factors CREB and CREM (see page 266), whereas others are mediated by the ability of the complex formed by desensitized β-adrenergic receptors and β-arrestin to serve as a platform for Ras-dependent mitogenic signaling (Luttrell et al., 1999). Together, these many mitogenic effects allow the sustained elevation of norepinephrine levels in heart failure to evoke a growth response in which the β-adrenergic effects of this mediator are synergistic with those of its α-adrenergic effects (Yamazaki et al., 1997). These growth-promoting effects are likely to stimulate remodeling and so probably play an important role in determining the poor prognosis in heart failure.

The "Generic" MAP Kinase Pathway

The signals transmitted by MAP kinase pathways reach the nucleus by a series of steps that resemble an American square dance; like a dancer, the signal moves gracefully along a series of partners. The early steps in this dance take place on a supporting structure, such as the plasma membrane, while later in the dance, the action moves through the cytosol, ending in the nucleus.

Common to MAP kinase pathways is activation of a serine/threonine kinase often referred to as *MAP kinase kinase kinase* (see Fig. 7-14). This name refers to the biological role of this protein kinase, which is to phosphorylate another kinase, called *MAP kinase kinase*. The latter then phosphorylates a third kinase, the *MAP kinase* that crosses the nuclear membrane to regulate gene expression. Different *MAP kinase kinase kinases*, *MAP kinase kinases*, and *MAP kinases* operate in the mitogenic and stress-activated pathways outlined in Fig. 7-14. These, and additional MAP kinase pathways not discussed in this text, are coupled by GTP-binding proteins in their initial phases, but because many other proteins participate in these signaling cascades, the exact functions of the G proteins differ markedly.

Mitogenic (Proliferative) Signaling by the "Classic" MAP Kinase Pathway

The MAP kinase-mediated signals that stimulate cell growth and proliferation are generally initiated by ligand binding to tyrosine kinase receptors. This causes the receptors to form an aggregate that, by activating their latent tyrosine kinase activity, autophosphorylates the receptor (Fig. 7-15). This phosphorylation reaction begins a series of aggregations, in which signaling proteins bind to one another, much as the partners in our dance join hands to form the square. Because the phosphoester groups represent newly formed "docking sites," autophosphorylation allows the receptors first to bind and then to phosphorylate *adaptor proteins* such as *Shc* (*src-homology*, so named because of its similarity to the gene *src*) and *Grb2* (*growth receptor binding protein*). The result is a multiprotein aggregate that is anchored along the inner surface of the plasma membrane (see Fig. 7-15) (for review, see Zhou et al., 1995). This receptor-adaptor protein aggregate then interacts with a guanine nucleotide-exchange factor called *Sos* (named after the drosophila mutant *son-of-sevenless*), which activates Ras by exchanging its bound GDP for GTP in a reaction analogous to that by which ligand-bound heptahelical receptors activate G_α (see Fig. 7-7B). Ras, which is central to many systems that control cell growth and proliferation (Boguski and McCormick, 1993), can be activated by many other signaling cascades.

The next reaction in the MAP kinase pathway occurs when the Ras-GTP complex activates a MAP kinase kinase kinase, such as *Raf-1* (see Figs. 7-14 and 7-15). This step in the signaling dance causes Raf-1, along with the Ras-GTP complex to which it is anchored, to be translocated to the plasma membrane (Leevers et al., 1994; Hall, 1994; Marshall, 1996). The activated Raf-1 then phosphorylates and activates the next partner in the dance, a MAP kinase kinase called *MEK-1* (*MAP kinase/ERK kinase*), also known in Tolkien's "orc language" as *MAKK (mitogen activated kinase kinase)*. Activated MEK-1 phosphorylates a MAP kinase called *ERK-2* (*extracellular-signal regulated kinase*), which moves to the nucleus to phosphorylate literally dozens of different transcription factors. This begins a new phase of the dance, which is discussed later under the heading "Transcription Factors."

MAP kinase pathways are activated not only by the tyrosine kinase receptors described in the preceding paragraph, but also by cell adhesion molecules and G protein-coupled receptors. Signaling by the latter can be coupled by G_α-GTP (Kolch et al., 1993) and free $G_{\beta\gamma}$, and by Ras that is activated by the internalized β-receptor–β-arrestin complex (Luttrell et al., 1999). Raf-1 can also be phosphorylated directly by protein kinase C.

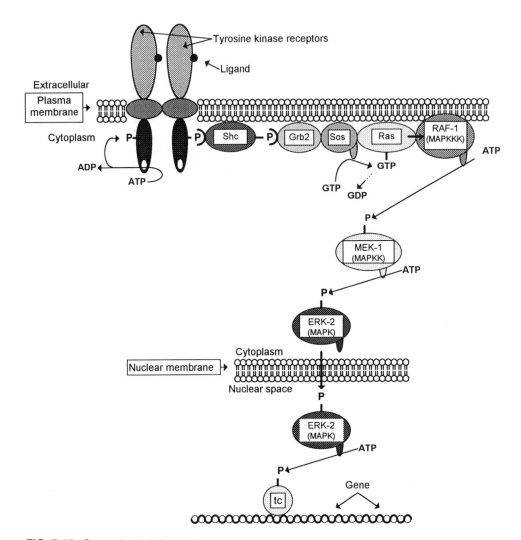

FIG. 7-15. Steps that link ligand-binding to a tyrosine kinase receptor and a MAP kinase-mediated signal that regulates gene expression. Binding of a ligand, such as a peptide growth factor, causes the tyrosine kinase receptors to form an aggregate that activates their latent tyrosine kinase activity. Autophosphorylation creates a "docking site" on the receptor that binds and then phosphorylates the adaptor protein Shc. This creates another docking site on Shc, which binds Grb2 to form a multiprotein aggregate along the inner surface of the plasma membrane. This aggregate then activates Sos, a guanine nucleotide-exchange factor that exchanges Ras-bound GDP for GTP. The activated Ras-GTP complex stimulates Raf-1, a MAP kinase kinase kinase (MAPKKK) that phosphorylates and activates the MAP kinase kinase (MAPKK) MEK-1, which then phosphorylates the MAP kinase (MAPK) ERK-2. Translocation of the latter to the nucleus allows the activated MAP kinase to phosphorylate nuclear transcription factors (tc). The latter then bind specific DNA sequences where they regulate gene expression.

Regulation of gene expression by MAP kinases allows a variety of signals to stimulate protein synthesis, initiate hypertrophy, and in proliferating cells, activate the cell cycle to induce mitosis. In the heart, Raf-1 mediates signals that favor reexpression of fetal genes, as well as those that cause hypertrophy (Thorburn et al., 1994). In view of the link between cell growth and cell death discussed in Chapter 6, it is not surprising that MAP kinases can also initiate programmed cell death (apoptosis). For these reasons, MAP kinase cascades probably play an important role in causing the Cardiomyopathy of Overload.

Stress-Activated MAP Kinase Pathways

MAP kinase pathways participate in cellular responses to inflammatory cytokines and to such stresses as viral infection, radiation, and toxins (for review, see Pelech and Charest, 1995; Canman and Kastan, 1996; Kyriakis and Avruch, 1996; Moriguchi et al., 1996; Force et al., 1996). Although there are many similarities between the mitogenic and stress-activated MAP kinase pathways, these two signal transduction cascades are regulated differently and activate different nuclear transcription factors.

Many stress-activated protein kinase systems are activated by ceramide, a lipid second messenger that is released from sphingomyelin, and many use the monomeric G protein *Rac*, which is related to Ras, to couple receptor-activation to downstream phosphorylations. The phosphorylations are catalyzed by stress-activated MAP kinase kinase kinases and MAP kinase kinases, which differ from those of the classical mitogenic MAP kinase pathways (Sánchez et al., 1994; Yan et al., 1994) (see Fig. 7-14). Stress-activated MAP kinase kinase kinases include *MEKK-1* (*MEK kinase-1*), whose function is analogous to that of Raf-1, and the MAP kinase kinase *SEK-1* (*SAPK/ERK kinase*, or *MKK-4*), whose function is analogous to that of MEK-1. An important MAP kinase in the stress-activated pathway is *c-Jun amino-terminal kinase* (*Jun kinase* or *JNK*), which phosphorylates the transcription factor *c-jun*. Once phosphorylated, stress-activated MAP kinases cross into the nucleus, where they activate transcription factors that differ from those activated by the mitogenic MAP kinases. This diversity allows each MAP kinase pathway to exert its own specific effects. Important actions of the stress-activated pathways include inhibition of cell proliferation and promotion of apoptosis, effects that differ from the stimulation of cell growth and division by mitogenic MAP kinases.

The MAP kinase pathways are not the only regulators of gene expression. Several other mitogenic mechanisms have already been discussed in this text; these include the cyclins discussed in Chapter 6, the JAK/STAT signaling system that is activated when inflammatory cytokines bind to their tyrosine kinase receptors (see Chapter 5), the transcription factor E2F whose availability is controlled by the pocket proteins, PK-C, intracellular steroid hormone receptors, the calcium-activated NF-AT3, and the cyclic AMP-response elements CREB and CREM mentioned earlier in this chapter. Many extracellular messengers operate through more than one signal transduction cascade; growth hormone, for example, activates both JAK/STAT and MAP kinase signaling systems (Wood et al., 1997), whereas nerve growth factor stimulates two different mitogenic MAP kinase pathways in signaling cascades that are coupled by different monomeric G proteins (York et al., 1998). This panoply of interlocking pathways provides both the flexibility and integration of gene expression that governs normal growth. In the patient with heart failure, these pathways probably contribute to a maladaptive growth response that plays an important role in the Cardiomyopathy of Overload (see Chapter 8).

PROLIFERATIVE SIGNALING BY INACTIVATED β-ADRENERGIC RECEPTORS

The ability of β-arrestin binding to phosphorylated β receptors has been mentioned at several points in this chapter because this may explain some of the beneficial effects of β blockers on long-term prognosis in heart failure. The recent observation that the β-receptor–β-arrestin complex interacts with members of the Src family of protein kinases to generate mitogenic signals (Luttrell et al., 1999) provides one of the more fascinating examples of integration in cell signaling. This mechanism appears to allow cells to modify their response to prolonged sympathetic stimulation by first downregulating the β receptor and then converting the downregulated receptor into a platform, or scaffold, upon which to assemble a signaling protein aggregate (Fig. 7-16). This aggregate, which has many similarities to that formed by the enzyme-linked receptors shown in Fig. 7-15, "tells" the cell that reliance on the short-term, cyclic AMP-mediated response to receptor activation no longer suffices, and that a growth signal is needed instead. Stated simplistically, this system indicates that the time for a stressed cell to run or fight has ended, and that to survive, the cell must grow its way out of trouble.

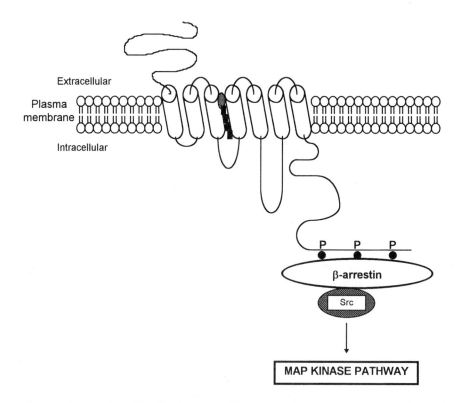

FIG. 7-16. Mechanism by which the inactivated β-adrenergic receptors can stimulate MAP kinase pathways. Phosphorylated, ligand bound receptors, bound to β-arrestin are translocated to clathrin-coated pits where they serve as a scaffold that activates members of the Src family of protein kinases. The latter then activated MAP kinase pathways that generate signals which modify cell growth.

TABLE 7-10. *Regulation of the protein composition of the heart*

Synthesis
  DNA transcription
    Selection of the DNA sequence to be read
    Transcription of the selected DNA sequence into a complementary RNA sequence
  RNA processing (alternative splicing)
    Selection and arrangement of exons to be spliced to form messenger RNA (mRNA)
  RNA export
    Selection and control of mRNA transport from the nucleus to the cytoplasm
  Translation
    Selection and control of mRNA translation into protein
Activation and inactivation (post-translational control)
  Modification of a protein that increases or decreases its activity, e.g., phosphorylation
  Protein interactions with other cell components, e.g., myosin binding to actin, troponin C binding to
  calcium
Breakdown
  RNA degradation
    Selection and control of mRNA breakdown, which turns off protein synthesis
  Protein degradation
    Selection and control of proteolysis, which removes proteins

REGULATION OF CELL COMPOSITION

Cell structure and composition are determined in part by the protein isoforms that are synthesized, by their rates of synthesis, by selective modification of formed proteins, and by the breakdown of individual proteins (Table 7-10). Protein synthesis, the focus of the present discussion, is determined largely by selection and transcription of the specific DNA sequences used as templates that encode complementary RNA sequences. The latter, called *primary RNA transcripts*, are often modified by *alternative splicing*, a "cut and paste" mechanism that, by rearranging the RNA sequence encoded by a specific DNA sequence, allows a single gene to encode several different messenger RNAs (mRNAs). Before the latter can participate in protein synthesis, the mRNA formed within the nucleus must be exported into the cytosol, where it is processed (translated) to encode its specific protein. Once a protein is synthesized, its activity can be regulated both by interactions with other cell components, as occurs when myosin interacts with actin and when troponin C binds calcium, or when the protein itself is modified, as occurs through the phosphorylations discussed in this and other chapters. Yet another determinant of the protein composition of a cell is the rate at which the individual proteins are broken down.

The following discussion highlights DNA transcription and DNA processing, the first two mechanisms listed in Table 7-10. For descriptions of the other processes mentioned in this table, and how they are regulated, refer to textbooks of molecular biology, which provide invaluable supplemental material for this chapter.

CONTROL OF GENE EXPRESSION

The final steps of the elaborate processes that control gene expression in eukaryotic cells take place in the nucleus. It is here that the signal transduction cascades discussed in this chapter regulate transcription of specific DNA base pair sequences. The processes select, transcribe, and process the information encoded in a gene to form the mRNA that moves back to the cytosol where it controls synthesis of the cell's protein machinery. These nuclear processes are as tightly regulated as the neurohumoral responses and signaling cascades discussed earlier in this text. Fortunately for the reader (as well as for the author!), the following discussion of transcriptional regulation within the nucleus is much less detailed than that of the extracellular messengers, their plasma membrane receptors, and the cytosolic signal transduction cascades that they control. This reflects my view that therapy targeted to gene transcription will play a lesser role in the management of heart failure than modification of the neurohumoral response and cytosolic signaling.

Promoter, Enhancer, and Repressor DNA Sequences in a Gene

Genomic DNA (the DNA found in chromosomes) not only contains the codes that determine the amino acid sequence of the cellular proteins but also includes many nucleic acid sequences that turn gene transcription on and off, and control transcription rate (see Fig. 7-15). These regulatory sequences, which do not encode protein structure, include *promoter* regions that are located at the 5′-end of the gene, "upstream" from the *start site* at which DNA transcription begins (see Fig. 7-17). Binding of the promoter to an appropriate transcription factor, along with other regulatory proteins, turns on the gene. One of the most important of these promoter regions is the *TATA box*, so named because its DNA sequence is made up of thymidine (T) and adenine (A) in the sequence TATA. This sequence probably represents a "weak" point in DNA structure; one at which the double helix is most readily unwound to separate the single-stranded DNA that is used for copying.

Transcription of a gene begins when its promoter region binds a highly regulated protein complex that includes, in addition to specific transcription factors and other regulators, members of a family of enzymes called *RNA polymerase* (for review, see Zawel and Reinberg, 1995). Many of the transcription factors discussed in this text generate a variety of regulatory aggregates that include RNA polymerases and a dazzling array of auxiliary factors. These aggregates, when bound to the promoter region of a gene, initiate and control DNA transcription (Zawel and Reinberg, 1995; Roberts and Green, 1995) when the activated RNA polymerase synthesizes an RNA whose sequence is determined by the DNA template. This RNA, which contains the information encoded in the gene downstream from the "start site" (Fig. 7-17), represents the primary RNA transcript that, after processing (see later text), is converted to the mRNA that is transported to the cytosol. Once it has reached the cytosol, mRNA serves as the template upon which ribosomes direct amino acid incorporation into newly formed proteins.

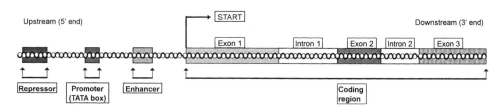

FIG. 7-17. Major regulatory sequences in genomic DNA. The protein is encoded by a coding region located downstream (toward the 3′ end of the DNA sequence) from a "START" sequence. Gene transcription is turned on when transcription factors and other proteins bind to a regulatory sequence, located at the 5′ end of the gene, called a promoter. The TATA box, which is made up of thymidine (T) and adenine (A), is one of the most important of these promoter regions. Transcription is regulated by enhancers, which activate, and repressors, which inhibit, gene expression. Enhancer and repressor sequences are found not only upstream from the start site, as shown in the figure, but also downstream, and even in the coding region. In the latter case, these regulatory sequences are found in introns, which represent DNA sequences that are not used to encode protein structure. The protein itself is encoded by mRNA transcribed from exons.

In addition to the promoter regions that turn on gene transcription, genomic DNA contains regulatory sequences that bind transcription factors, which control the rate of gene expression. These regulatory DNA sequences include *enhancer* regions and *repressor* regions, sequences that increase and decrease the rate of gene expression, respectively. Regulatory sequences are not only found on the upstream 5′-end of the gene, as shown in Fig. 7-17, but can also be located downstream from the 3′-end of the transcribed region of the gene, and within unexpressed DNA sequences located between coding regions of the gene (introns). Transcriptional regulation generally involves cooperative interactions among transcription factors, RNA polymerases, and other regulators that, in controlling the expression of a single gene, often bind to several regulatory DNA sequences. In some cases, a single transcription factor aggregate binds simultaneously to several regions of a single gene.

RNA Processing and Alternative Splicing

Although the primary RNA transcript is generally an accurate transcript of the DNA sequence of the gene, not all of the RNA encoded by genomic DNA is used to direct protein synthesis. Large segments of the primary transcript, called *introns*, are often eliminated before the remaining RNA sequences, made up of the expressed *exons*, are assembled into the mRNA that is exported from the nucleus to provide the template for protein synthesis (Fig. 7-18).

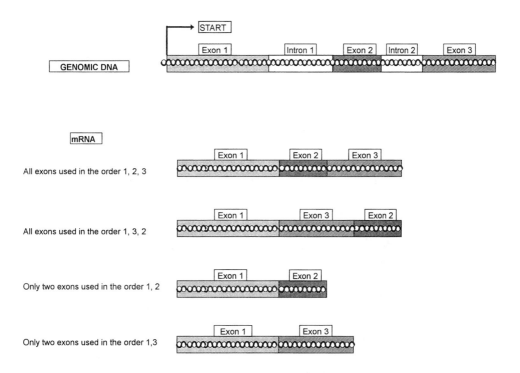

FIG. 7-18. Alternative splicing in a gene that contains three exons. Shown are four messenger RNAs (mRNA) formed by elimination of introns, followed by selection and rearrangement of exons. The four examples in this figure are only a few of the possible products of alternative splicing in that one, two, or all three of these exons can be combined in additional combinations and permutations.

The ability of cells to eliminate introns and to select and arrange exons, generally called *alternative splicing*, provides yet another means for regulating gene expression. Some simple examples of this mechanism are illustrated in Fig. 7-18, which shows how a gene containing three exons can encode four different mRNAs; this illustration is by no means exhaustive in that the three exons can be used in many additional permutations and combinations. Some genes contain tens of exons, so that alternative splicing provides an elaborate mechanism for generating many different protein isoforms from a single DNA sequence.

Transcription Factors

Key to the regulation of gene expression are the transcription factors that recognize and bind to specific DNA sequences. Transcription factors are proteins and phosphoproteins that can turn on a gene by binding to its promoter, accelerate its expression by binding to an enhancer sequence, or slow its transcription by binding to a repressor sequence (see Fig. 7-17). The transcription factors discussed in this text represent only a small sample of the enormous number of different molecules that regulate gene expression.

A key feature of the transcription factors is their ability to select a specific DNA sequence and then regulate its expression. This specificity is made possible by different structural motifs that provide the tight "fit" needed for a transcription factor to select its target gene (Papavassiliou, 1995). Transcription factor structures include the *helix-loop-helix*, which was encountered in the discussion of the myogenic determinants, and the *helix-turn-helix* found in homeobox regulators. A *zinc finger* structure, which uses an atom of zinc to orient the various domains of the transcription factor, occurs in steroid and thyroid hormone receptors. A fourth important structure, the *leucine zipper*, is found in many of the dimeric transcription factors that mediate the immediate-early gene response in the overloaded heart (see later text). One of these leucine zipper transcription factors was encountered in the earlier discussion of c-*jun*, which is synthesized by the stress-activated MAP kinase called Jun kinase (see Fig. 7-13). The "zipper" in these transcription factors is provided by a series of leucine residues that form parallel chains of hydrophobic bonds, which link members of this family to one another.

Transcription factors generally operate as dimers, in which each subunit binds to one of the two DNA strands in a selected region of a chromosome. This interaction resembles a "body lock," in which a wrestler holds an opponent firmly between his knees. Cooperative interactions between a transcription factor and its gene not only allow the transcription factor to regulate gene expression, but also make it possible for regulatory regions of the gene to modify the actions of the transcription factor (Lefstin and Yamamoto, 1998). The resulting allosteric interactions between genes and transcription factors permit a single transcription factor to interact sequentially with several genes to generate a coordinated growth response.

Transcription factors can be activated by *post-translational modification* of an existing inactive form of the factor (e.g., by phosphorylation), or they can be synthesized *de novo* in response to one of the signaling cascades described earlier in this chapter. Posttranslational regulators include nuclear transcription factors that are phosphorylated by MAP kinase pathways and PK-C. *CREB* and *CREM (cyclic AMP receptor element-binding protein* and *cyclic AMP receptor element modulator*, respectively), are activated by cyclic AMP-dependent protein kinases (Comb et al., 1986; Montminy et al., 1986; Delegeane et al., 1987; Tsukada et al., 1987; Roesler et al., 1988; Habener, 1990; Horiuchi et al., 1991, Lucas and Granner, 1992; for review, see Meyer and Habener, 1993; Marx, 1993; Monaco et al., 1997; Johnson et al., 1997), and so allow β-adrenergic stimuation to regulate cell growth. The latter may play an important role in maladaptive hypertrophy, as evidenced by the beneficial actions of β blockade in patients with heart failure.

Another mechanism for transcription factor activation is exemplified by E2F, which remains inactive as long as it is bound to a pocket protein, becoming activated when phosphorylation of the binding-protein releases E2F from its pocket. Still other transcription factors, such as the intracellular steroid receptors, are activated when they bind to a specific ligand that enters the cell. The latter are called *hormone receptor elements* or *HREs* because they bind directly to hormones that cross the plasma membrane. The possibility that steroid receptor activation contributes to the maladaptive growth of the failing heart is suggested by a recent clinical trial that showed improved survival in patients given spironolactone, a drug that blocks the binding of aldosterone to the intracellular receptors that mediate the effects of this mineralocorticoid (see Chapter 9).

Oncogenes and Protooncogenes

Genes whose activation causes uncontrolled cell growth and proliferation are called *oncogenes*, whereas *protooncogenes* are normal cellular genes that, when mutated, generate a product that induces malignant transformation. The term protooncogene is often used in referring to genes, such as c-*myc*, c-*fos*, and c-*jun*, which are rapidly activated in response to stress. Oncogenes related to these normal cell regulators are found in some viruses; in the examples just provided, these are called v-*myc*, v-*fos*, and v-*jun*. Other protooncogenes, when mutated, can induce malignant transformation. These include genes that encode tyrosine kinase receptors, G proteins such as Ras, pocket proteins, steroid receptors, and enzymes that participate in MAP kinase pathways, such as Raf. Because the term protooncogene has such a broad meaning, its use is avoided in the present text.

RESPONSE OF THE MYOCARDIUM TO STRESS

A large number of genes become activated when cardiac myocytes are subjected to a stress, such as ischemia, stretch, or increased developed tension (see Table 7-11) (for reviews, see Chien et al., 1991, 1993; Komuro and Yazaki, 1993; Yamazaki et al., 1995; Sadoshima and Izumo, 1997; Hefti et al., 1997). The first genes to be upregulated, called *immediate-early response genes*, are not normally transcribed in the resting (G$_0$) phase of the cell cycle. The rapidity with which these genes become activated, in some cases within minutes after a cardiac myocyte is overloaded (Starksen et al., 1986; Izumo et al., 1987; Mulvagh et al., 1987; Kumoro et al., 1988; Izumo et al., 1988), means that activation does not require protein synthesis. Instead, most immediate-early genes are activated by phosphorylations and other post-translational modifications. If the stress is sustained, additional genes, called *late-response genes*, become activated in reactions that do depend on the synthesis of new proteins. Many late-response genes are activated by transcription factors whose synthesis is stimulated by the immediate-early genes. Both the immediate-early and late-response genes are important in adaptive hypertrophy. They are also likely to play a pathogenic role in heart failure, where some may cause cell elonga-

TABLE 7-11. *Stress-activated genes*

Immediate-early response genes: do not require *de novo* protein synthesis e.g., c-*myc*, c-*fos*, c-*jun*, *hsp*-70.
Late response genes: activated by transcription factors synthesized in the immediate-early response e.g., genes that encode cytoskeletal and myofibrillar proteins, mitochondrial proteins, synthetic enzymes, cyclins and Cdks, additional transcription factors

tion, whereas others stimulate apoptosis and other maladaptive features of the Cardiomyopathy of Overload (see Chapter 8).

Immediate-Early Response Genes

Mediators of the neurohumoral response, the inflammatory cytokines, and the peptide growth factors and cell adhesion molecules all use signaling pathways discussed in this chapter to activate the immediate-early response (for review, see Vincent et al., 1993; Hefti et al., 1997). One of the most important activators of the immediate-early response in the overloaded heart is cell stretch, which by deforming adhesion molecules, stimulates MAP kinases and other mitogenic pathways (Komuro and Yazaki, 1993; Yamazaki et al., 1995; Sadoshima and Izumo, 1997). A similar complement of immediate-early genes is activated when the heart is made ischemic (Brand et al. 1992, Knöll et al., 1994). This stress response is extraordinarily complex, in that it is accompanied by the activation of more than 100 different genes. These include *ras*, which encodes the monomeric GTP-binding protein Ras; the nuclear transcription factors c-*myc*, c-*fos*, and c-*jun*, which encode the corresponding leucine zipper transcription factors; and *hsp-70*, which encodes a heat shock protein (see later text).

The sequential rise and fall in the levels of the mRNA encoded by these "stress" genes demonstrates that instead of responding in a monotonic fashion, the many genes that participate in the immediate-early response are programmed to follow individual time courses. Various genes are activated at different rates during the first minutes and hours after the onset of the stress, and then are shut off at different times over the next few hours or days. In addition to these temporal heterogeneities, there are spatial heterogeneities in the immediate-early response. These are evidenced by the appearance of the mRNAs encoding different protein isoforms at different times in various regions of the overloaded heart (Schiaffino et al., 1989).

The rich control of the immediate-early response is exemplified by c-Myc, one of the nuclear transcription factors expressed in proliferating cells (for review, see Henriksson and Lüscher, 1996). Because c-Myc induces the transcription of genes whose protein products regulate the cell cycle (Thompson, 1998), it is not surprising that in G_0, the quiescent state of the cell cycle, levels of the c-Myc protein are quite low and its mRNA (c-*myc*) virtually undetectable. Increased expression of the c-Myc protein in malignant cells is associated with continuous cell cycling. In the heart, c-Myc not only activates the hypertrophic process but also leads to preferential expression of fetal genes. This is not surprising because this transcription factor inhibits expression of the adult phenotype during skeletal muscle myogenesis (Miner and Wold, 1991). Reversion to the fetal phenotype in overloaded hearts, therefore, is due in part to the ability of c-Myc, along with other mediators of the immediate-early response, to inhibit synthesis of protein isoforms that characterize the adult phenotype in terminally differentiated cardiac myocytes. Another role of c-Myc in the response to stress is its ability to initiate programmed cell death, an effect that is due in part to increased expression of the transcription factor p53, which provides a powerful stimulus for apoptosis (see Chapter 6).

Heat Shock Proteins

Among the first genes to be activated by stress are genes that encode members of a family of proteins called *heat shock proteins* (for review, see Craig, 1993; Knowlton, 1995; Bukau and Horwich, 1998). This term reflects the appearance of these proteins shortly after cells are exposed to elevated temperatures. The rapid upregulation of the genes that encode these proteins is remarkable because even a single stretch of the adult rat heart can increase expression of Hsp-70 (Knowlton et al., 1991).

Heat shock proteins are also called *molecular chaperones* because of their ability to bind, and thereby stabilize, hydrophobic surfaces that become exposed in partially denatured proteins (Hartl, 1996). Like the elderly aunt described in Chapter 6 who protects a susceptible youngster from associating with undesirable companions, heat shock proteins prevent the irreversible aggregations that denature damaged proteins. In addition to inhibiting protein denaturation in stressed cells, heat shock proteins promote refolding of damaged proteins, aid the natural folding of newly synthesized proteins, and facilitate protein transport across membranes. Their effects on protein conformation allow heat shock proteins to regulate cellular function; by modifying the biological activity of transcription factors, they may also regulate gene expression. Upregulation of members of the Hsp-70 family (so named because their molecular weight is about 70 kDa) as part of the immediate-early response in the pressure-overloaded heart, therefore, not only plays a protective role but may also influence the growth response.

Late Response Genes

The immediate-early response, while important in the initial response of the heart to stress, is only transient, being followed by the more sustained activation of a different complement of genes called the *late-response genes*. The genes expressed in this later phase require the synthesis of new proteins and so differ from the genes expressed in the immediate-early response. Late-response genes encode mitochondrial proteins, cytoskeletal and myofibrillar proteins, synthetic enzymes, nonhistone chromosomal proteins, some of the cyclins and Cdks discussed in Chapter 6 and additional transcription factors (Lanahan et al., 1992; Vincent et al., 1993). Many of the late-response genes expressed by the overloaded heart encode fetal proteins and protein isoforms normally found in the fetal heart during development (see later text). Replacement of the adult cardiac myosin heavy chain isoform with the fetal isoform, for example, plays an important role both in reducing energy consumption and depressing contractility in the failing heart. Another reversion to the fetal phenotype is reduced incorporation of calcium pump ATPase molecules into sarcoplasmic reticulum membranes, a response that slows relaxation. Cell cycle stimulation, another consequence of the late response in overloaded cardiac myocytes, probably plays an important role in determining the poor prognosis in patients with heart failure because efforts to "push" terminally differentiated cardiac myocytes out of G_0 increase their susceptibility to apoptosis.

Reexpression of the Fetal Phenotype

One of the remarkable features of the growth response of the overloaded heart is the reappearance of patterns of gene expression normally seen in fetal life. The functional consequences of this reversion to the "fetal phenotype" are complex. For example, expression of the low ATPase fetal myosin heavy chain replaces the higher ATPase myosin normally found in the adult heart. This isoform shift has both beneficial and detrimental effects. By slowing the turnover of myosin cross-bridges, this substitution has a negative inotropic effect that exacerbates the hemodynamic abnormalities caused by chronic overloading. However, this isoform shift also reduces the rate of ATP hydrolysis by the heart's contractile machinery, which has an energy-sparing effect that can be beneficial to an overloaded, energy-starved heart. Reversion to the fetal phenotype in the overloaded heart also has important effects on energy production, notably to reduce the utilization of fatty acids as the source for metabolic energy (for review, see van Bilsen et al., 1998). Changes in key ion channels synthesized in the hypertrophied heart (Ten Eick et al., 1992; Rosen et al., 1999) may play an important role in arrhythmogenesis.

OVERVIEW AND SUMMARY

In setting the stage for the next chapter, which highlights the relevance of maladaptive growth in the patient with heart failure, this overview of cellular regulation concludes with a few generalizations. Most important is that the terminally differentiated cardiac myocyte can be viewed as a cell with few options other than to contract and relax. Like a stolid ox, our cardiac myocytes spend their lifetimes pulling a burden. The remarkable durability of these myocytes reflects the fact that, as long as their activity is restricted to the task of contracting and relaxing, these cells survive for decades, sometimes for more than a century. This durability, however, comes with a price, which is that stimuli that modify this routine can prove fatal. If, for example, a heart is paced continuously at a rate more rapid than is natural, it soon begins to fail, and its cells begin to die. Similarly, sustained mechanical overload shortens cardiac myocyte survival. This means that, even though the heart normally beats without pause for decades, this activity must remain within limits. Forcing a heart to exceed its limits sets into motion a series of responses that, while initially compensatory, eventually destroy the cardiac pump. We return to this important concept in the Chapter 8, in the discussion of Cardiomyopathy of Overload.

A second overarching concept that has been highlighted in this chapter is that even the simplest intervention that modifies cellular function evokes a multiplicity of responses. This is seen in the branching and overlapping of the many signal transduction cascades discussed in this text. Even a stimulus as simple as an increase in muscle length evokes not only a change in cardiac performance (Starling's Law of the Heart), but also a multigene response. For more than 150 years, since the discovery of the length-tension relationship, stretching a muscle was recognized to increase its ability to do work. Elucidation of the function of the integrins and other cell adhesion molecules, however, has made this story vastly more complex. It has become clear that stretch also generates a powerful signal for cell growth.

Yet another principle set forth in this chapter is that cell signaling rarely proceeds in a "straight line," as depicted in Fig. 7-1. Instead, as shown in Figs. 7-2 through 7-4, almost all signals lead to an impressive array of cellular responses. One of the important corollaries to this generalization, from the viewpoint of the heart failure patient, is that efforts to modify cell signaling so as to do good, perhaps invariably also do harm. Signal transduction should therefore be viewed as a floodlight, rather than a spotlight. According to this analogy, the patient with a damaged heart calls upon compensatory responses to help stay on the safest path while avoiding the many pitfalls and dangers that lurk alongside the road. However, the beam of the "compensatory torch" is generally too broad, and so not only helps the patient avoid danger but unfortunately also awakens dormant monsters whose appearance on the scene can prove fatal. The challenge in modifying cell signaling, therefore, is best met with an understanding of both the benefits and dangers that can accompany the evoked responses. In heart failure, this is best accomplished by intelligent and informed use of available drugs, along with monitoring the individual responses so as to reduce suffering and prolong survival with the least likelihood of awakening the many demons that threaten these patients. This is not an easy task because, as we have learned from recent clinical trials, what is obvious is often not important, and what is important is not always obvious.

BIBLIOGRAPHY

Alberty B, Bray D, Lewis J, Raff M, Roberts K, Watson JD (1994). *Molecular Biology of the Cell,* 3rd ed. Garland, New York.

Bugaisky L, Zak R (1986). Biological mechanisms of hypertrophy. In Fozzard H, Haber E, Katz A, Jennings R, Morgan HE, eds. *The Heart and Cardiovascular System.* Raven Press, New York, pp 1491–1506.

Bugaisky L, Gupta M, Gupta MG, Zak R (1992). Cellular and molecular mechanisms of hypertrophy In Fozzard H, Haber E, Katz A, Jennings R, Morgan HE, eds. *The Heart and Cardiovascular System,* 2nd ed. Raven Press, New York, pp 1621–1640.

Calladine CR, Drew HR (1992). *Understanding DNA.* Academic Press, London.

Kupfer J, Rubin SA (1998). The molecular and cellular biology of heart failure. In Hosenpud JG, Greenberg B, eds. *Congestive Heart Failure.* Springer-Verlag, New York, pp. 17–53.

Roberts R, Schneider MD (1990). *Molecular Biology of the Cardiovascular System.* Wiley-Liss, New York.

Swynghedauw B, ed (1990). *Cardiac Hypertrophy and Failure.* INSERM, Paris.

Watson S, Arkinstill S (1994). *The G-Protein Linked Receptor Facts Book.* Academic Press, London.

REFERENCES

Bading H, Ginty DD, Greenberg M (1993). Regulation of gene expression in hippocampal neurons by distinct calcium signaling pathways. *Science* 260:181–186.

Berridge M (1997). The AM and FM of calcium signaling. *Nature* 386:759–760.

Beznak M (1964). Hormonal influences in regulation of cardiac performance. *Circ Res* 15(Suppl 2):141–150.

Boguski MS, McCormick F (1993). Proteins regulating Ras and its relatives. *Nature* 366:643–654.

Böhm M, Eschenhagen T, Gierschik P, Larisch K, Lensche H, Mende U, Schmitz W, Schnabel P, Scholz H, Steinfah M, Erdmann E (1994). Radioimmunochemical quantification of $Gi\alpha$ in right and left ventricle from patients with ischaemic and dilated cardiomyopathy and predominant left ventricular failure. *J Mol Cell Cardiol* 26:133–149.

Bourne HR (1995). Team blue sees red. *Nature* 376:727–729.

Bowling N, Walsh RA, Song G, Estridge T, Sandusky GE, Fouts RL, Mintze K, Pickard T, Roden R, Bristow MR, Sabbah HN, Mizrahi JL, Gromo G, King GL, Vlahos CJ (1999). Increased protein kinase C activity and expression of Ca^{2+} sensitive isoforms in the failing human heart. *Circulation* 99:384–391.

Brand T, Shrma HS, Fleischmann KE, Duncker DJ, McFalls EO, Verdouw PD, Schaper W (1992). Proto-oncogene expression in porcine myocardium subjected to ischemia and reperfusion. *Circ Res* 71:1351–1360.

Bukau B, Horwich AL (1998). The Hsp70 and Hsp60 chaperone machines. *Cell* 92:351–366.

Cachero TG, Moroelli AD, Peralta EG (1998). The small GTP-binding protein RhoA regulates a delayed rectifier potassium channel. *Cell* 93:1077–1085.

Canman CE, Kastan MB (1996). Three paths to stress relief. *Nature* 384:213–214.

Chien KR, Knowlton KU, Zhu H, Chien S (1991). Regulation of cardiac gene expression during myocardial growth and hypertrophy: molecular studies of an adaptive physiologic response. *FASEB J* 5:3037–3046.

Chien KR, Zhu H, Knowlton KU, Miller-Hance W, van-Bilsen M, O'Brien TX, Evans SM (1993). Transcriptional regulation during cardiac growth and development. *Annu Rev Physiol* 55:77–95.

Clapham DE, Neer EJ (1997). G protein $\beta\gamma$ subunits. *Annu Rev Pharmacol* 37:167–203.

Comb M, Birnberg NC, Seasholtz A, Herbert E, Goodman HM (1986). A cyclic AMP- and phorbol-ester inducible DNA element. *Nature* 323:353–356.

Cook S, McCormick F (1993). Inhibition by cAMP of *ras*-dependent activation of *raf. Science* 262:1069–1072.

Cook S, McCormick F (1994). Ras blooms on sterile ground. *Nature* 369:361–362.

Craig EA (1993). Chaperones: helpers along the pathways to protein folding. *Nature* 260:1902–1904.

Crespo P, Xu N, Simonds WF, Gutkind JS (1994). Ras-dependent activation of MAP kinase pathway mediated by G-protein $\beta\gamma$ subunits. *Nature* 369:418–420.

Crespo P, Xu N, Simonds WF, Gutkind JSEvans RM (1988). The steroid and thyroid receptor superfamily. *Science* 240:889–895.

Daaka Y, Luttrell LM, Lefkowitz RJ (1997). Switching of coupling of the β_2-adrenergic receptor to different G proteins by protein kinase A. *Nature* 390:88–91.

Danielsen W, V der Leyen H, Meyer W, Neuman J, Schmitz W, Scholz H, Starbutty J, Stein J, Döring V, Kalmár P (1989). Basal and isoprenaline-stimulated cAMP content in failing versus non-failing human cardiac preparations. *J Cardiovasc Pharmacol* 14:171–173.

DebBurman SK, Ptasienski J, Benovic JL, Hosey MM (1996). G protein-coupled receptor kinase GRK-2 is a phospholipid-dependent enzyme that can be conditionally activated by G protein $\beta\gamma$ subunits. *J Biol Chem* 271:22552–22562.

Delegeane AM, Ferland LH, Mellon PL (1987). Tissue-specific enhancer of the human glycoprotein hormone α-subunit gene: dependence on cyclic AMP-inducible elements. *Mol Cell Biol* 7:3994–4002.

Dostal DE, Hunt RA, Kule CE, Bhat GJ, Karoor V, McWhinney CD, Baker KM (1997). Molecular mechanisms of angiotensin II in modulating cardiac function: intracardiac effects and signal transduction pathways. *J Mol Cell Cardiol* 29:2893–2902.

Egan SE, Weinberg RA (1993). The pathway to signal achievement. *Nature* 365:781–783.

Ehrlich BE, Watras J (1988). Inositol 1,4,5-trisphosphate activates a channel from smooth muscle sarcoplasmic reticulum. *Nature* 336:583–586.

Eschenhagen T, Mende U, Nose M, Schmitz W, Scholz H, Haverich A, Hirt S, Döring V, Kalmar P, Höppner W, Seitz H-J (1992). Increased messenger RNA level of the inhibitory G protein α subunit $G_{i\beta-2}$ in human end-stage heart failure. *Circ Res* 70:688–696.

Everett AW. Clark WA, Chizzonite RA, Zak R (1983). Changes in synthesis rates of α and β myosin heavy chains in rabbit heart after treatment with thyroid hormone. *J Biol Chem* 258:2421–2425.

Farnsworth CL, Freshney NW, Rosen LB, Ghosh A, Greenberg ME, Feig LA (1995). Calcium activation of Ras mediated by neuronal exchange factor Ras-GRF. *Nature* 376:524–527.

Feldman AM, Cates AE, Veazey WB, Hershberger RE, Bristow MR, Baughman KL, Baumgartner W, Van Dop C (1988). Increase of the 40,000-mol wt pertussis toxin substrate (G protein) in the failing human heart. *J Clin Invest* 82:189–197.

Force T, Avruch JA, Bonventre JY, Kyriakis JM (1996). Stress-activated protein kinases in cardiovascular disease. *Circulation* 78:947–953.

Funder JW (1993). Mineralocorticoids, glucocorticoids, receptors and response elements. *Science* 259:1132–1133.

Gotoh Y, Nishida E (1995). Activation mechanism and function of the MAP kinase cascade. *Mol Reprod Dev* 42:486–492.

Graves LM, Bornfeldt KE, Krebs EG (1997). Historical perspectives and new insights involving the MAP kinase cascades. *Adv Second Mess Phosphoprotein Res* 31:49–61.

Gray PC, Scott JD, Catterall WA (1998). Regulation of ion channels by cAMP-dependent protein kinase and A-kinase anchoring proteins. *Curr Opin Neurobiol* 8:330–334.

Gruver CL, DeMayo F, Goldstein MA, Means AR (1993). Targeted developmental overexpression of calmodulin induces proliferative and hypertrophic growth of cardiomyocytes in transgenic mice. *Endocrinology* 133:376–388.

Gudermann T, Schöneberg T, Schultz G (1997). Functional and structural complexity of signal transduction via G-protein-coupled receptors. *Annu Rev Neurosci* 20:399–427.

Habener JF (1990). Cyclic AMP response element binding proteins: a cornucopia of transcription factors. *Mol Endocrinol* 4:1087–1094.

Hall A (1994). A biochemical function for Ras—at last. *Science* 264:1413–1414.

Hartl FU (1996). Molecular chaperones in cellular protein folding. *Nature* 381:571–580.

Hefti MA, Harder BA, Eppenberger HM, Schaub MC (1997). Signaling pathways in cardiac myocyte hypertrophy. *J Mol Cell Cardiol* 29:2873–2892.

Heilbrunn SM, Shah P, Bristow MR, Valentine HA, Ginsburg R, Fowler MB (1989). Increased β-receptor density and improved hemodynamic response to catecholamine stimulation during long-term metoprolol therapy in heart failure from dilated cardiomyopathy. *Circulation* 79:483–490.

Henriksson M, Lüscher B (1996). Proteins of the Myc network: essential regulator of cell growth and differentiation. *Adv Cancer Res* 68:109–182.

Herbette LG, Mason RP (1992). Techniques for determining membrane and drug-membrane structures: a reevaluation of the molecular and kinetic basis for the binding of lipid-soluble drugs to their receptors in heart and brain. In Fozzard H, Haber E, Katz AM, Jennings R, Morgan HE, eds. *The Heart and Cardiovascular System*, 2nd ed. Raven Press, New York, pp 417–462.

Horiuchi M, Nakamura N, Tang S-S, Barrett G, Dzau VJ (1991). Molecular mechanism of tissue-specific regulation of mouse renin gene expression by cyclic AMP. *J Biol Chem* 266:16247–16254.

Insel PA, Ransnäs LA (1988). G proteins and cardiovascular disease. *Circulation* 78:1511–1513.

Irvine R (1996). Taking stock of PI-PLC. *Nature* 380:581–583.

Izumo S, Nadal-Ginard B, Mahdavi V (1988). Protooncogene induction and reprogramming of cardiac gene expression produced by pressure overload. *Proc Nat Acad Sci U S A* 85:339–343.

Izumo S, Nadal-Ginard B, Mahdavi V (1990). The thyroid hormone receptor α gene generates functionally different proteins isoforms by alternative splicing. In Roberts R, Schneider MD. *Molecular Biology of the Cardiovascular System*. Wiley-Liss, New York, pp 112–123.

Izumo S, Lompré AM, Matsuoka R, Kren G, Schwartz K, Nadal-Ginard B, Mahdavi V (1987). Myosin heavy chain messenger RNA and protein isoform, transitions during cardiac hypertrophy. *J Clin Invest* 79:970–977.

Janknecht R, Hunter T (1996). A growing coactivator network. *Nature* 383:22–23.

Johnson CM, Hill CS, Chawla S, Treisman R, Bading H (1997). Calcium controls gene expression via three distinct pathways that can function independently of the ras/mitogen-activated protein kinases (ERKs) signaling cascade. *J Neurosci* 17:6189–6202.

Katz AM, Adler PN, Watras J, Messineo FC, Takenaka H, Louis CF (1982). Fatty acid effects on calcium influx and efflux in sarcoplasmic reticulum vesicles from rabbit skeletal muscle. *Biochim Biophys Acta* 687:17–26.

Klausner RD, Kleinfeld AM, Hoover RL, Karnovsky MJ (1980). Lipid domains in membranes. Evidence derived from structural perturbations induced by free fatty acids and lifetime heterogeneity analysis. *J Biol Chem* 255:1286–1295.

Knöll R, Arras M, Zimmerman R, Schaper J, Schaper W (1994). Changes in gene expression following short coronary occlusions studied in porcine hearts with run-on assays. *Cardiovasc Res* 28:1062–1069.

Knowlton AA, Eberli FR, Brecher P, Romo GM, Owen A, Apstein CS (1991). A single myocardial stretch or decreased systolic fiber shortening stimulates the expression of the heat shock protein 70 in the isolated, erythrocyte-perfused rabbit heart. *J Clin Invest* 88:2018–2025.

Knowlton AA (1995). The role of heat shock proteins in the heart. *J Mol Cell Cardiol* 27:121–131.

Kolch W, Heidecker G, Kochs G, Hummel R, Vahadi H, Mischak H, Finkenzeller G, Marme D, Rapp UR (1993). Protein kinase C_α activates RAF-1 by direct phosphorylation. *Nature* 364:249–252.

Komoro I, Yazaki Y (1993). Control of cardiac gene expression by mechanical stress. *Annu Rev Physiol* 55:55–75.

Komoro I, Yazaki Y (1994). Intracellular signaling pathways in cardiac myocytes induced by mechanical stress. *Trends Cardiovasc Med* 4:117–121.

Komuro I, Kurabayashi M, Takaku F, Yazaki Y (1988). Expression of cellular oncogenes in the myocardium during the developmental stage and pressure-overloaded hypertrophy of the rat heart. *Circ Res* 62:1075–1079.

Krontiris TG (1995). Oncogenes. *N Engl J Med* 333:303–306.

Kyriakis JM, Avruch J (1996). Sounding the alarm: protein kinase cascades activated by stress and inflammation. *J Biol Chem* 271:24313–24316.

Lanahan A, Williams JB, Sanders LK, Nathans D (1992). Growth factor-induced delayed early response genes. *Mol Cell Biol* 12:3919–3929.

Laugwitz K-L, Allgeier A, Offermanns S, Spicher K, Van Sande J, Dumont JE, Schultz G (1996). The human thyrotropin receptor: a heptahelical receptor capable of stimulating members of all four G-protein families. *Proc Acad Sci U S A* 93:116–120.

Leevers SJ, Paterson HF, Marshall CJ (1994). Requirement for Ras in Raf activation is overcome by targeting Raf to the plasma membrane. *Nature* 369:411–414.

Lefkowitz RJ, Pitcher J, Krueger K, Daaka Y (1997). Mechanisms of β-adrenergic receptor desensitization and resensitization. *Adv Pharmacol* 42:416–420.

Lefstin JA, Yamamoto KR (1998). Allosteric effects of DNA on transcriptional regulators. *Nature* 392:885–888.

Lengsfeld M, Morano I, Ganten U, Ganten D, Rüegg JC. Gonadectomy and hormonal replacement changes systolic blood pressure and ventricular myosin isoenzyme pattern of spontaneously hypertensive rats. *Circ Res* 63:1090–1094.

Lewis TS, Shapiro PS, Ahn NG (1998). Signal transduction through MAP kinase cascades. *Adv Cancer Res* 74:49–139.

Liu M, Simon MI (1996). Regulation by cyclic AMP-dependent protein kinase of a G-protein-mediated phospholipase C. *Nature* 382:83–87.

Lucas PC, Granner DK (1992). Hormone response domains in gene transcription. *Annu Rev Biochem* 61:1131–1173.

Luttrell LM, Biesen TV, Hawes BE, Koch WJ, Krueger KM, Touhara K, Lefkowitz RJ (1997). G-protein-coupled receptors and their regulation. Activation of the MAP kinase signaling pathway by G-protein-coupled receptors. *Adv Second Messenger Phosphoprotein Res* 31:263–277.

Luttrell LM, Ferguson SSG, Daaka Y, Miller WEE, Maudsley S, Della Rocca GJ, Lin F-T, Kawakatsu H, Owada K, Luttrell DK, Caron MG, Lefkowitz RJ (1999). β-arrestin-dependent formation of β_2 adrenergic receptor-src protein kinase complexes. *Science* 283:655–661.

Maack T (1992). Receptors of atrial natriuretic factor. *Annu Rev Physiol* 54:11–27.

Marsh JD, Lehmann MH, Ritchie RH, Gwathmey JK, Green GE, Schiebinger RJ (1998). Androgen receptors mediate hypertrophy of cardiac myocytes. *Circulation* 98:256–261.

Marshall CJ (1996). Raf gets it together. *Nature* 383:127–128.

Marx J (1993). Two major signaling pathways linked. *Nature* 262:988–990.

McDonough PM, Hanford DS, Sprenkle AB, Mellon NR, Glembotski CC (1997). Collaborative roles for c-Jun N-terminal kinase, c-Jun, serum response factor, and Sp 1 in calcium-regulated myocardial gene expression. *J Biol Chem* 272:24046–24053.

Meyer TE, Habener JF (1993). Cyclic adenosine $3',5'$-monophosphate response element binding protein (CREB) and related transcription-activated deoxyribonucleic acid-binding proteins. *Endocrinol Rev* 14:269–290.

Miner JH, Wold BJ (1991). c-*myc* inhibition of MyoD and myogenin-initiated myogenic differentiation. *Mol Cell Biochem* 11:2842–2851.

Molkentin JD, Lu J-R, Antos CL, Markham B, Richardson J, Robbins J, Grant SR, Olson EN (1998). A calcineurin-dependent transcriptional pathway for cardiac hypertrophy. *Cell* 93:215–228.

Monaco L, Lamas M, Tamai K, Lalli E, Zazopoulos E, Penna L, Nantel F, Foulkes NS, Mazzucchelli C, Sassone-Corsi P (1997). Coupling transcription to signaling pathways. cAMP and nuclear factor cAMP-responsive element modulator. *Adv Second Mess Phosphoprotein Res* 31:64–74.

Montminy MR, Sevarino KA, Wagner JA, Mandel G, Goodman RH (1986). Identification of a cyclic-AMP-responsive element within the rat somatostatin gene. *Proc Nat Acad Sci U S A* 83:6682–6686.

Moriguchi T, Gotoh Y, Nishida E (1996). Roles of the MAP kinase cascade in vertebrates. *Adv Pharmacol* 36:121–137.

Mulvagh SL, Michael LH, Perryman MB, Roberts R, Schneider MD (1987). A hemodynamic load *in vivo* induces cardiac expression of the cellular oncogene c-*myc*. *Biochem Biophys Res Comm* 147:627–636.

Nash JA, Hammond HK, Saffitz JE (1996). Cellular compartmentalization of $G_s\alpha$ in canine myocytes and its redistribution in heart failure. *Am J Physiol* 271:H2209–H2217.

Neer EJ (1995). Heterotrimeric G proteins: organizers of transmembrane signals. *Cell* 80:249–257.

Neumann J, Schmitz W, Scholz H, von Meyernick L, Döring V, Kalmar P (1988). Increase in myocardial G_i-proteins in heart failure. *Lancet* ii:936–937.

Nishizuka Y (1995). Protein kinase C and lipid signaling for sustained cellular responses. *FASEB J* 9:484–496.

Papavassiliou AG (1995). Transcription factors. *N Engl J Med* 332:45–47.

Pelech SL, Charest DL (1995). MAP kinase-dependent pathways in cell cycle control. *Prog Cell Cycle Res* 1:33–52.

Ping P, Hammond HK (1994). Diverse G protein and βadrenergic receptor mRNA expression in normal and failing porcine hearts. *Am J Physiol* 267:H2079–H2085.

Rannels DE, McKee EE, Morgan HE (1977). Regulation of protein synthesis and degradation in heart and skeletal muscle. In Litwack G, ed. *Biochemical Actions of Hormones.* Academic Press, New York, pp 135–195.

Rao A, Luo C, Hogan PG (1997). Transcription factors of the NFAT family regulation and function. *Annu Rev Immunol* 15:707–747.

Roberts SGE, Green MR (1995). Dichotomous regulators. *Nature* 375:105–106.

Roesler WJ, Vandenbark GR, Hanson RW (1988). Cyclic AMP and the induction of eukaryotic gene transcription. *J Biol Chem* 263:9063–9066.

Rosen LB, Ginty DD, Weber MJ, Greenberg M (1994). Membrane depolarization and calcium influx stimulate MEK and MAP kinase via activation of Ras. *Neuron* 12:1207–1221.

Rosen MR, Cohen IS, Danilo P Jr, Steinberg SF (1998). The heart remembers. *Cardiovasc Res* 119:643–647.

Roth DA, Urasawa K, Helmer GA, Hammond HK (1993). Down regulation of cardiac GTP-binding proteins in right atrium and left ventricle in pacing-induced congestive heart failure. *J Clin Invest* 91:939–949.

Sadoshima J, Izumo S (1997). The cellular and molecular response of cardiac myocytes to mechanical stress. *Annu Rev Physiol* 59:551–571.

Sadoshima J, Qiu Z, Morgan JP, Izumo S (1995). Angiotensin II and other hypertrophic stimuli mediated by G-protein-coupled receptors activate tyrosine kinase, mitogen-activated protein kinase, and 90 kD S6 kinase in cardiac myocytes: the critical role of Ca^{2+}-dependent signaling. *Circ Res* 76:1–15.

Sakata Y, Hoit BD, Liggett SB, Walsh RA, Dorn GW II (1998). Decompensation of pressure-overload hypertrophy in Gαq-overexpressing mice. *Circulation* 97:1488–1495.

Sánchez I, Hughes RT, Mayer BJ, Yee K, Woodgett JR, Avruch J, Kyriakis JM, Zon LI (1994). Role of SAPK/ERK kinase-1 in the stress-activated pathway regulating transcription of c-Jun. *Nature* 372:794–798.

Schiaffino S, Samuel JL, Sassoon D, Lompre AM, Garner I, Marotte F, Buckingham M, Rappaport L, Schwartz K (1989). Nonsynchronous accumulation of α-skeletal actin and β-myosin heavy chain mRNAs during early stages of pressure-overloaded-induced cardiac hypertrophy demonstrated by *in situ* hybridization. *Circ Res* 64:937–948.

Schnabel P, Böhm M, Gierschik P, Jakobs KH, Erdmann E (1990). Improvement of cholera toxin-catalyzed ADP ribosylation by endogenous ADP-ribosylation factor from bovine brain provides evidence for an unchanged amount of $G_{s\alpha}$ in failing human myocardium. *J Mol Cell Cardiol* 22:73–82.

Schnabel P, Gäs H, Nohr T, Camps M, Böhm M (1996). Identification and characterization of G protein-regulated phospholipase C in human myocardium. *J Mol Cell Cardiol* 28:2419–2427.

Simpson PC (1999). β-protein kinase C and hypertrophic signaling in human heart failure. *Circulation* 93:334–337.

Starksen NF, Simpson PC, Bishopric N, Coughlin SR, Lee WMF, Escobedo JA, Williams LT (1986). Cardiac myocyte hypertrophy is associated with c-*myc* protooncogene expression. *Proc Nat Acad Sci U S A* 83:8348–8350.

Steinberg SF, Goldberg M, Rybin VO (1995). Protein kinase C isoform diversity in the heart, *J Mol Cell Cardiol* 27: 141–153.

Sugden PH, Clerk A (1998). "Stress-responsive" mitogen-activated protein kinases (c-jun N-terminal kinases and p38 mitogen-activated protein kinases) in the myocardium. *Circ Res* 83:345–352.

Svetson BR, Kong X, Lawrence JC (1993). Increasing cyclic AMP attenuates activation of mitogen-activated protein kinase. *Proc Nat Acad Sci U S A* 90:10305–10309.

Tada M, Kirchberger MA, Iorio JM, Katz AM (1975). Control of cardiac sarcolemmal adenylate cyclase and sodium, potassium-activated adenosine triphosphatase activities. *Circ Res* 36:8–17.

Taylor SJ, Chae HZ, Rhee SG, Exton JH (1991). Activation of β1 isozyme of phospholipase C by α subunits of the Gq class of G proteins. *Nature* 350:516–518.

Ten Eick RE, Whalley DW, Rasmussen HH (1992). Connections: heart disease, cellular electrophysiology, and ion channels. *FASEB J* 6:2568–2580.

Thompson EB (1998). The many roles of c-Myc in apoptosis. *Annu Rev Physiol* 60:575–600.

Thompson MA, Ginty DD, Bonni A, Greenberg ME (1997). L-type voltage-sensitive Ca^{2+} channel activation regulates c-*fos* transcription at multiple levels. *J Biol Chem* 272:4224–4235.

Thorburn J, McMahon M, Thorburn A (1994). Raf-1 kinase activity is necessary but not sufficient for cellular morphology changes associated with cardiac myocyte hypertrophy. *J Biol Chem* 269:30580–30586.

Timmerman LA, Clipstone NA, Ho SN, Northrop JP, Crabtree GR (1996). Rapid shuttling of NF-AT in discrimination of Ca^{2+} signals and immunosuppression. *Nature* 383:837–840.

Trumpp-Kallmeyer S, Hoflack J, Bruinvels A, Hilbert M (1992). Modeling of G-protein-coupled receptors: application to dopamine, adrenaline, serotonin, acetylcholine, and mammalian opsin receptors. *J Med Chem* 35:3448–3462.

Tsukada T, Fink JS, Mandel G, Goodman RH (1987). Identification of a region in the human vasoactive intestinal polypeptide gene responsible for regulation by cyclic AMP. *J Biol Chem* 262;8743–8747.

van Biesen T, Lutterell LM, Hawes BE, Lefkowitz RJ (1996). Mitogenic signaling via G Protein-coupled receptors. *Endocrinol Rev* 17:698–714.

van Bilsen M, van der Vusse GJ, Renemann RS (1998). Transcriptional regulation of metabolic processes: implications for cardiac metabolism. *Pflügers Archiv Eur J Physiol* 437:2–4.

van Hoof C, Goris J, Merlevede W (1993). Phosphotyrosine protein phosphatases: master key enzymes in signal transduction. *News Physiol Sci* 38:3–7.

Vincent S, Marty L, Le Gallic L, Jeanteur P, Fort P (1993). Characterization of late response genes sequentially expressed during renewed growth of fibroblastic cells. *Oncogene* 8:1603–1610.

Vojtek AB, Cooper JA (1995). Rho family members: activators of MAP kinase cascades. *Cell* 82:527–529.

Wess J (1997). G-protein-coupled receptors: molecular mechanisms involved in receptor activation and selectivity of G-protein recognition. *FASEB J* 11:346–354.

Whitmarsh AJ, Shore P, Sharrocks AD, Davis RJ (1995). Integration of the MAP kinase signal transduction pathways at the serum response element. *Science* 269:403–407.

Wood TJJ, Haldosen L-A, Sliva D, Sundström M, Norstedt G (1997). Stimulation of kinase cascades by growth hormone: a paradigm for cytokine signaling. *Prog Nucl Acid Res* 57:73–94.

Yamazaki T, Komuro I, Yazaki Y (1995). Molecular mechanism of cardiac cellular hypertrophy by mechanical stress. *J Mol Cell Cardiol* 27:133–140.

Yamazaki T, Komuro I, Zou Y, Kudoh S, Shiojima I, Hiroi Y, Mizuno T, Aikawa R, Takano H, Yazaki Y (1997). Norepinephrine induces the *raf*-1 kinase/mitogen-activated protein kinase cascade through both α_1- and β-adrenoreceptors. *Circulation* 95:1260–1268.

Yan M, Dai T, Deak JC, Kyriakis JM, Zon LI, Woodget JR, Templeton DJ (1994). Activation of stress-activated protein kinase by MEKK1 phosphorylation of its activator SEK1. *Nature* 372:798–800.

York RD, Yao H, Ellig CL, Echert SP, McClewsky EW, Stork PJS (1998). Rap 1 mediates sustained MAP kinase activation induced by nerve growth factor. *Nature* 392:622–626.

Zawel L, Reinberg D (1996). Common themes in assembly and function of eukaryotic transcription complexes. *Annu Rev Biochem* 64:533–561.

Zhou M-M, Ravichandran KS, Olejniczak ET, Petros AM, Meadows RP, Sattler M, Harlan JE, Wade WS, Burakoff SJ, Feslik SW (1995). Structure and ligand recognition of the phosphotyrosine binding domain of Shc. *Nature* 378:584–592.

Zwick E, Daub H, Aoki N, Yamaguchi-Aoki Y, Tinhofer I, Maly K, Ullrich A (1997). Critical role of calcium-dependent epidermal growth factor receptor transactivation in PC12 cell membrane depolarization and bradykinin signaling. *J Biol Chem* 272:24767–24770.

8

Maladaptive Hypertrophy and the Cardiomyopathy of Overload: Familial Cardiomyopathies

One thing seems certain, namely that chronic overload of the heart does lead even- tually to heart failure even when the myocardium is normal at the start. How this failure comes about is a question that needs settling. Perhaps the solution to this last problem, as much as anything else, will go far to advance our knowledge about heart failure.

L. N. Katz (1964).

Chapter 1 reviewed the way that the great clinician-pathologists of the 18th and 19th centuries came to recognize both the beneficial and harmful consequences of overload-induced cardiac hypertrophy. Following Morgagni, who in the late 18th century postulated that, when blood flow through the heart was obstructed, the "more frequent and stronger actions" of the heart increased its thickness, thoughtful 19th century clinicians stressed the ability of chronic overload to cause cardiac enlargement. The initial adaptive hypertrophic response to overload was often likened to the skeletal muscle enlargement caused by chronic exercise, such as in the legs of a dancer or the upper extremities of a laborer. Less obvious, but apparent to the keen clinical observers of the late 19th century, was that cardiac hypertrophy had long-term, maladaptive, consequences. Schroetter, for example, noted in 1876 that although hypertrophy "may exist for many years . . . it certainly leads to . . . fatty degeneration and subsequent dilatation." Similarly, Paul wrote in 1884, "It has frequently been said that the heart hypertrophies in order to establish a sort of compensation. . . . This view would be correct if the hypertrophy remained stationary; but experience has shown that the excess of work imposed upon the heart finally deteriorates its fibres." The view that adaptive hypertrophy led, after time, to a maladaptive response was clearly stated at the end of the 19th century by Osler, who described three stages in the hypertrophic response to overload: a period of "development," followed by one of "full compensation," that ended in "broken compensation [which] commonly takes place slowly and results from degeneration and weakening of the heart muscle" (See Chapter 1 for references to these and other descriptions.)

The modern study of adaptive and maladaptive hypertrophy can be traced to the work of Meerson, who in the 1950s and 1960s carried out a series of experiments whose results are summarized in a now classical paper (Meerson, 1961) and text (Meerson, 1983). Using as his experimental model the acute pressure overload caused by aortic banding, Meerson reexamined Osler's three phases in the hypertrophic response to overload (Table 8-1). As had been noted clinically, Meerson found that the acute imposition of an

TABLE 8-1. *Three stages in the heart's response to sustained overload*

Stage	Duration	Response	Manifestations
1	Days	Development (Osler) Transient breakdown (Meerson)	Pulmonary congestion, low cardiac output, acute LV dilatation, early hypertrophy
2	Weeks	Full compensation (Osler) Stable hyperfunction (Meerson)	Less pulmonary congestion, increased cardiac output, established (adaptive) hypertrophy
3	Months or years	Broken compensation (Osler) Exhaustion and progressive cardiosclerosis (Meerson)	Progressive LV failure and dilatation (remodeling), maladaptive hypertrophy leading to cell death and fibrosis

overload was followed by a tripartite response. Immediately after awakening from anesthesia, the animals exhibited acute left heart failure, with pulmonary congestion and low cardiac output. After several days without specific therapy, the animals improved because their hearts had begun to hypertrophy. However, this phase, which Meerson called "stable hyperfunction" (analogous to Osler's "full compensation"), did not last more than a few weeks. Over the following months, the animals began to deteriorate, first exhibiting evidence of progressive left ventricular failure and finally dying of this condition. Examination of the hearts at this stage showed not only progressive cellular hypertrophy but also evidence for cell death and extensive fibrosis. These observations were the basis for my father's comment, at the head of this chapter, that understanding how overload damaged the heart could provide the key to understanding heart failure.

A clinical counterpart to Meerson's experiment came to my attention during the early 1970s when I was at Mount Sinai Hospital in New York City. I vividly recall two patients who, several months earlier, had been admitted to small suburban hospitals complaining of severe shortness of breath. The chest radiographs in both patients showed pulmonary infiltrates that had been interpreted as pneumonia. Both had responded slowly to antibiotics and supportive therapy, including oxygen, and both were eventually discharged, having improved considerably. However, neither regained their normal state of health. Eventually, both patients experienced increasing dyspnea and, on reexamination, a loud systolic murmur was heard for the first time. Repeat chest radiographs showed obvious cardiac enlargement, which led to their referral to Mount Sinai with a diagnosis of mitral insufficiency. In both cases, review of the earlier chest radiographs demonstrated that the illness originally diagnosed as "pneumonia" had been, in fact, acute pulmonary edema. Subsequent surgery revealed that both had had ruptured mitral valve chordae tendinae.

The spontaneous improvement following a sudden hemodynamic overload in these patients is consistent with the natural history described in Table 8-1. The improvement of the acute left ventricular failure caused by chordal rupture could not be attributed to cardiac therapy, which these patients had not received, nor to lessening of the mitral regurgitation, which is not a feature of this valve abnormality. One explanation for the improvement, not documented but almost certainly present in both patients, is left atrial dilatation. The growth response initiated by atrial stretch, which is analogous to that seen in a volume-overloaded ventricle, increases the capacity of this chamber to accommodate the blood that regurgitates through the leaky mitral valve, which, in turn, reduces left atrial pressure and alleviates pulmonary congestion. A more important explanation for the spontaneous improvement is development of left ventricular hypertrophy, which, as stated by Osler, allows "the heart's vigor [to meet the increased] requirements of the circulation." In accord with the observations of the 19th century clinician-pathologists and the work of Meerson, the compensation was only temporary. Both patients deteriorated rapidly, and had it not been possible to replace their mitral valves, it is unlikely that either would have survived more than a year after the initial event.

Deterioration of the hypertrophied heart (stage 3 in Table 8-1) is a major problem in most patients with heart failure. A simple explanation for this deterioration, that the hypertrophic response cannot alleviate the overload on the individual sarcomeres, was effectively ruled out many decades ago, when several groups calculated wall stress in patients with aortic stenosis (Sandler and Dodge, 1963; Hood et al., 1968; Grossman et al., 1975). All found that hypertrophy, by increasing wall thickness and reducing cavity size, could return systolic wall stress almost to normal levels. Only after the heart began to fail did wall stress, and thus sarcomere overload, increase. Convincing evidence that myocardial deterioration, rather than persistence of an uncompensated overload, is the major cause of the progressive deterioration of the overloaded heart is provided by the universal clinical observation that valve replacement cannot restore health to patients who have had a long-standing hemodynamic overload. Even when a damaged valve is replaced with a well-functioning prosthetic valve, patients do not recover if the operation is delayed beyond a "point of no return." This occurs because, with time, the major problem shifts from the defective valve to the heart muscle, which becomes irreversibly damaged by excessive and prolonged overload. These and other findings demonstrate that chronic overload is as damaging to the heart as a toxin or a virus, an interpretation that led me to coin the term "Cardiomyopathy of Overload" to describe this condition (Katz, 1990; 1994).

HOW FAST DOES THE OVERLOADED HEART FAIL? NATURAL HISTORY

Survival after the onset of symptoms in most clinical trials of therapy for heart failure is short, averaging less than 5 years. Longer periods of time, however, often elapse between the onset of cardiac overloading and the appearance of the clinical syndrome that is recognized as heart failure. This was apparent in the years before open heart surgery, when it was possible to observe the natural history of many forms of structural heart disease. Paul Wood, in the second edition of his classic *Diseases of the Heart and Circulation* (1956), states that, in rheumatic aortic incompetence, in which the left ventricle is volume-overloaded, average life expectancy after the development of a hemodynamically significant lesion is 20 to 30 years. Furthermore, as noted by Wood, "exercise tolerance remains remarkably good until the end." As a trainee in Wood's clinic in London in 1960, I saw several individuals who had remained asymptomatic for more than 20 years with "wide open" aortic insufficiency, as evidenced by dilated hearts and aortic diastolic pressures that were between 0 and 20 mmHg. The prognosis in aortic stenosis, as noted by Wood, is more dependent on the severity of the lesion. Patients with moderate stenosis, with only slight slowing of the upstroke of the peripheral pulse, moderately delayed aortic valve closure, and moderate left ventricular hypertrophy (in 1956 determined by electrocardiography [ECG] because there were no echocardiograms) had life expectancies of 10 to 20 years. Patients with severe aortic stenosis, evidenced by fully developed physical signs and severe ECG changes "[could] not be expected to survive more than 5 to 10 years," even when asymptomatic. Survival after the onset of symptoms was even shorter, generally a year or two. Hypertension, which differs from aortic stenosis because the elevated aortic diastolic pressure increases coronary perfusion, has a better prognosis than aortic stenosis, except that hypertension damages other organs and causes stroke and renal failure. Overall, it is probably fair to state that patients with a modest hemodynamic overload can remain asymptomatic for many years, often more than a decade. However, once symptoms develop, average survival is about 5 years (Fig. 8-1).

Wood's meticulously collected data show that prognosis in patients with a left ventricular pressure overload is worse than that in those with a volume overload, a fact that is also well documented in patients with congenital heart disease and either right ventricular pressure or volume overload. The volume overload caused by an atrial septal defect, in which right ventricular stroke volume is often about three times normal, is remarkably well tolerated; patients in whom pulmonary hypertension does not develop can have a normal life expectancy, sometimes dying at an advanced age of noncardiac causes. Right ventricular pressure overload, as seen in pulmonary valve stenosis, had a much worse prognosis in the era before this lesion could be repaired surgically; in patients whose pulmonary artery pressures were three to five times normal, death usually occurred from right ventricular failure between ages 30 and 35 years.

In developed countries, where the major cause of heart failure is left ventricular damage caused by myocardial infarction, survival can be predicted from the severity of the left ventricular dysfunction, which in these patients is readily estimated by measuring ejection fraction. In the usual clinical trial in heart failure, which enrolls patients with low ejection fraction (systolic dysfunction), who are generally men with an average age of about 60 years, 50% survival rate is about 5 years. The prognosis is not much different in members of this population who have ischemic heart disease and those with idiopathic dilated cardiomyopathy. Less is known about prognosis in the rapidly growing population

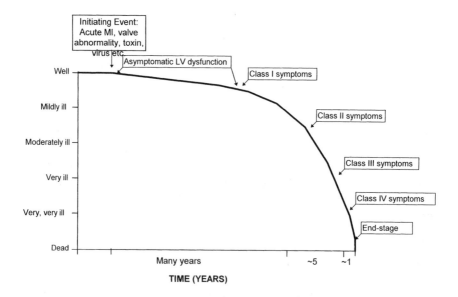

NATURAL HISTORY OF CARDIAC OVERLOAD

FIG. 8-1. Heart failure is a progressive, lethal syndrome characterized by accelerating deterioration. Following a period of asymptomatic left ventricular dysfunction that can last more than a decade, survival after the onset of significant symptoms averages about 5 years. The actual rate of deterioration is highly variable and depends on the nature and cause of the overload, the age and sex of the patient, and many other factors.

of patients whose heart failure is associated with a low ejection fraction (diastolic dysfunction), most of whom are older women, in their 70s. The prognosis appears to be somewhat better in diastolic than in systolic dysfunction, possibly because remodeling is not a prominent feature in the former group.

Is There a "Transition" from Cardiac Hypertrophy to Heart Failure?

Much has been written about a "transition" from hypertrophy to heart failure—from the early stage characterized by asymptomatic left ventricular dysfunction to the later stages that are dominated by worsening hemodynamic abnormalities. A central assumption implicit in the view of a transition from hypertrophy to failure is that these hearts pass some sort of a milestone, after which the patient's symptoms can no longer be held in check by adaptive hypertrophy. An alternative view is that no such milestone exists, so that there is no transition; instead, the natural history in these patients is characterized by "progression."

My own opinion is that deterioration of the hypertrophied heart is most correctly viewed as a progression and that the apparent transition from hypertrophy to failure is determined largely by noncardiac factors, mainly the fluid retention that occurs when the kidneys are stimulated by the hemodynamic defense reaction. In the experimental heart failure induced by pressure overload, for example, maladaptive features of hypertrophy are present, and progress, long before the development of symptomatic heart failure (Onodera et al., 1998). Another problem with the concept of a transition is that *hypertrophy* describes the heart's architecture, whereas *failure* represents a hemodynamic syndrome. Most important, there is no transition if this term is used to describe a point of no return; instead, patients with advanced heart failure readily move into and out of clinical heart failure. This chapter is being written during the holiday season from November to the end of December, where the "holiday meal" highlights the ease with which patients can go from a symptom-free life to one with significant clinical disability. Worsening occurs because of the huge sodium intake that accompanies an American turkey dinner, with its salt-rich stuffing and gravy, not to mention the salted Brussels sprouts, carrots, and mashed potatoes. The holiday meal can expand circulating blood volume to such an extent that these patients develop severe dyspnea and even pulmonary edema. This apparent transition to heart failure is readily reversed by diuretic therapy and a more judicious diet. Furthermore, the improvement can be maintained for years with a prudent salt intake, diuretics, and appropriate therapy with angiotensin-converting enzyme (ACE) inhibitors and β blockers. Yet maladaptive hypertrophy continues to progress in these patients, even though effective therapy can for a time alleviate and, in many patients, even eliminate the clinical manifestations of heart failure. Failure to appreciate the progressive deterioration of the overloaded heart throughout this course is one of the major reasons for the inadequate therapy commonly offered to these patients.

Another objection to the idea of a "transition" is that it implies that life cannot return to normal once a patient has experienced an episode of severe heart failure. Although this was once the case, modern therapy makes it overly gloomy to talk of a transition or "point of no return."

In the last analysis, of course, this distinction is really a matter of terminology. Whether worsening heart failure occurs by a *transition* or a *progression* is largely a matter of definition—in either case, the Cardiomyopathy of Overload does worsen, but much can be done to improve both symptoms and prognosis.

TABLE 8-2. *Possible mechanisms for the Cardiomyopathy of Overload*

Progressive dilatation (remodeling)
    Altered myocyte phenotype (cell elongation)
    Fiber slippage
    Fibrosis
Necrosis (accidental cell death)
    Inflammation, cytokines
    Free radicals
    Calcium overload
    Energy starvation
      Increased energy demands
      Decreased energy supply
        Inadequate nutrient coronary flow
        Fewer capillaries
        Mitochondrial DNA damage
        Decreased creatine phosphokinase (phosphocreatine shuttle)
Apoptosis (programmed cell death)

MECHANISMS BY WHICH CHRONIC OVERLOADING CAN INDUCE THE CARDIOMYOPATHY OF OVERLOAD

At least three general mechanisms can explain the progressive deterioration of the overloaded heart: progressive dilatation (remodeling), necrosis, and apoptosis (Table 8-2). None is simple and all overlap, one with another. Furthermore, overload establishes a number of vicious cycles (Fig. 8-2). The following discussion, while in many places spec-

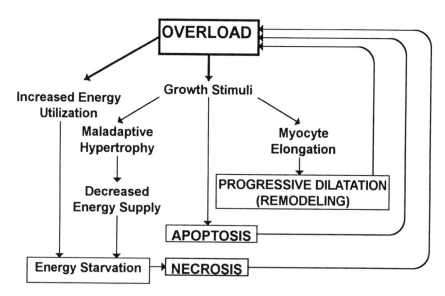

FIG. 8-2. Some of the vicious cycles that operate in the overloaded heart. Overload both increases energy utilization and stimulates growth (dark arrows). The former contributes directly to a state of energy starvation, which is made worse by several consequences of maladaptive hypertrophy that decrease energy supply. The latter include myocyte elongation, which causes remodeling, a progressive dilatation that increases wall tension so as to increase the overload. Growth stimuli also promote apoptosis, which by decreasing the number of viable cardiac myocytes, increases the load on those that survive. Hypertrophy also causes architectural changes that reduce the energy supply to working cardiac myocytes.

ulative, builds on these concepts by linking the pathophysiology and molecular biology of cell regulation presented in earlier chapters of this text to recent clinical insights regarding heart failure. The resulting portrayal of heart failure as a molecular disorder of the myocardial cell can, it is hoped, provide a framework for understanding this clinical syndrome, and for designing therapeutic strategies that can help these patients.

PROGRESSIVE DILATATION (REMODELING)

Cardiac dilatation, the first of the three general mechanisms that damage the failing heart (see Table 8-2), is not a stable condition, but instead progresses steadily and inexorably. In other words, dilatation begets more dilatation in a vicious cycle that represents a major cause of the Cardiomyopathy of Overload (Fig. 8-3). This vicious cycle allows any disease that causes the heart to dilate to initiate a remodeling process that worsens steadily and, if not halted, eventually kills the patient.

A major exception to this generalization is seen in the "athlete's heart," a physiologic hypertrophy that is initiated during brief periods of intense physical activity, when adrenergic stimulation is accompanied by reduced peripheral resistance. This phenotype of hypertrophy carries none of the adverse long-term implications of pathologic hypertrophy. Although the reasons are not well understood, the differences probably arise because the molecular signals initiated by intermittent exercise-induced overload are not the same as those which cause the Cardiomyopathy of Overload, in which growth-promoting stimuli impinge on the heart 24 hours a day, 7 days a week. In the latter, the heart deteriorates progressively until either the load is removed or the patient dies.

Deleterious Effects of Dilatation

According to Starling's Law of the Heart, dilatation increases the ability of the heart to pump blood, whereas according to the Law of Laplace, dilatation increases wall tension, which as discussed below both reduces ejection and increases the energy cost of the work performed. The Law of Laplace states that the tension in the walls of a chamber like the heart (T) is directly proportional to the pressure within the cavity (P) and the radius (R), according to the relationship $T \alpha P \times R$. Thus, dilatation of the failing heart increases the force that must be generated by its sarcomeres to achieve a given level of cavity pressure.

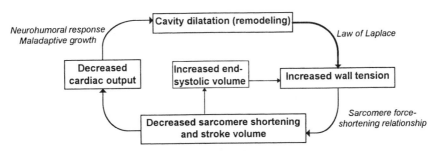

FIG. 8-3. Cavity dilatation establishes a vicious cycle that increases wall tension (dark arrow), which decreases sarcomere shortening and stroke volume. The latter increase end-systolic volume and decrease cardiac output, which cause further cavity dilatation. The last step in this vicious cycle is amplified when the neurohumoral response to the decrease in cardiac output stimulates further dilatation (remodeling).

Increased wall tension also reduces sarcomere shortening. Concentric hypertrophy, by increasing wall thickness, alleviates some of these maladaptive effects. Because the Law of Laplace for a thick-walled chamber states that $T = P \times R/h$, where h is wall thickness, the increased wall thickness reduces the tension on the individual sarcomeres.

The Law of Laplace has important consequences in the dilated heart, most of which are deleterious. In the first place, much as pulling a heavy trailer shortens the range of an automobile, increased sarcomere tension decreases the heart's ability to eject. This contributes to the vicious cycle shown in Fig. 8-3, in which cavity dilatation increases wall tension, which decreases sarcomere shortening and stroke volume, which leaves behind a greater end-systolic volume, which adds further to cavity dilatation. This vicious cycle reduces cardiac output and so amplifies the hemodynamic defense reaction discussed in Chapter 4. One maladaptive effect of many mediators of this neurohumoral response is to stimulate the mitogenic pathways described in Chapters 6 and 7, which helps to explain why cavity dilatation is progressive. Stretch also stimulates cell adhesion molecules to activate mitogenic pathways, which provides another stimulus that increases progressive cavity dilatation.

The Law of Laplace also states that dilatation reduces the ability of the failing heart to generate pressure. This adverse effect stimulates the hemodynamic defense reaction to constrict vascular smooth muscle and so increase peripheral resistance. The result is an increase in left ventricular afterload that both reduces stroke work and causes a further increase in wall tension. This establishes yet another vicious cycle (Fig. 8-4), in which the hemodynamic defense reaction initiated by impaired pump performance increases peripheral resistance, which increases afterload, which further decreases ejection, which causes further dilatation by increasing end-systolic (residual) volume. Decreased ejection, by causing cavity dilatation, also increases wall tension, which worsens pump performance by reducing sarcomere shortening. The decreased stroke volume further impairs pump performance (see Fig. 8-4).

Two of the steps shown in Fig. 8-4 stimulate maladaptive growth of the failing heart. The first is the worsening pump performance, which by activating the hemodynamic defense reaction releases mediators that activate mitogenic pathways. The second is the

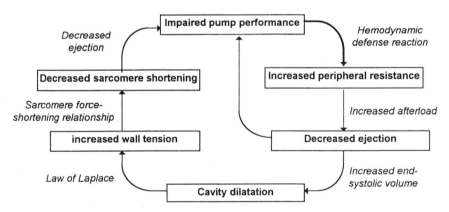

FIG. 8-4. A vicious cycle is initiated when impaired cardiac pumping causes the hemodynamic defense reaction to increase peripheral resistance. The increased afterload decreases ejection, which further impairs pump performance and causes cavity dilatation. The latter, according to the Law of Laplace, increases wall tension, which further impairs pump performance.

ability of increased wall tension and stretch to activate mitogenic signals generated by cell adhesion molecules. These signals, by promoting cell elongation, contribute to the vicious cycles in which progressive cavity dilatation in the failing heart increases wall tension.

Dilatation has adverse effects on the energetics of the failing heart that may be as important as the increased wall tension and reduced ejection discussed in the preceding paragraphs. The reason is that even the normal heart is "on the edge" in terms of its ability to generate the large amounts of high-energy phosphate needed to pump blood. One manifestation of the precarious balance between energy production and energy consumption is the almost complete extraction of oxygen by the normal heart, which is reflected in the very low oxygen content of coronary venous blood. Any abnormality that increases energy demands, therefore, can worsen this balance, especially in the failing heart where energy production is impaired.

The energetics of the normal heart are also precarious because of the low efficiency of cardiac contraction. The mechanical efficiency of the normal heart, which can be estimated as the proportion of the chemical energy generated from oxidative metabolism that is converted into mechanical work, is generally less than 15%. It is also well established that more energy is required to increase systolic pressure than to increase ejection (Evans and Matsuoka, 1915). In the failing heart, energy demands are increased by cavity dilatation and the high peripheral resistance, both of which reduce efficiency by increasing wall tension. A simple way to understand the inefficiency caused by increased wall tension is to compare the heart to a spring. According to this analogy, expending energy to develop wall tension during isovolumic contraction is like using energy to stretch the spring; in both cases, much of this energy is degraded to heat when tension decreases. The amount of this energy wastage is directly proportional to load, both on the spring and on the heart. Normally, some of the potential energy stored in the heart's elasticities can be converted to useful work as the sarcomeres shorten during ejection. In the dilated heart, however, both sarcomere shortening and ejection are impaired because of the increased wall tension (see earlier discussion). As a result, conversion of this potential energy to useful work is reduced. These problems are especially deleterious in end-stage heart failure, where energy production can be severely impaired, and energy reserves exhausted. The adverse energetics associated with ventricular dilatation are discussed later in this chapter, when the role of energy starvation in causing calcium overload and necrosis in the failing heart is explored.

Cell Elongation, Progressive Dilatation, and Remodeling

Maladaptive growth and changing myocyte phenotype play an important role in causing the progressive dilatation (remodeling) of the failing heart. The strongest evidence for a causal link between changes in cardiac myocyte phenotype and the Cardiomyopathy of Overload is the increased cell length seen in patients with systolic dysfunction, whether caused by ischemic heart disease or by a dilated cardiomyopathy (Beltrami et al., 1994; Gerdes and Capasso, 1995; Zafeiridis et al., 1998). The changes in cell morphology that accompany systolic dysfunction are quite different from those seen in diastolic dysfunction (pressure overload), in which the major abnormality is increased cell thickness rather than cell elongation. These phenotypic differences indicate that increased systolic wall stress activates signal transduction systems which increase cell *width* by causing new sarcomeres to be added in parallel, whereas diastolic stretch increases cell *length* when new sarcomeres are added in series (Fig. 8-5).

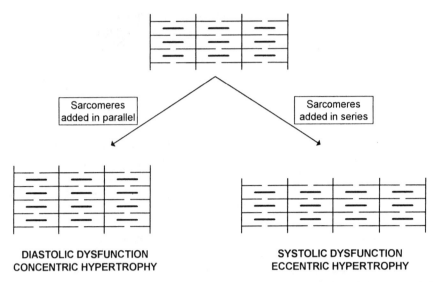

DIASTOLIC DYSFUNCTION
CONCENTRIC HYPERTROPHY

SYSTOLIC DYSFUNCTION
ECCENTRIC HYPERTROPHY

FIG. 8-5. Myocyte thickening (seen in diastolic dysfunction and concentric hypertrophy) and myocyte elongation (seen in systolic dysfunction and eccentric hypertrophy) are due in part to different patterns of myocyte hypertrophy. Diastolic dysfunction occurs when sarcomeres are added in parallel (left); systolic dysfunction occurs when they are added in series (right).

The existence of these different phenotypes provides solid evidence that specialized signaling pathways can activate different patterns of myocyte growth in the overloaded human heart. This has been demonstrated in cultured neonatal cardiac myocytes, in which myocyte thickening and elongation are controlled by different signaling pathways (Wollert et al., 1996). Cardiotrophin-1, a cytokine, causes cells to become longer, whereas the α_1-adrenergic agonist phenylephrine, which binds to G protein-coupled receptors, causes the cells to become thicker. These findings could be explained if stimulation of a stress-activated MAP kinase by the cytokine caused sarcomeres to be added in series to increase cell length and so stimulate eccentric hypertrophy, whereas stimulation of a mitogenic MAP kinase pathway by phenylophrine led to sarcomere addition in parallel, which increased cell thickness and caused concentric hypertrophy. Such an interpretation is premature because both cardiotrophin-1 and phenylephrine can activate additional signal transduction pathways. Also, these data are probably not directly relevant to clinical heart failure because the responses of the adult heart to these and other extracellular messengers differ from those of neonatal cardiac myocytes. Despite these uncertainties, the study of Wollert et al. (1996) represents a watershed because it implies that agents targeted to specific signal transduction systems can selectively modify the pattern of myocyte hypertrophy.

An ideal agent for the treatment of systolic dysfunction would reverse, or at least inhibit, progressive dilatation (remodeling). Remarkably, there is already evidence that such agents already exist. These are the nitrates, converting enzyme inhibitors, and β-adrenergic blockers, which as discussed in Chapter 9, inhibit remodeling of the failing heart. Further characterization of the signal transduction pathways that control the different patterns of sarcomere addition shown in Fig. 8-5 is likely to provide a foundation for the development of more specific, and more potent, means to block the progressive dilation of the failing heart.

Fiber Slippage

Another mechanism that has been proposed to explain remodeling is slippage of groups of sarcomeres or cells past one another (Fig. 8-6). This mechanism was suggested many years ago, when the number of fiber layers was found to remain unchanged in the eccentrically hypertrophied, failing left ventricle (Linzbach, 1960). Fiber slippage probably occurs in acute ventricular dilatation, such as immediately after valve rupture, and may be a cause for the infarct expansion that is sometimes seen in the first few days after an acute myocardial infarction (Hutchins and Bulkley, 1978; Olivetti et al., 1990). The role of fiber slippage in the slower remodeling of the failing heart, however, is less clear because this syndrome is accompanied by myocyte elongation (Gerdes and Capasso, 1995).

Role of Nonmyocytes

Although about 75% of the normal mass of the heart is cardiac muscle, the predominant cell type are nonmyocytes, which include fibroblasts, endocardial and epicardial cells, and the smooth muscle and endothelial cells found in the coronary vessels. Nonmyocytes represent approximately two thirds of the cells found in the atria and ventricles (for review, see Weber and Brilla, 1991), an apparent discrepancy that is readily explained by their much smaller size.

The proportion of nonmyocytes is increased in the failing heart, in large part because of the ability of these cells to divide. Unlike adult cardiac myocytes, which have virtually no capacity to proliferate, nonmyocytes readily enter the cell cycle and undergo normal mitosis. It is not surprising, therefore, that cardiac myocyte hypertrophy and fibroblast proliferation are independently controlled (Weber and Brilla, 1991). Differences in the signaling systems that control myocyte hypertrophy and the proliferation of many different types of nonmyocyte explain one major difference between the pathologic hypertrophy seen in failing hearts, in which fibrosis is a prominent feature, and the physiologic hypertrophy of the athlete's heart, in which there is little or no abnormal fibrosis (Weber and Brilla, 1991).

In addition to producing the extracellular matrix proteins that maintain the heart's architecture, nonmyocytes generate a number of signaling molecules. These include angiotensin II, peptide growth factors, cytokines, and other neurohumoral mediators. All of these extracellular messengers, as noted in earlier chapters, are able to modify gene expression in cardiac myocytes by paracrine signaling. Distortion of nonmyocytes can also distort, and so activate, cell adhesion molecules on the cardiac myocytes. Nonmyocyte activation and proliferation, therefore, are likely to play an important role in the maladaptive growth response that accompanies the Cardiomyopathy of Overload.

Fibrosis

Severe heart failure is accompanied by an increased amount of interstitial fibrous tissue in the walls of the heart (Caspari et al., 1977; Schaper et al., 1991; Weber et al., 1994; Marijianowski et al., 1995). Not only is there a greater collagen content in the failing heart but also the nature of the collagen changes. The most dramatic abnormality is seen in end-stage heart failure, in which a rigid type I collagen replaces the more elastic type III collagen (Weber et al., 1988; Chapman et al., 1990; Marijianowski et al., 1995). These changes are partly responsible for the reduced compliance and impaired filling seen in patients with dilated ventricles. The role of fibrosis in mild heart failure is less clear. In hearts that have large, remote infarcts, increased collagen deposition in the noninfarcted regions could be an early manifestation of the diffuse fibrotic process seen in end-stage

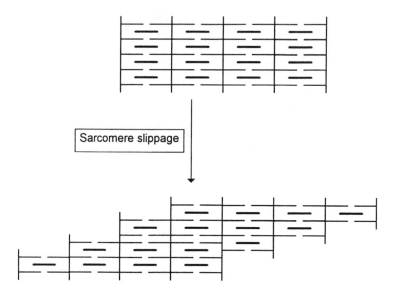

Sarcomere slippage

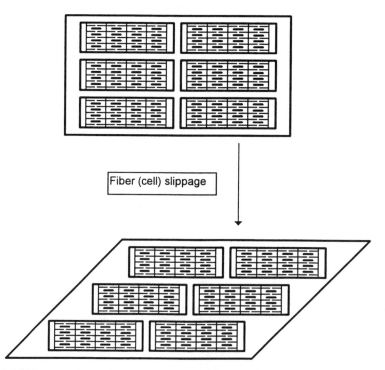

Fiber (cell) slippage

FIG. 8-6. Myocyte elongation can result from slippage. This can occur when sarcomeres (top) or cells (bottom) slip longitudinally by one another.

heart failure. However, this could also represent a patchy fibrosis caused by collagen deposition in localized areas of ischemic necrosis (Marijianowski et al., 1997).

Several stimuli have been suggested to increase the amount of fibrous tissue in the failing heart (Table 8-3). One mechanism is the actions of many peptide growth factors that stimulate growth and proliferation, which can be secreted by both myocytes and nonmyocytes. These peptides include TGF-β_1, a major promoter of fibrosis, whose levels are increased in the failing heart. Elevations of TGF-β_1 are greater in myocytes than in nonmyocytes and are more marked in pressure overload than in volume overload hypertrophy (Calderone et al., 1995). It is not clear, however, whether TGF-β_1 participates in pathogenic fibrosis that injures the heart, or whether instead, this peptide growth factor acts as part of a healing process. The latter appears to be the case in a genetic rat model of hypertrophy, in which genes that encode extracellular matrix proteins, notably TGF-β_1, were upregulated only in the later stages of this condition, after the animals exhibited evidence for heart failure (Boluyt et al., 1994).

Angiotensin II provides another stimulus for fibrosis. This peptide acts directly to promote fibrosis (Crawford et al., 1994), and indirectly to regulate the levels of additional signaling molecules that regulate tissue repair (for review, see Weber, 1997). Aldosterone, a steroid whose production is stimulated by the renin-angiotensin system, has been suggested to play a major role in stimulating fibrosis of the failing heart, so that inhibition of aldosterone-induced fibrosis may account for some of the beneficial effects of ACE inhibitors in heart failure (for review, see Weber and Brilla, 1991). This view is supported by the ability of the converting enzymes to increase the levels of kinins, which have counterregulatory effects that generally oppose the actions of angiotensin II, including inhibition of collagen accumulation in the overloaded heart (Wollert et al., 1997).

Another mechanism that can lead to fibrosis in the failing heart is the inflammatory response discussed in Chapter 5. Locally produced cytokines can activate macrophages and monocytes, which then attract and activate fibroblasts (for review, see Weber, 1994). Perhaps the most important cause of this inflammatory response, and thus fibrosis of the failing heart, is necrosis, which evokes an inflammatory response that leads to a robust fibrotic reaction.

The role of fibrosis in the failing heart, as discussed earlier, remains unclear. Collagen deposition can have adverse effects, but because fibrosis prevents tissue stretch, this process could be compensatory if deposition of extracellular matrix proteins provided structural support after cardiac myocytes are lost through necrosis. Evidence for the latter interpretation is found in studies of late reperfusion after myocardial infarction, at a time when cells are no longer viable. Even though there is little or no myocardial cell salvage in these patients, the increased fibrous tissue deposition caused by reperfusion creates a strong scar that reduces infarct expansion (Pfeffer and Braunwald, 1990; Topol et al., 1992). The alternative view, that fibrous tissue deposition is among the pathogenic

TABLE 8-3. *Mediators and mechanisms that can contribute to fibrosis of the failing heart*

Promoters of fibrosis
  Peptide growth factors (e.g., TGF-β)
  Inflammatory cytokines
  Angiotensin II
  Aldosterone
  Necrotic cell death
Inhibitors of fibrosis
  Kinins (bradykinin)

mechanisms that contribute to maladaptive hypertrophy, is suggested by evidence that collagen can encase or even strangle normal myocytes (Weber et al., 1988). Extracellular collagen deposition can also contribute to arrhythmogenesis by increasing extracellular electrical resistance. One answer to this question may lie in the ability of treatments that inhibit fibrosis, notably ACE inhibitors and aldosterone receptor blockers, to prolong survival in patients with heart failure.

NECROSIS (ACCIDENTAL CELL DEATH)

Necrosis, the "accidental" cell death generally associated with injury and plasma membrane rupture, probably plays an important role in the failing heart (see Table 8-2). Although its quantitative importance is not known, the extensive fibrosis seen in end-stage heart failure, especially after long-standing pressure overload, is probably the result of significant myocyte necrosis. Potential causes include the actions of the cytokines and free radicals, energy starvation, and calcium overload. Hemodynamic overloading itself can cause necrosis by several mechanisms (Fig. 8-7). These include maladaptive consequences of the hypertrophic process, which can worsen energy starvation by reducing energy production and increasing energy expenditure. Dilatation (remodeling), as noted earlier, also increases energy demands.

Inflammation, Cytokines, Free Radicals

The inflammatory response that is induced by overload, may play an important role in causing necrotic cell death in the failing heart. This response, which is mediated by cytokines such as TNF-α, is activated both by elevated circulating levels of these peptides and by autocrine and paracrine effects of locally secreted cytokines. Cytokines release re-

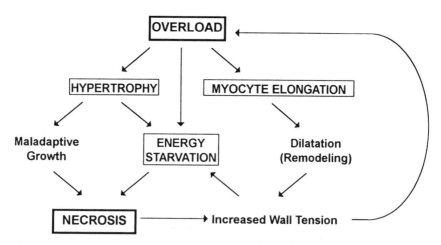

FIG. 8-7. Overload can cause necrosis by mechanisms that include maladaptive consequences of the hypertrophic process and energy starvation. The latter can result from architectural changes that decrease energy supply and increase energy demands. These mechanisms contribute to a number of vicious cycles, notably the ability of myocyte elongation and necrotic cell death to increase wall tension, which further increase myocyte overload.

active oxygen species and free radicals, such as NO (nitric oxide), all of which can cause membrane damage. The resulting loss of plasma membrane integrity represents a major feature of necrosis.

Energy Starvation

It is likely that failing hearts contain many energy-starved myocytes, resulting both from an increase in energy demand and a reduced capacity for energy production. A major cause for increased energy demands is hemodynamic overloading, which is exacerbated when the hemodynamic defense reaction increases preload and afterload, and increases the heart's inotropy, lusitropy, and chronotropy. The ability of the failing heart to meet these increased energy demands is made difficult by inadequate nutrient coronary flow and fewer capillaries, fibrosis, an increased distance for oxygen diffusion to the core of hypertrophied myocytes, mitochondrial abnormalities, and reduced levels of creatine phosphokinase that impair high-energy phosphate transfer via the phosphocreatine shuttle. In addition to impairing function, energy starvation causes calcium overloading of cardiac myocytes, which can be a major cause of cell death in the energy-starved heart.

The most important effects of energy starvation in a failing heart are to reduce allosteric effects of adenosine triphosphate (ATP) that accelerate ion fluxes through ion channels, ion exchangers, and ion pumps, and to decrease the free energy released during hydrolysis of the terminal ("high-energy") phosphate bond of ATP. Attenuation of the allosteric effects of ATP can worsen the hemodynamic abnormalities by slowing the calcium fluxes responsible for both contraction and relaxation, whereas the major effect of reduced free energy from ATP hydrolysis is to impair calcium removal from the cytosol by the calcium pump of the sarcoplasmic reticulum (Tian et al., 1996). Both of these effects increase cytosolic calcium, which accelerates ATP hydrolysis by the other calcium-activated systems found within cells (Fig. 8-8). This increases the calcium overload, which establishes yet another vicious cycle that further worsens the energy starvation in a failing heart.

Calcium Overload

Calcium overload is probably the most dangerous consequence of energy starvation in the failing heart. In addition to increasing diastolic tension, calcium overload is central to several vicious cycles by which energy starvation leads to necrosis (see Fig. 8-8). Calcium overloading increases energy expenditure because this cation activates a number of energy-requiring processes, the most important of which are the ATP-consuming interactions between actin and myosin. Increased cytosolic calcium also reduces energy production by dissipating the electrochemical gradient across the mitochondrial inner membrane, which uncouples oxidative phosphorylation. Together, the ability of calcium overload to accelerate energy consumption and slow energy production can cause an explosive increase in cytosolic calcium that leads to membrane rupture and cell necrosis.

Increased cytosolic calcium also activates signaling pathways that stimulate cell growth and proliferation. In addition to contributing to remodeling, these calcium-activated signals can cause apoptosis, a third potential cause of cell death in the failing heart.

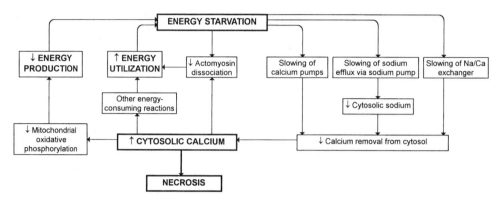

FIG. 8-8. Energy starvation, by increasing cytosolic calcium, establishes several vicious cycles that can cause cardiac myocyte necrosis. By inhibiting the sodium/calcium exchanger, the sodium pump, and the calcium pumps of the sarcoplasmic reticulum and plasma membrane, energy starvation impairs calcium removal from the cytosol. The result is an increase in cytosolic calcium that inhibits actomyosin dissociation, which in addition to impairing relaxation, increases energy consumption so as to worsen energy starvation. Mitochondrial oxidative phosphorylation is inhibited by increased cytosolic calcium, so that calcium overload also decreases energy production. As calcium overload worsens, these vicious cycles amplify one another, leading eventually to necrosis of the energy-starved cells.

APOPTOSIS (PROGRAMMED CELL DEATH)

Apoptosis, as described in Chapter 6, can be viewed as an "abortive form of mitosis" because the same signals that stimulate cell division also lead to programmed cell death. One of the major "benefits" of apoptosis is that it eliminates cells without inducing a fibrotic reaction, which distinguishes this type of cell death from necrosis. Apoptosis plays an essential role in embryonic development, where it provides for the removal of unneeded and imperfectly formed cells. Apoptotic cell death is also vital in proliferating tissues, such as the hematopoietic system, gut, and glandular tissue, where this process eliminates damaged, potentially malignant cells. In the terminally differentiated cells of the adult heart, however, apoptosis is a calamity. The reason is simply that heart muscle has little or no ability to regenerate.

A recent controversy has arisen between those who emphasize the possibility that adult cardiac myocytes can reenter the cell cycle and undergo mitosis (Anversa and Kajstura, 1998) and those who emphasize the limits of the capacity of these cells to proliferate (Soonpa and Field, 1998). A reading of the early literature on this subject (for review, see Rumyantsev, 1977) indicates that both views are correct. Severely overloaded cardiac myocytes do make abortive attempts at proliferation, but this proliferative response cannot regenerate a significant amount of functioning heart muscle. Furthermore, although overload has long been known to lead to the appearance of a few mitotic figures, efforts at cell division in the heart do not end well. This is clearly seen in the description provided in Table 8-4, which is taken from Ring (1950), who describes the abortive nature of this proliferative response in the hearts of adult rabbits and cats. The tissue studied was taken from the edge of an experimental infarct, where mitotic figures often appeared within the uninfarcted myocytes, sometimes in groups of adjacent cells. Mitosis probably occurred most frequently at this site because the mechanical stresses that deform cell adhesion molecules are maximal along the border between

TABLE 8-4. *Morphologic findings in regenerating myocardial tissue along the border of an experimental infarct in the rabbit**

Day 4:	. . . the ends of the peripheral muscle are surrounded by macrophages.
Day 5:	. . . the line of division between muscle and fibrous tissue is well marked. The ends of the muscle are discrete, usually striated to their terminations and occasionally expanded...occasional mitotic figures are seen.
Days 7–9:	. . . the terminal transverse striation is lost, but the ends...present short thin buds, often with a longitudinal chain of two or three nuclei.
Day 13:	. . . the tips of the muscle fibers are rounded and often enclosed by a new formation of fibrous tissue. Even where the muscle ends are free, however, no further growth of fibres occurs, in spite of the marked vascularity of the region at this stage.
Day 16:	. . . there is renewed activity in the connective tissue around the ends of the fibres. Occasional mitotic figures in muscle nuclei are seen, while the connective tissue nuclei appear grouped in large numbers around the terminations of the muscle. This activity is followed by a more extensive deposition of fibrous tissue around the muscle tips, which enables the latter to obtain a more direct insertion into the main fibrous mass....While the hyperchromatic nuclei and pronounced fibrillar characteristics of these strands suggest that this is new muscle, the ends show no signs of growth. These fibers are seen on reconstruction of the whole lesion to be on the edge of an area of muscle absorption and in no place continuous with normal muscle.

*Citations are from Ring (1950).

viable uninfarcted muscle and necrotic cells. Even though there is an excellent blood supply at the edge of the infarct, the attempts at myocyte proliferation were abortive; aside from the "budding" of a few new cells, there was no evidence for significant regeneration of new, viable myocardium (Ring, 1950). These observations, based on relatively simple technology (the light microscope), but interpreted using the most elegant of analytic instruments (the human brain), are likely to apply also to the failing heart, in which attempts at mitosis lead to little, if any, useful regeneration. As noted by Anversa and Kajstura (1998), these findings are relevant to heart failure mainly because they highlight the possibility that both the amount and quality of cardiac myocyte regeneration could be increased.

The ability of overload to induce apoptotic death of cardiac myocytes probably occurs when efforts to force a terminally differentiated adult cardiac myocyte into the cell cycle make the cell vulnerable to this form of cell death (Walsh and Perlman, 1997). One way to visualize this process is to equate the terminally differentiated cardiac myocyte and an individual who has chosen a monastic life; both give up the challenges of a worldly life—including the joys of procreation—to concentrate on a single task. In the case of the heart, this task is to beat without pause. A schematic view of how this choice may come about and how the attempt to reenter the cell cycle could lead both to apoptosis and necrosis is provided in Fig. 8-9.

It is apparent that hypertrophy shortens the lifespan of the human heart and that in laboratory animals this adverse outcome is due in part to degeneration of the overloaded cardiac myocytes (Meerson, 1961). Beginning in the mid-1990s, descriptions of apoptosis in hypertrophied hearts began to appear, although methodologic problems discussed in Chapter 6 often caused overestimates of the extent of apoptosis. The quantitative importance of the apoptotic process in heart failure, therefore, remains uncertain. Although apoptosis provides an attractive explanation for the Cardiomyopathy of Overload, the evidence that this process plays a major role in the deterioration shown in Fig. 8-1 is not now compelling.

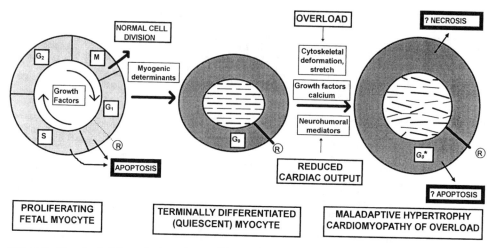

FIG. 8-9. Terminal differentiation of a proliferating fetal myocyte and maladaptive hypertrophy of an adult myocyte represent major transitions that are controlled by different transcription factors. The transition from the proliferating fetal myocyte to the terminally differentiated adult myocyte, which is initiated by the myogenic determinants, causes the myocyte to withdraw from the cell cycle into a quiescent phase called G_0. Accompanying the cessation of cell cycling is a reduced susceptibility to apoptosis, which occurs toward the end of G_1 and the beginning of the S phases. This transition is not reversible in that the capacity for normal cell division cannot be regained by renewed stimuli for myocyte growth. For this reason, mitogenic stimuli such as cytoskeletal distortion, stretch, release of cytokines and other growth factors, neurohumoral stimulation, and increased cellular calcium, all of which occur when the heart is overloaded, cannot restore the ability of cardiac myocytes to divide normally. In the adult heart, these growth-promoting stimuli cause myocyte hypertrophy, but stimuli that increase in cell size have maladaptive consequences. The latter include disorganization of cellular architecture, a tendency for energy starvation that leads to calcium overload and necrosis, and efforts to reenter the cell cycle that increase vulnerability to programmed cell death (apoptosis).

AN OVERVIEW OF CELL SIGNALING

Four simplified figures are included at this point to help the reader integrate abnormal mitogenic signaling and the pathogenesis of the Cardiomyopathy of Overload. These figures, which illustrate the variety of stimuli and signaling cascades that regulate cell growth, summarize material presented in earlier chapters in an abbreviated format. Shown are the growth regulatory effects of a cytokine (Fig. 8-10), a β-adrenergic agonist (Fig. 8-11), an α-adrenergic agonist (Fig. 8-12), and a cell adhesion molecule (Fig. 8-13). These figures, which should be viewed mainly as summaries, are intended to illustrate areas that hold some promise in developing therapy that can slow, and possibly reverse, the Cardiomyopathy of Overload.

FAMILIAL CARDIOMYOPATHIES

The last decade has seen a rapid growth of knowledge of heritable disorders that cause heart failure. Although the clinical manifestations of these pathophysiologic entities are often the same as those in the more common forms of heart failure, the underlying etiologic mechanisms are distinct. The familial cardiomyopathies are discussed at this point because new information about their molecular causes is identifying parallels between overload-induced hypertrophy (the Cardiomyopathy of Overload) and the growing number of inherited molecular disorders that cause the heart to fail.

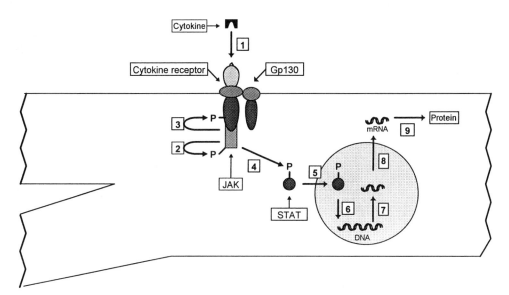

FIG. 8-10. Some steps in the transmission of a cytokine-mediated growth signal. Cytokine-binding to its receptors (1) causes the latter to form aggregates that often include an additional protein called gp130. These aggregates then incorporate tyrosine kinase called JAK, which can catalyze three different tyrosine phosphorylations: autophosphorylation of JAK (2), phosphorylation of the receptor (3) and gp130 (not shown), and phosphorylation of the transcription factor STAT (4). The phosphorylated STAT translocates to the nucleus (5) where it binds to and activates specific DNA sequences (6). This results in gene transcription (7), export of the newly formed mRNA (8), and protein synthesis (9).

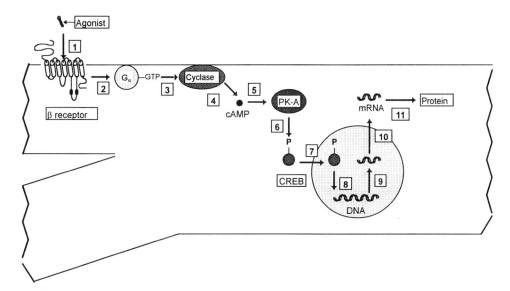

FIG. 8-11. Some steps in the transmission of a growth signal initiated by the binding of a β agonist to its receptor. Binding of the agonist to its receptor (1) activates the G-proteins, which as shown in the figure causes GTP to bind to G_α (2). The activated G_α then activates adenylyl cyclase (3), which stimulates cyclic AMP production (4). The latter activates protein kinase A (PKA) (5), a serine/threonine kinase that catalyzes a number of phosphorylations, including that of a cyclic AMP-receptor binding protein (CREB) (6). The latter translocates to the nucleus (7) where it binds to and activates specific DNA sequences (8). This results in gene transcription (9), export of the newly formed mRNA (10), and protein synthesis (11).

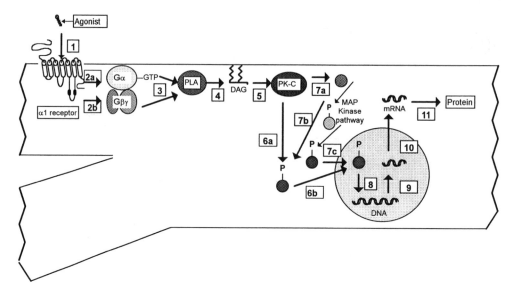

FIG. 8-12. Some steps in the transmission of the growth signal initiated by the binding of an α_1-agonist to its receptor. Binding of the agonist to its receptor (1) activates the G-proteins, which both causes GTP to bind to G_α (2a), and to dissociate from $G_{\beta\gamma}$ (2b). Both of the latter can activate phospholipase A (PLA) (3), which releases diacyl glycerol (DAG) from membrane lipids (4). The latter then activates protein kinase C (PKC) (5), a serine/threonine kinase that can phosphorylate and activate transcription factors directly (6a) or stimulate a MAP kinase pathway (7a). The latter activates additional transcription factors (7b) that translocate to the nucleus (7c) along with the transcription factors directly phosphorylated by PKC (6b) where both bind to and activate specific DNA sequences (8). This results in gene transcription (9), export of the newly formed mRNA (10), and protein synthesis (11).

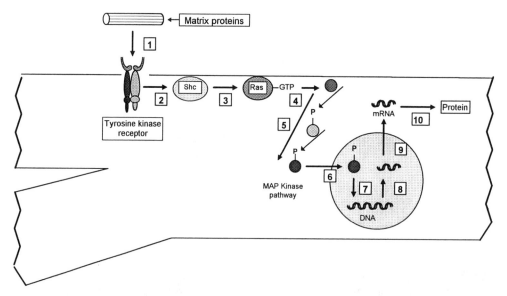

FIG. 8-13. Some steps in the transmission of the growth signal initiated by the activation of a cell adhesion molecule when it binds to the extracellular matrix. Binding of the matrix protein to a cell adhesion molecule (1), here labeled a tyrosine kinase receptor because of its ability to catalyze intracellular phosphorylations, activates the coupling protein Shc (2), which causes GTP to bind to Ras, a monomeric G protein (3). The latter then activates a MAP kinase pathway (4), which phosphorylates transcription factors (5) that translocate to the nucleus (6). The phosphorylated transcription factors bind to and activate specific DNA sequences (7) that stimulate gene transcription (8), export of the newly formed mRNA (9), and protein synthesis (10).

TABLE 8-5. *Classification and molecular abnormalities in the familial cardiomyopathies*

Hypertrophic cardiomyopathy* (mainly myofibrillar abnormalities)
β-Myosin heavy chain
Myosin binding protein C
Troponin T
Troponin I
Ventricular myosin regulatory light chain
Ventricular myosin essential light chain
α-Tropomyosin
Dilated cardiomyopathy (? mainly cytoskeletal abnormalities)
Dystrophin-sarcoglycan complex (Duchenne, Becker, Limb-Girdle muscular dystrophy)
Laminin (merosin)
Vinculin and metavinculin
Desmin
Mitochondrial proteins
Frataxin (Friedreich's ataxia)
Protein kinase (myotonic dystrophy)
Emerin (Emery-Dreifuss muscular dystrophy)
Restrictive cardiomyopathy (? cytoskeletal abnormalities)
Desmin
Amyloid

*Listed in approximate order of frequency; the last four appear to be rare.

The familial cardiomyopathies, like the "inborn errors of metabolism" that were characterized earlier in the 20th century, are providing valuable insights regarding disease mechanisms. Identification of molecular abnormalities that may contribute to the progressive deterioration of the failing heart has led to major advances in current understanding of the mechanisms by which overload damages normal heart muscle. In the case of the familial cardiomyopathies, the challenge is to understand how a specific molecular disorder causes the heart to fail. Although only a decade has passed since the first molecular cause of a familial cardiomyopathy was reported (Geisterfer-Lowrance et al., 1990), literally dozens of mutations involving most of the myofibrillar proteins and many cytoskeletal proteins are known to cause the heart to fail.

Familial cardiomyopathies can be divided into three classes (Table 8-5). The first to be characterized at a molecular level were the hypertrophic cardiomyopathies, which are generally caused by mutations involving the myofibrillar proteins. Least common are the restrictive cardiomyopathies, about which little is known except that some are caused by mutation of a cytoskeletal protein. Familial dilated cardiomyopathies, once thought to be uncommon, if not rare, are emerging as a major cause of the "idiopathic dilated cardiomyopathies." The following discussion, which highlights the molecular abnormalities responsible for the cardiomyopathies, deals briefly with some clinical features of this syndrome. More detailed descriptions of the clinical manifestations and management of this syndrome are found in standard textbooks.

Hypertrophic Cardiomyopathies

By definition, a hypertrophic cardiomyopathy occurs when the heart hypertrophies without an obvious cause. Bell, in 1802, described hearts that were "dense, firm, thick in substance, but [with small cavity]…dilated without, but…contracted within" in which there was "no ossification of the valves, no straightening of the aorta, nor any other obstruction to excite the heart" that could explain the thickened ventricular walls. We have come to know that many of these patients had hypertensive heart disease, in which increased afterload provided the stimulus that caused the heart's walls to thicken. More recently, concentric hypertrophy was found in patients with normal blood pressure. Attention was initially directed to obstruction of the left ventricular outflow tract, between the hypertrophied septum and the anterior leaflet of the mitral valve. The common finding of outflow obstruction in these hearts led to the widespread use of such terms as "idiopathic hypertrophic subaortic stenosis" (IHSS) and "hypertrophic obstructive cardiomyopathy" (HOCM). Whereas obstruction to blood flow from the left ventricle into the aorta can represent a major pathophysiologic abnormality in some patients, it is apparent that the underlying disorder is diastolic dysfunction that is caused by inappropriate concentric hypertrophy of the left ventricle.

Clinical Features

Hypertrophic cardiomyopathies can be diagnosed at any age; in general, the earlier this syndrome becomes manifest, the worse the prognosis (for review, see Spirito et al., 1997). The first manifestation can be sudden death, resulting, most likely, from disorganized depolarization of the thick-walled ventricle. Dyspnea, a common symptom, is due to impaired filling of the concentrically hypertrophied left ventricle. Angina pectoris, the chest pain syndrome that arises in an energy-starved heart, is also common because coronary perfusion can be limited by massive hypertrophy and increased intramyocardial tension. Syncope (fainting) and presyncope (light-headedness), which generally occur during exertion, can be caused when the reduced stroke volume significantly lowers low cardiac output. Syncope can also be due to an arrhythmia, in which case this symptom may herald sudden death. Physical findings include a collapsing arterial pulse, caused by the very brief period at the onset of systole when the "muscle-bound" left ventricle rapidly ejects its limited stroke volume. The decreased left ventricular compliance can cause a fourth heart sound (S4 or atrial sound). A systolic, ejection-type murmur is often heard; this is most commonly caused when the anterior leaflet of the mitral valve approaches a thickened interventricular septum to narrow the outflow tract of the left ventricle. The murmur is typically increased by maneuvers that decrease left ventricular preload and so reduce left ventricular volume; these include the Valsalva maneuver and rising from a squatting position. Conversely, the murmur is usually decreased by maneuvers that increase left ventricular preload, such as leg raising or handgrip. Squatting also reduces the intensity of the murmur because it increases the afterload on the left ventricle, and so alleviates left ventricular outflow tract obstruction.

Asymmetrical left ventricular hypertrophy can distort the electrocardiogram so that, in some patients, in addition to the features of left ventricular hypertrophy, one often sees deep, broad Q waves ("pseudoinfarction patterns") in various leads. Complex ventricular ectopy also occurs.

The "gold standard" for diagnosis of hypertrophic cardiomyopathy was, until recently, the echocardiogram, which typically shows left ventricular hypertrophy with a small left ventricular cavity. The decreased end-diastolic volume often increases ejection fraction. The pattern of left ventricular hypertrophy can be global, but more commonly there are localized areas of wall thickening. These are generally seen in the interventricular septum, but other areas of the left ventricle can also be thickened disproportionally. The distribution of localized areas of hypertrophy can vary in patients who share a common genotype. Systolic anterior motion (SAM) of mitral valve brings this structure into contact with the septum during ejection, which causes the outflow tract obstruction.

The prognosis in these patients depends on the molecular abnormality (Rosenzweig et al., 1991). In some families, most members affected with the genetic abnormality die suddenly before adulthood; whereas in other families, the affected individuals may live to old age with slowly progressing left ventricular failure. The severity of heart failure symptoms, degree of left ventricular hypertrophy, and extent of outflow tract obstruction are not good predictors of survival, but when these are minimal, this implies a more favorable prognosis. Major predictors of a poor prognosis include some genotypes, a young age at diagnosis, and the occurrence of syncope and severe arrhythmias.

Pathologic and Pathophysiologic Features

Patients with hypertrophic cardiomyopathies have hypertrophied ventricles with thick walls and a small cavity (concentric hypertrophy). The wall thickening is often asymmetrical, commonly with prominent hypertrophy of the interventricular septum. The role of a systolic pressure gradient between the left ventricular cavity and the aorta is controversial because cavity obliteration, rather than outflow tract obstruction, can be the major cause of the reduced stroke volume in some patients. In addition to thickened muscle fibers, microscopic examination demonstrates myofibrillar disarray, in which the parallel arrangement and alignment of sarcomeres in adjacent myocytes is distorted. The massive hypertrophy impairs left ventricular filling (diastolic dysfunction) and can cause these hearts to be energy starved. The latter, which is caused by the massive wall thickening and increased myocyte diameter, can lead to myocardial cell necrosis and fibrosis. The latter abnormalities, along with the thickened wall, increase the vulnerability of these hearts to arrhythmias.

Molecular Abnormalities

Most hypertrophic cardiomyopathies are caused by mutation of genes that encode myofibrillar proteins (for review, see Priori et al., 1999). This syndrome has also been seen in patients with Friedreich's ataxia, Turner's and Noonan's syndromes, Fabry's disease, and neurofibromatosis (O'Rourke et al., 1994); an early report that this condition can be caused by an abnormality in L-type calcium channels (Wagner et al., 1989) has not been confirmed.

More than 100 different mutations have been identified in at least seven different myofibrillar proteins (see Table 8-5). The frequency of these different genotypes depends on the country or region in which these patients are located. In approximate order of frequency, mutations are found in β-myosin heavy chain, myosin binding protein C, troponin T, troponin I, ventricular myosin regulatory light chain, ventricular myosin essential light chain, and α-tropomyosin. The last four appear to be rare. Most of these mutations cause the proteins to be truncated, generally because of missense mutations. Errors in splicing and deletions are also found, but duplications and insertions are rare. The mutated proteins are generally stable, and some, notably β-myosin heavy chain mutations, give rise to "poison polypeptides," which, when incorporated into the sarcomere, impair its function. Others, notably the myosin binding protein C mutations, create a "haploinsufficiency" in which there is not enough of the normal peptide to maintain function. In some cases, the abnormal proteins interfere with normal sarcomere assembly.

The "penetrance" of these mutations can vary, even for a given mutation in a given family in which some affected individuals die at a young age and others who are less severely affected survive much longer. The clinical severity generally increases with increasing age and may be greater in male patients. The echocardiographic distribution and severity of the hypertrophy can differ dramatically among individuals with the same genotype, even in siblings.

β-Myosin Heavy Chain Mutations

Mutations in the β-myosin heavy chain, the first molecular abnormality to have been identified in this syndrome (Geisterfer-Lowrance et al., 1990), are the most extensively studied of these molecular abnormalities (for review, see Marian and Roberts, 1995; Bonne et al., 1998). A causal link between the β-myosin heavy chain gene mutations and the human disease has been confirmed in transgenic mice, in which a hypertrophic cardiomyopathy that reproduces the clinical phenotype develops when they express these genes (Vikstrom et al., 1996; Geisterfer-Lowrance et al., 1996). The specific mutation in this protein plays an important role in determining prognosis; for example, replacement of arginine with glutamine at position 403 is associated with a much worse prognosis than either replacement of valine with methionine at position 606 (Epstein et al., 1992; Watkins et al., 1992) or replacement of arginine with glutamine at position 256 (Fananapazir and Epstein, 1994). Because the changes in this protein generally weaken the muscle by reducing ATPase activity and shortening velocity (Lankford et al., 1995), hypertrophy has been suggested to represent a compensation for depressed contractility. The latter interpretation is supported by evidence that expression of both c-H-*ras* and c-*myc* are upregulated in the hearts of patients with hypertrophic cardiomyopathy (Kai et al., 1998) because both of these growth factors participate in overload-induced hypertrophy and cause reversion to the fetal phenotype.

Myosin-Binding Protein C Mutations

Although there is a clear association between myosin-binding protein C mutations and hypertrophic cardiomyopathy, the causal mechanisms are less well understood than those involving the β-myosin heavy chains. Myosin-binding protein C mutations, which include insertions, deletions, and point mutations, generally produce a relatively benign clinical syndrome that appears late in life and has a relatively good prognosis (Nimura et al., 1998). This protein does not participate in shortening and force-generation, but instead serves mainly to support sarcomeric structure by binding myosin in the thick filaments to the titin filaments that maintain sarcomeric structure.

α-Tropomyosin, Troponin T, Troponin I, and Myosin Light Chain Mutations

A number of mutations that cause hypertrophic cardiomyopathy have been found in tropomyosin and troponin, the regulatory proteins of the thin filament (Thierfelder et al., 1994; Bonne et al., 1998). The link between most of these mutations and the abnormal growth, however, is not apparent. Increased calcium sensitivity of the myofibrils might stimulate growth by impairing relaxation; alternatively, the abnormal growth stimulus might occur if the normal stoichiometry among these regulatory proteins were to be disrupted so as to decrease force generation. The identification of a "hot spot" in the α-tropomyosin gene is of interest because different mutations at this site, which normally encodes aspartate, lead to a variable hypertrophic response but a relatively benign clinical prognosis (Coviello et al., 1997). A similar hot spot may exist in troponin T, where mutations again cause a variable, and sometimes more serious, prognosis than mutations involving tropomyosin (Forissier et al., 1996). At this time, little is known of the causal links between specific mutations and the clinical diseases.

Dilated Cardiomyopathies

In the modern industrialized world, about half of the patients with heart failure are found to be suffering from systolic dysfunction (eccentric hypertrophy), in which the major cause of the dilated heart and low ejection fraction is prior myocardial infarction (ischemic heart disease). The most common etiology of this form of heart failure was once volume overloading, in which dilation was caused by a leaky valve (mitral or aortic insufficiency), but with the virtual disappearance of rheumatic and syphilitic heart disease, these causes have become uncommon. Other causes include toxins, such as ethanol, and anthracyclines, such as doxorubicin, that are used to treat malignancies (for review, see Singal and Iliskovic, 1998); lists of these agents, along with metabolic disorders, such as hemochromatosis, are found in standard textbooks of medicine and cardiology. There remains a large population with systolic dysfunction and a low ejection fraction, about 30% to 35% of the patients with this form of heart failure, who are often said to suffer from an idiopathic dilated cardiomyopathy (IDC or DCM). The term idiopathic reflects our ignorance of causation because this Greek word can be loosely translated as "unknown mechanism" or, more literally, "caused within" or "self caused." Because "idiopathic" simply states that the etiology is unknown, the present text refers to this type of heart failure as *dilated cardiomyopathy*.

The terminology in this field is rather unsatisfactory. In 1980, the World Health Organization and International Society and Federation of Cardiology agreed on the simple overall classification of cardiomyopathies in Table 8-5: dilated, hypertrophic, and restrictive cardiomyopathies (WHO/ISFC, 1980). This brief and thoughtful report defines cardiomyopathies as "heart muscle diseases of unknown cause" and so excludes from this diagnosis all known causes of heart failure, which were called "specific heart muscle disease." Coronary, hypertensive, valvular, and congenital heart diseases were not considered to be cardiomyopathies because their causes are known. "Heredofamilial diseases" were listed among the "specific" diseases, but in the following discussion, they are considered to be cardiomyopathies. Some of the remaining specific diseases, including infective, metabolic, and deficiency diseases, and the heart failure associated with systemic diseases, are listed in Table 8-6.

TABLE 8-6. *Specific heart muscle diseases**

Infective diseases
   Viral (e.g., coxsackie), protozoal (e.g., Chagas' disease)
Metabolic diseases
   Thyrotoxicosis
General system diseases
   Lupus
Sensitivity and toxic reactions
   Cobalt, anthracyclines

---

*This classification excludes heart disease of known cause, notably hypertensive, coronary (ischemic), valvular, and congenital heart diseases.

Until recently, viral infections were generally believed to be responsible for most cases of dilated cardiomyopathy. There is no doubt that viral infection can cause *acute myocarditis*, but this often severe form of heart failure is uncommon. Furthermore, the pathogenic role of viral infection in chronic dilated cardiomyopathy is less clear than was once believed. Acute viral myocarditis may not, in fact, often progress to chronic DCM, because most patients with active myocarditis recover completely (for review, see O'Connell, 1997). Furthermore, despite widely accepted morphologic criteria for the diagnosis of myocarditis (Aretz et al., 1986), generally referred to as the "Dallas Classification System" or "Dallas Criteria," the role of viral infection in causing these morphologic findings is far from established. Serologic studies, recombinant DNA analyses, and gene amplification by the polymerase chain reaction have identified portions of viral genome in the hearts of a significant fraction of these patients (for review, see Kawai and Abelmann, 1987; Kawai, 1999), but there is evidence that these viruses are not active participants in the pathogenesis of the dilated cardiomyopathies, but instead are "innocent bystanders." The latter interpretation is suggested by the finding that the prevalence of enteroviral genome in biopsy samples from patients with "specific" forms of heart disease is the same as in those with dilated cardiomyopathies (Keeling et al., 1992).

Knowledge of the etiology of dilated cardiomyopathy has been greatly advanced by evidence that up to one third of patients with this condition have an inherited disorder (Keeling et al., 1995; Grünig et al., 1998; Baig et al., 1998). The ability to identify molecular causes of disease is progressing rapidly, in part because of the Human Genome Project. Recent data indicate that the number of underlying molecular abnormalities will be much higher—informal conversations at recent meetings (1998) suggest that as many as 50% of patients with dilated cardiomyopathies have a familial disorder, and one speculation that was presented in a corridor conversation is that as many as 90% may be familial in etiology!

Several chromosomal loci for gene abnormalities that cause dilated cardiomyopathies have been identified. One common phenotype, which begins as conduction system disease, appears to arise from mutations on chromosomes 1p-1q, 1q-32, 3p25-p22, 10q21-23, and 9q13-22. The gene involved in another phenotype, which is associated with mitral valve prolapse, is found on chromosome 10, whereas *metavinculin*, an alternatively transcribed product of the gene that encodes vinculin, has been found to be absent in one patient with dilated cardiomyopathy (Maeda et al., 1997). However, as of early 1999, few gene products have been identified in the human disease.

Much more is known about transgenic mice in which dilated cardiomyopathy can be caused by abnormalities involving several known proteins, many of which are cytoskeletal. A causal link between cytoskeletal abnormalities and dilated cardiomyopathies is also seen clinically in skeletal muscle dystrophies, notably the proteins of the dystrophin-sarcoglycan complex. Mutations in this array of proteins, which links actin filaments within cells to laminin in the extracellular matrix (Fig. 8-14), cause several forms of skeletal muscular dystrophy. Dystrophin abnormalities are responsible for *Duchenne muscular dystrophy*, a milder *Becker muscular dystrophy*, and the devastating *severe childhood autosomal recessive muscular dystrophy*. Abnormalities in other proteins of this complex have been identified, or implicated, in *limb-girdle muscular dystrophies* and *congenital muscular dystrophy* (for review, see Duggan et al., 1997; Ozawa et al., 1998; Towbin, 1998). All of these diseases, which are manifest primarily in skeletal muscle, can affect the heart, sometimes severely. Mutations in dystrophin (Mutoni et al., 1993; Yoshida et al., 1993; Ortiz-Lopez et al., 1997) and dystrophin-linked glycoproteins (Fadic et al., 1996), which occur in the hearts of these patients, have been shown to cause di-

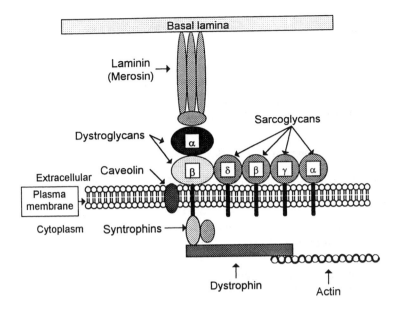

THE PLASMA MEMBRANE-DYSTROPHIN CYTOSKELETON

FIG. 8-14. Major proteins of the dystrophin cytoskeleton, which links actin within the cell to the basal lamina of the extra extracellular matrix, include the cytosolic proteins dystrophin and syntrophins, which form connections across the plasma membrane through the sarcoglycans, dystroglycans, and caveolin. The latter are attached to extracellular matrix proteins, including laminin (merosin).

lated cardiomyopathies. Another X-linked syndrome, *Emery-Dreifuss muscular dystrophy*, has been associated with defects in *emerin*, a cytoskeletal protein associated with the desmosomes and fascia adherens in the intercalated disc (Cartegni et al., 1997). Other cytoskeletal proteins whose mutations have been implicated as causes of dilated cardiomyopathy include desmin (which is also associated with restrictive cardiomyopathies), laminin (or merosin), and vinculin (for review, see Towbin, 1998). A clue as to the mechanism responsible for the progressive dilatation in these syndromes (see Chapter 6) is the participation of these proteins in signaling by the cell adhesion molecules.

The list of proteins in which mutations have been linked with the dilated cardiomyopathies extends beyond the cytoskeletal proteins, and includes *mitochondrial dystrophies* (Dionisi-Vici et al., 1997), which are caused by abnormalities in an acetylhydrolase that destroys oxygen free radicals (Ichihara et al., 1998), and the *Holt-Oram Syndrome*, which is due to abnormalities in as yet unidentified gene products (Basson et al., 1997). *Myotonic dystrophy*, which is caused by the insertion of multiple repeats of triplet base sequences into the untranslated region of a protein kinase gene (for review, see Hamshere et al., 1996; Korade-Mirnics et al., 1998), is also associated with a cardiomyopathy. Similarly, *Friedreich's ataxia*, which is associated with hypertrophic cardiomyopathy, is caused by expansion of a repeat of the trinucleotide GAA within a nuclear gene that encodes a mitochondrial protein called *frataxin* (Beal, 1998; Schapira, 1998; Schols et al., 1997). Frataxin participates in mitochondrial iron transport, so that when its function is impaired, iron accumulates within mitochondria; this causes the generation of oxygen free radicals that impair oxidative phosphorylation and damage cells. Many features of this syndrome, however, remain unexplained, notably the mechanism for the common association of this syndrome with hypertrophic cardiomyopathy (Child et al., 1986; Gunal et al., 1996).

Although some of the aforementioned work remains to be confirmed and the clinical significance of many recently reported gene abnormalities remains to be established, it is likely that a number of additional gene abnormalities will be found to play a major role in the pathogenesis of the "idiopathic" dilated cardiomyopathies.

Restrictive Cardiomyopathies

The restrictive cardiomyopathies, which are characterized by impaired ventricular filling without inappropriate hypertrophy, occur when the compliance of the heart is reduced (for review, see Kushwaha et al., 1997). Causes of this rare cardiomyopathy include idiopathic fibrosis (endomyocardial fibroelastosis) and amyloid deposition. Abnormal aggregates of the cytoskeletal protein *desmin* have been reported to cause a restrictive cardiomyopathy sometimes referred to as *desmin cardiomyopathy* (see Abraham et al., 1998), and there is one report of a familial restrictive cardiomyopathy caused by desmin accumulation (Zachara et al., 1997). Abnormalities in this cytoskeletal protein have also been associated with dilated cardiomyopathies (Muntoni et al., 1997; Lobrinus et al., 1998).

CONCLUSION

This chapter, in discussing possible causes of the progressive deterioration of the overloaded heart along with a rapidly increasing number of recognized molecular disorders that cause the heart to fail, highlights the central theme of this text—that knowledge of the molecular structure of the failing heart, the signal transduction systems that modify this structure, and the mechanisms that regulate myocardial cell growth and death, may hold the key to understanding the causes of the poor prognosis in patients with heart failure. As discussed in Chapter 9, therapeutic strategies based on this understanding have, over the past decade, come to occupy a central position in the management of this syndrome. The remarkable convergence of molecular biology, on the one hand, and clinical trials, on the other, is having a major impact on our ability to control symptoms, prolong life expectancy, and reduce costs in the rapidly growing population of patients who suffer from heart failure.

BIBLIOGRAPHY

Katz AM (1992). *Physiology of the Heart*, 2nd ed. Raven Press, New York.

REFERENCES

Abraham SC, DeNofrio D, Loh E, Minda JM, Tomaszewski JE, Petra GG, Reynolds C (1998). Desmin myopathy involving cardiac, skeletal, and vascular smooth muscle: report of a case with immunoelectronmicroscopy. *Hum Pathol* 29:876–882.

Anversa P, Kajstura J (1998). Ventricular myocytes are not terminally differentiated in the adult mammalian heart. *Circ Res* 83:1–14.

Aretz Ht, Billingham ME, Edwards WD, Factor SM, Fallon JT, Fenoglio JJ Jr, Olsen EGJ, Schoen FJ (1986). Myocarditis. A histopathologic definition and classification. *Am J Cardiovasc Pathol* 1:3–14.

Baig MK, Goldman JH, Caforio ALP, Coonar AS, Keeling PJ, McKenna WJ (1998). Familial dilated cardiomyopathy: cardiac abnormalities are common in asymptomatic relatives and may represent early disease. *J Am Coll Cardiol* 31:195–201.

Beal MF (1998). Mitochondrial dysfunction in neurodegenerative diseases. *Biochim Biophys Acta* 1366:211–213.

Beltrami CA, Finato N, Rocco M, Feruglio GA, Puricelli C, Cigola E, Quaini F, Sonnenblick EH, Olivetti G, Anversa P (1994). Structural basis for end-stage failure in ischemic cardiomyopathy in humans. *Circulation* 89:151–163.

Boluyt MO, O'Neill L, Meredith AL, Bing OH, Brooks WW, Conrad CH, Crow MT, Lakatta EG (1994). Alterations in cardiac gene expression during the transition from stable hypertrophy to heart failure: marked upregulation of genes encoding matrix components. *Circ Res* 75:23–32.

Bonne G, Carrier L, Richard P, Hainque B, Schwartz K (1998). Familial hypertrophic cardiomyopathy. From mutations to functional defects. *Circ Res* 83:580–593.

Calderone A, Takahashi N, Izzo NJ Jr, Thaik CM, Colucci WS (1995). Pressure- and volume-induced left ventricular hypertrophies are associated with distinct myocyte phenotypes and differential induction of peptide growth factor mRNAs. *Circulation* 92:2385–2390.

Cartegni L, di Barletta MR, Barresi R, Squarzoni S, Sabatelli P. Maraldi N, Mora M, Di Blasi C, Cornelio F, Merlini L, Villa A, Cobianchi F, Toniolo D (1997). Heart-specific localization of emerin: new insights into Emery-Dreifuss muscular dystrophy. *Hum Mol Genet* 6:2257–2264.

Caspari PG, Newcomb M, Gibson K, Harris P (1977). Collagen in the normal and hypertrophied human ventricle. *Cardiovasc Res* 11:554–558.

Chapman D, Weber KT, Eghbali M (1990). Regulation of fibrillar collagen types I and III and basement membrane type IV collagen gene expression in pressure overloaded rat myocardium. *Circ Res* 67:787–794.

Child JS, Perloff JK, Bach PM, Wolfe AD, Perlman S, Kark RA (1986), Cardiac involvement in Friedreich's ataxia: a clinical study of 75 patients. *J Am Coll Cardiol* 7:1370–1378.

Coviello DA, Maron BJ, Spirito P, Watkins H, Vosberg H-P, Thierfelder L, Schoen FJ, Seidman JG, Seidman CE (1997). Clinical features of hypertrophic cardiomyopathy caused by mutation of a "hot spot" in the alpha-tropomyosin gene. *J Am Coll Cardiol* 29:635–640.

Crawford DC, Chobanian AV, Brecher P (1994). Angiotensin II-induced fibronectin expression associated with cardiac fibrosis in the rat. *Circulation* 74:727–739.

Dionisi-Vici C, Ruitenbeek W, Fariello G, Bentlage H, Wanders RJ, Schagger H, Bosman C, Piantadosi C, Sabetta G, Bertini E (1997). New familial mitochondrial encephalopathy with macrocephaly, cardiomyopathy, and complex 1 deficiency. *Ann Neurol* 42:661–665.

Duggan DJ, Gorospe JR, Fanin M, Hoffman EP, Angelini C (1997). Mutations in the sarcoglycan genes in patients with myopathy. *N Engl J Med* 336:618–624.

Epstein N, Cohn GM, Fananapazir L (1992). Differences in clinical expression of hypertrophic cardiomyopathy associated with two distinct mutations in the β-myosin heavy chain gene: a 908$^{Leu \rightarrow Val}$ mutation and a 403$^{Arg \rightarrow Gln}$ mutation. *Circulation* 86:345–352.

Evans DC, Matsuoka Y (1915). The effect of various mechanical conditions on the gaseous metabolism and efficiency of the mammalian heart. *J Physiol (Lond)* 49:378–405.

Fadic R, Sunada Y, Waclawik AJ, Buck S, Lewandoski PJ, Campbell KP, Lotz BP (1996). Brief report: deficiency of a dystrophin-associated glycoprotein (adhalin) in a patient with muscular dystrophy and cardiomyopathy. *N Engl J Med* 334:362–366.

Fananapazir L, Epstein N (1994). Genotype-phenotype correlations in hypertrophic cardiomyopathy. Insights provided by comparisons of kindreds with distinct and identical β-myosin heavy chain gene mutations. *Circulation* 89:22–32.

Forissier J-F, Carrier L, Farza H, Bonne G, Bercovici J, Richard P, Hainque B, Townsend PJ, Yacoub MH, Fauré S, Dubourg O, Millaire A, Hagège AA, Desnos M, Komajda M, Schwartz K (1996). Codon 102 of the cardiac troponin T gene is a putative hot spot for mutations in familial hypertrophic cardiomyopathy. *Circulation* 94:3069–3073.

Geisterfer-Lowrance AAT, Kass S, Tanbigawa G, Vosberg H-P, McKenna W, Seidman CE, Seidman JG (1990). A molecular basis for familial hypertrophic cardiomyopathy: a β cardiac myosin heavy chain gene missense mutation. *Cell* 62:999–1006.

Geisterfer-Lowrance AAT, Christie M, Conner DA, Ingwall JS, Schoen FJ, Seidman CE, Seidman JG (1996). A mouse model of familial hypertrophic cardiomyopathy. *Science* 272:731–734.

Gerdes AM, Capasso JM (1995). Editorial review: structural remodeling and mechanical dysfunction of cardiac myocytes in heart failure. *J Mol Cell Cardiol* 27:849–856.

Grossman W, Jones D, McLaurin LP (1975). Wall stress and patterns of hypertrophy in the human left ventricle. *J Clin Invest* 56:56–64.

Grünig E, Tasman JA, Kücherer H, Franz W, Kübler W, Katus HA (1998). Frequency and phenotypes of familial dilated cardiomyopathy. *J Am Coll Cardiol* 31:186–194.

Gunal N, Saraclar M, Ozkutulu S, Senocak F, Topaloglu H, Karaaslan S (1996). Childhood onset of Friedreich's ataxia. *Acta Pediatr Jpn* 38:308–311.

Hamshere MG, Brook JD (1996). Myotonic dystrophy, knockouts, warts and all. *Trends Genet* 12:332–334.

Hood WP Jr, Rackley CE, Rolett EL (1968). Wall stress in the normal and hypertrophied human left ventricle. *Am J Cardiol* 22:550–558.

Hutchins GM, Bulkley BH (1978). Infarct expansion versus extension: two different complications of acute myocardial infarction. *Am J Cardiol* 41:1127–1132.

Ichihara S, Yamada Y, Yokota M (1998). Association of a G$^{994} \rightarrow$T missense mutation in the plasma platelet-activating factor acetylhydrolase gene with genetic susceptibility to nonfamilial dilated cardiomyopathy in Japanese. *Circulation* 98:1881–1885.

Kai H, Muraishi A, Sugiu Y, Nishi H, Seki Y, Kuwaraha F, Kimura A, Kato H, Imaiziumi T (1998). Expression of proto-oncogenes and gene mutation of sarcomeric proteins in patients with hypertrophied cardiomyopathy. *Circ Res* 83:594–601.

Katz AM (1996). Calcium channel diversity in the cardiovascular system. *J Am Coll Cardiol* 28:522–529.

Katz AM (1990). Cardiomyopathy of overload: a major determinant of prognosis in congestive heart failure. *N Engl J Med* 322:100–110.

Katz LN (1964). Heart failure. Introduction. In: Andrus EC, Maxwell CH, eds. *The Heart and Circulation,* Vol 1, Research. FASEB, Washington, DC, pp 532–557.

Kawai C (1999). From myocarditis to cardiomyopathy: mechanisms of inflammation and cell death. Learning from the past for the future. *Circulation* 99:1091–1100.

Kawai C, Abelmann WH (1987). *Pathogenesis of Myocarditis and Cardiomyopathy. Cardiomyopathy Update 1.* University of Tokyo Press, Tokyo.

Keeling PJ, Jeffery S, Caforio ALP, Taylor R, Bottazzo GF, Davies MJ, McKenna WJ (1992). The prevalence of enteroviral genome within the myocardium from patients with idiopathic dilated cardiomyopathy and controls by the polymerase chain reaction. *Br Heart J* 68:554–559.

Keeling PJ, Gang Y, Smith G, Seo H, Bent SE, Murday V, Caforio ALP, McKenna WJ (1995). Familial dilated cardiomyopathy in the United Kingdom. *Br Heart J* 73:417–421.

Korade-Mirnics Z, Babitzke P, Hoffman E (1998). Myotonic dystrophy: molecular windows on a complex etiology. *Nucl Acid Res* 26:1363–1368.

Kushwaha SS, Fallon JT, Fuster V (1997). Restrictive cardiomyopathy. *N Engl J Med* 336:267–276.

Lankford EB, Epstein N, Fananapazir L, Sweeny HL (1995). Abnormal contractile properties of muscle fiber expressing β-myosin heavy chain gene mutations in patients with hypertrophic cardiomyopathy. *J Clin Invest* 95:1409–1414.

Linzbach AJ (1960). Heart failure from the point of view of quantitative anatomy. *Am J Cardiol* 5:370–382.

Maeda M, Holder E, Lowes B, Valent S, Bies RD (1997). Dilated cardiomyopathy associated with deficiency of the cytoskeletal protein metavinculin. *Circulation* 95:17–29.

Marian AJ, Roberts R (1995). Recent advances in the molecular genetics of hypertrophic cardiomyopathy. *Circulation* 92:1336–1347.

Marijianowski MMH, Teeling P, Mann J, Becker AS (1995). Dilated cardiomyopathy is associated with an increase in the type I/type III collagen ratio: a quantitative assessment. *J Am Coll Cardiol* 25:1263–1272.

Marijianowski MMH, Teeling P, Becker AS (1997). Remodeling after myocardial infarction in humans is not associated with interstitial fibrosis of noninfarcted myocardium. *J Am Coll Cardiol* 30:76–82.

Meerson FZ (1961). On the mechanism of compensatory hyperfunction and insufficiency of the heart. *Cor et Vasa* 3:161–177.

Meerson FZ (1983). *The Failing Heart: Adaptation and Deadaptation.* Raven Press, New York.

Muntoni F, Cau M, Ganau A, Congiu R, Arvedi G, Mateddu A, Marrosu MG, Canchetti C, Realdi G, Cao A, Melis MA (1993). Deletion of the dystrophin muscle promoter region associated with X-linked dilated cardiomyopathy. *N Engl J Med* 329:921–925.

Muntoni F, DiLenarda A, Porcu M, Sinagra G, Mateddu A, Marrosu G, Ferlini A, Cau M, Milasin J, Ganau A, Melis MA, Marrosu MG, Canchetti C, Sanna A, Falaschi A, Camerini F, Giacca M, Mestroni L (1997). Dystrophin gene abnormalities in two patients with idiopathic dilated cardiomyopathy. *Heart* 78:608–612.

Nimura H, Bachinski LL, Sangwatanaroj S, Watkins H, Chudley AE, McKenna W, Kristinsson A, Roberts R, Sole M, Maron B, Seidman JG, Seidman CE (1998). Mutations in the gene for cardiac myosin-binding protein C and late-onset familial hypertrophic cardiomyopathy. *N Engl J Med* 338:1248–1257.

O'Connell JB (1998). Diagnosis and medical treatment of inflammatory cardiomyopathy. In Topol EJ, ed. *Textbook of Cardiovascular Medicine.* Lippincott-Raven, Philadelphia, pp 2309–2326.

Olivetti G, Capasso JM, Sonnenblick EH, Anversa P (1990). Side-to-side slippage of myocytes participates in ventricular wall remodeling acutely after myocardial infarction in rats. *Circ Res* 67:23–34.

Onodera T, Tamura T, Said S, McCune SA, Gerdes AM (1998). Maladaptive remodeling of cardiac myocyte shape begins long before failure in hypertension. *Hypertension* 32:753–757.

O'Rourke RA, Silverman ME, Schlant RC (1994). General examination of the patient. In Schlant RC, Alexander RW, eds. *The Heart,* 8th ed. McGraw Hill, New York, pp 217–251.

Ortiz-Lopez R, Li H, Su J, Goytia V, Towbin JA (1997). Evidence for a dystrophin missense mutation as a cause of X-linked dilated cardiomyopathy. *Circulation* 95:2434–2440.

Ozawa E, Noguchi S, Mizuno Y, Hagiwara Y, Yoshida M (1998). From dystrophinopathy to sarcoglycanopathy: evolution of a concept of muscular dystrophy. *Muscle Nerve* 21:421–436.

Pfeffer MA, Braunwald E (1990). Ventricular remodeling after myocardial infarction. Experimental observations and clinical implications. *Circulation* 81:1161–1172.

Priori SG, Barhanin J, Hauer RNW, Haverkamp W, Jongsma HJ, Kleber AG, McKenna WJ, Roden DM, Rudy Y, Schwartz K, Schwartz P, Towbin JA, Wilde AM (1999). Genetic and molecular basis of cardiac arrhythmias: impact on clinical management. Parts I and II. *Circulation* 99:518–528.

Ring PA (1950). Myocardial regeneration in experimental lesions of the heart. *J Pathol Bact* 62:21–27.

Rosenzweig A, Watkins H, Hwang D-S, Miri M, McKenna W, Traill TA, Seidman JG, Seidman CE (1991). Preclinical diagnosis of familial hypertrophic cardiomyopathy by genetic analysis of blood lymphocytes. *N Engl J Med* 325:1753–1760.

Rumyantsev PP (1977). Interrelations of the proliferation and differentiation of processes during cardiac myogenesis and regeneration. *Int Rev Cytol* 51:187–273.

Sandler H, Dodge HT (1963). Left ventricular tension and stress in man. *Circ Res* 13:91–104.

Schaper J, Froede R, Hein St, Buck A, Hashizume H, Speiser B, Friedl A, Bleese N (1991). Impairment of the myocardial ultrastructure and changes of the cytoskeleton in dilated cardiomyopathy. *Circulation* 83:504–514.

Schapira AH (1998). Mitochondrial dysfunction in neurodegenerative disorders. *Biochim Biophys Acta* 1366: 225–233.

Schols L, Amoiridis G, Przuntek H, Frank G, Epplan JT, Epplen C. Friedreich's ataxia. Revision of the phenotype according to molecular genetics. *Brain* 120:2131–2140.

Singal PK, Iliskovic N (1998). Doxorubicin-induced cardiomyopathy. *N Engl J Med* 339:900–905.

Soonpa MH, Field LH (1998). Survey of studies examining mammalian cardiomyocyte DNA synthesis. *Circ Res* 83:15–26.

Spirito P, Seidman CE, McKenna WJ, Maron BJ (1997). The management of hypertrophic cardiomyopathy. *N Engl J Med* 336:775–785.

Thierfelder L, Watkins H, McRae C, Lamas R, McKenna W, Vosberg H-P, Seidman JG, Seidman CE (1997). α-Tropomyosin and cardiac troponin T mutations cause familial hypertrophic cardiomyopathy: a disease of the sarcomere. *Cell* 77:701–712.

Tian R, Ingwall JS (1996). Energetic basis for reduced contractile reserve in isolated rat hearts. *Am J Physiol* 270 (*Heart Circ Physiol* 39):H1207–H1216.

Topol EJ, Califf RM, Vandormael M, Grimes CL, George BS, Sanz ML, Wall T, O'Brien M, Schwaiger M, Aguirre FV, et al (1992). A randomized trial of late reperfusion therapy for acute myocardial infarction. Thrombolysis and angioplasty in myocardial infarction-6 study group. *Circulation* 85:2090–2099.

Towbin JA (1998). The role of cytoskeletal proteins in cardiomyopathies. *Curr Opinion Cell Biol* 10:131–139.

Vikstrom KL, Factor SM, Leinwand LA (1996). Mice expressing mutant myosin heavy chains are a model for familial hypertrophic cardiomyopathy. *Mol Med* 2:556–557.

Wagner JA, Sax FL, Weisman HF, Porterfield J, McIntosh C, Weisfeldt ML, Snyder SH, Epstein SE (1989). Calcium-antagonist receptors in the atrial tissue of patients with hypertrophic cardiomyopathy. *N Engl J Med* 320:755–761.

Walsh K, Perlman H (1997). Cell cycle exit upon myogenic differentiation. *Curr Opin Genet Dev* 7:597–602.

Watkins H, Rosenzweig A, Hwang D–D, Levi T, McKenna W, Seidman CE, Seidman JG (1992). Characteristics and prognostic implications of myosin missense mutations in familial hypertrophic cardiomyopathy. *N Engl J Med* 326:1108–1114.

Weber KT, Brilla CG (1990). Pathological hypertrophy and cardiac interstitium. Fibrosis and the renin-angiotensin-aldosterone system. *Circulation* 83:1849–1865.

Weber KT (1997).Extracellular matrix remodeling in heart failure. A role for de novo angiotensin II generation. *Circulation* 96:4065–4082.

Weber KT, Janicki JS, Schroff SG, Pick R, Chen RM, Bashey RI (1988). Collagen remodeling of the pressure-overloaded, hypertrophied nonhuman primate myocardium. *Circ Res* 62:757–765.

Weber KT, Sun T, Tyagi SC, Cleutjens JPM (1994). Collagen network of the myocardium: function, structural remodeling and regulatory mechanisms. *J Mol Cell Cardiol* 26:279–292.

WHO/ISFC (1980). Report of the WHO/ISFC task force on the definition and classification of cardiomyopathies. *Br Heart J* 44:672–673.

Wollert KC, Taga T, Saito M, Narazaki M, Kishimoto T, Glembotski CC, Vernallis AB, Heath JK, Pennica D, Wood WI, Chien KR (1996). Corticotrophin-1 activates a distinct form of cardiac muscle cell hypertrophy. Assembly of sarcomeric units in series via gp130/leukemia inhibitory factor receptor-dependent pathways. *J Biol Chem* 271: 9535–9545.

Wollert KC, Studer R, Doerfer K, Schieffer E, Holubarsch C, Just H, Drexler H (1997). Differential effects of kinins on cardiomyocyte hypertrophy and interstitial collagen matrix in the surviving myocardium after myocardial infarction in the rat. *Circulation* 95:1910–1917.

Wood P (1956). *Diseases of the Heart and Circulation*, 2nd ed. JB Lippincott, Philadelphia.

Yoshida K, Ikeda S, Nakamura A, Kagoshima M, Takeda S, Shoji S, Yanagisawa N (1993). Molecular analysis of the Duchenne muscular dystrophy gene in patients with Becker muscular dystrophy presenting with dilated cardiomyopathy. *Muscle Nerve* 16:1161–1166.

Zachara E, Bertini E, Lioy E, Boldrini R, Prati PL, Bosman C (1997). Restrictive cardiomyopathy due to desmin accumulation in a family with evidence of autosomal dominant inheritance. *Gior Ital Cardiol* 27:436–442.

Zafeiridis A, Jeevanandam V, Houser SR, Margulies KB (1998). Regression of left ventricular hypertrophy following left ventricular assist device support. *Circulation* 98:656–662.

9

Therapeutic Strategies
for Managing Heart Failure

The hallmark of the cardiologist is the skill with which he recognizes and treats all aspects of heart failure. However, no physician should undertake the treatment of heart failure without a thorough understanding of what is and what is not heart failure; the importance, in achieving an optimal therapeutic success, of identifying both the nature of the underlying heart disease and the factors immediately responsible for precipitating heart failure; the drugs and other measures effective in the management of heart failure, and their integration into a sound rationale of therapy; *and the harm that may be caused by therapy injudiciously or erroneously applied.*

E. N. Silber and L. N. Katz (1975)

what a young woman says to her eager lover should be written on the wind, and on the surface of a swift-flowing stream.

Catullus, *Poem 70;* trans. P. B. Katz

The quotations that head this chapter define both the major objective and the major challenge in writing this text. The objective, emphasized at many points in earlier chapters, is to provide the foundation upon which to build a "thorough understanding of what *is* and what *is not* heart failure." Integration of molecular mechanisms and clinical features in this syndrome provides an essential background for the basic scientist seeking to advance our knowledge of the pathophysiology and pharmacology of heart failure. This integration is equally important for the health care practitioner who must approach these patients with the pathophysiologic understanding needed for optimal management of this syndrome.

Recent developments have demonstrated that heart failure can no longer be treated by measures that simply alleviate signs and symptoms. The reason is that there are many drugs which, when given over the long term, make patients feel better, reduce the need for hospitalization, and improve prognosis. Yet these same drugs can have opposite short-term effects and initially make patients worse. Conversely, the benefits of a surprisingly large number of drugs that make patients feel better and improve objective measurements of pump performance can last only a short time; in many cases, after a few days or weeks, the benefits disappear and are replaced by an accelerated clinical deterioration that worsens misery, adds to cost, and shortens survival. These counterintuitive patterns illustrate a general rule in heart failure: *what is obvious is often not important, and what is important is often not obvious.*

Treatment of heart failure requires the integration of a vast body of knowledge of both pathophysiology and pharmacology. Those who manage this syndrome must understand the nature of the underlying heart disease, the neurohumoral response to impaired pump function, the actions of a growing number of therapeutic agents and, above all, how these interact one with another in the individual patient. The vast body of information that is summarized in this text has become an essential foundation for developing the "sound rationale of therapy" mentioned at the head of this chapter. If this understanding is lacking, efforts at clinical management will fall far short of optimum. Yet gaining such an understanding has become a daunting challenge because this field is changing so rapidly that, in the words of Catullus' lover, new information seems almost to be "written on the wind, and on the surface of swift-flowing water." What is learned can easily be lost in a flood of new material, much of which falls out of date within a few years.

This chapter is intended to provide an overview of recent trends in the management of heart failure, highlighting the growing impact of information derived from the basic sciences. Detailed treatment plans, along with discussions of various drugs, are found in the authoritative chapters on this subject in most medicine, cardiology, and heart failure texts. Readers are also referred to the many articles on this rapidly changing subject that appear regularly in leading journals, recent reviews, and essays (Eichhorn and Bristow, 1996; Cohn, 1996; Califf and Gheorghiade, 1998; Stevenson et al., 1998), and two consensus reports (Remme, 1997; Packer and Cohn, 1999). The goal of this chapter, therefore, is to provide a mechanistically based overview of therapy that integrates recent discoveries in molecular biology with the traditional approaches based on the paradigms of organ physiology and cell biochemistry. Because therapy of heart failure must begin by addressing the problems caused by the impaired pump function, which are most troublesome to these patients, our discussion opens with an examination of the hemodynamics of heart failure. The review of therapy directed to such biochemical abnormalities as the depressed contractility in the cells of the failing heart is short, largely because of disappointing long-term results of inotropic agents. The chapter ends with an effort to integrate recent discoveries in molecular biology with new approaches to therapy, using as an impetus the ability of this paradigm to explain unexpected results of several recent clinical trials. Our goal, therefore, is not to provide a "care path" for the treatment of this condition but instead to integrate the six paradigms discussed in Chapter 1, highlighting newly emerging concepts that appear to hold the key to future advances in the management of heart failure.

THE DIAGNOSIS

The first step in developing a therapeutic plan for any condition is making a correct diagnosis. There is little value in using a strategy describing the management of heart failure to treat fluid accumulation in a patient whose major problem is renal failure or hepatic cirrhosis, which, like heart failure, can cause anasarca. Similarly, the management of breathlessness requires a correct diagnosis because there are many causes of dyspnea besides left ventricular failure. A careful history and thorough physical examination can provide invaluable clues to the causes of these and other signs and symptoms that are commonly seen in heart failure. Measurement of jugular venous pressure, for example, remains the "gold standard" in defining a cardiac cause for edema; except in patients who have recently received a diuretic, the finding of a normal venous pressure virtually "rules out" backward failure of the right heart. Conversely, heart failure caused by a "silent" myocardial infarction should be a leading diagnostic consideration in a patient who, before the onset of worsening dyspnea, had experienced an episode of severe chest pain.

Once the diagnosis of heart failure is entertained, special tests are needed to confirm this hypothesis, and to identify the cause for this syndrome. Currently, key tests focus on the architecture of the heart, although there is considerable value in hemodynamic measurements. A distinction between "high output failure" and "low output failure" can be made on the basis of the contour of the arterial pulse; in low output failure, the pulse is small, whereas a large "bounding" pulse suggests high output failure. Although this distinction is rather dated, largely because virtually all heart failure is characterized by a low cardiac output, the unusual patient with high output failure is still seen. Nutritional deficiencies such as beriberi are rare in developed countries, and "routine" laboratory examinations pick up the occasional high output heart failure caused by anemia. "Masked" hyperthyroidism, sometimes seen in the elderly, must be considered, as should the rare occurrence of an arteriovenous shunt. More than 30 years ago, after joining the faculty at a major academic health center, I inherited a heart failure patient who had a huge jaw tumor for which surgery had been refused. For almost 2 years I treated this patient, whose working diagnosis was "ischemic heart disease," continuing the strategy of the cardiologist whom I had replaced without giving much thought to this diagnosis. It was only after I had become troubled by the fact that this lady had a normal electrocardiogram and a bounding pulse that I took a moment to feel her jaw. The latter, which was about the size of a melon, was quite warm, which on reflection made it obvious that her problem was high output failure resulting from arteriovenous shunting in the tumor. Anecdotes such as this illustrate the importance of a careful, *and thoughtful*, history and physical examination.

Imaging of the heart, which has emerged as a critical tool for the diagnosis of heart failure, distinguishes between systolic and diastolic dysfunction. Invasive left ventriculography is much less convenient than echocardiography and nuclear imaging of the labeled blood pool inside the heart (the "MUGA"); all allow ejection fraction to be determined with considerable accuracy. The echocardiogram, because it is neither invasive nor exposes the patient to ionizing radiation, is especially useful in establishing the diagnosis when heart failure is suspected, although this test is too expensive for screening. Because hemodynamic overloading of the ventricles stimulates the expression of genes that encode the natriuretic peptides (see Chapter 4), elevated plasma levels of these peptides appear likely to provide an accurate, and cost-effective, means to screen for heart failure in the general population (McDonagh et al., 1998; Clerico et al., 1998; Meada et al., 1998). Early results of such screening have been quite revealing because they indicate that, in a large population, many individuals with significant left ventricular dysfunction are not correctly diagnosed, which means that they cannot be treated appropriately, and that others who are diagnosed as having heart failure are, in fact, suffering from other illnesses.

Echocardiography has proven invaluable in assessing the severity of left ventricular systolic dysfunction because it provides accurate measurements of ejection fraction. Although the extent to which left ventricular ejection is impaired correlates poorly with the severity of symptoms (Benge et al., 1980; Franciosa et al., 1981; Lipkin and Poole-Wilson, 1986; Volterrani et al., 1994), ejection fraction provides an excellent predictor of mortality rate (Gradman et al., 1989). For this reason, there is a growing consensus that an echocardiogram should be obtained in virtually every individual suspected of having heart failure, both to classify the syndrome and establish prognosis. Use of this expensive test for routine follow-up, however, is more difficult to justify.

In contrast to patients with systolic dysfunction, in which measurement of ejection fraction represents a "gold standard" for both diagnosis and prognosis, noninvasive testing is less useful in those with diastolic dysfunction. This is because the major architectural abnormality in these patients is concentric hypertrophy, which means that ejection fraction can be normal or only slightly depressed. In fact, diastolic dysfunction can be difficult to diagnose, and almost impossible to quantify, unless left ventricular filling pressure is measured directly, which requires cardiac catheterization. The need for better means to identify and evaluate patients with diastolic dysfunction adds to the attractiveness of biochemical tests for screening.

"CURABLE" FORMS OF HEART FAILURE

Although most patients who suffer from heart failure in developed countries have a progressive disease, one must be on the alert for the occasional patient in whom this condition can be "cured." Etiologies such as hyperthyroidism, vitamin deficiency, and hemochromatosis are rare, but they should always be considered lest a treatable cause be overlooked. Chronic alcoholism is associated with dilated cardiomyopathy, so that exposure to this (and other) toxic substances should, where possible, be eliminated. Valvular heart disease, once the major cause of heart failure, is now uncommon; major exceptions are bacterial endocarditis, often seen in intravenous drug users, and the increasing number of elderly patients with calcific aortic stenosis. These and other forms of structural heart disease are readily diagnosed at the bedside by a thoughtful physical examination—exceptions, where the characteristic murmurs become almost inaudible, such as severe mitral stenosis with pulmonary hypertension and end-stage aortic stenosis, are rarely seen.

An important treatable cause of heart failure in developed countries is that caused by "hibernating" myocardium. This condition is seen in patients with coronary heart disease in whom large regions of the left ventricle are sufficiently underperfused to impair function, but who receive enough blood supply to maintain viability (Rahimtoola, 1989, 1997; Heusch, 1998; Wijns et al., 1998). This condition is not common, but because coronary revascularization can restore full health to individuals who appear to be suffering from severe, and even end-stage heart failure, the diagnosis of hibernating myocardium must always be considered.

Another treatable cause of heart failure is hypertension. This condition plays an important etiologic role in the diastolic dysfunction seen in the elderly. The increased afterload associated with elevated blood pressure also worsens the clinical manifestations of systolic dysfunction, and so represents an indication for vasodilator therapy (see later text).

It is becoming increasingly important to consider coronary artery occlusive disease among the treatable causes of heart failure. Dramatic improvements in risk factor modification are altering the natural history of ischemic heart disease, which is a major cause of heart failure in the industrialized world. Appropriate management of such risk factors as smoking, diabetes mellitus, hypertension, hyperlipidemias, and elevated homocysteine levels can prevent both worsening heart failure and the *de novo* appearance of heart failure caused by coronary artery atherosclerosis.

Mitral insufficiency can represent a major complication of systolic dysfunction when dilatation of the mitral annulus impairs valve closure. Valve replacement in these patients, although hazardous, may be necessary. Such leaks can be palliated by "unloading" the heart with vasodilators, which decreases the systolic pressure that forces blood backward into the left atrium, and by reducing ventricular volume, which can improve mitral valve closure. Much of the putative benefit of ventriculectomy (the "Batista procedure"), in which a wedge of the left ventricle is removed to reduce left ventricular volume, may be due to the ability of this operation to reduce mitral insufficiency.

Tachycardia-induced heart failure, although rare, does occur, and treatment of incessant tachycardias can alleviate the manifestations of heart failure in an occasional patient. Because sinus tachycardia is common in patients with heart failure, efforts to slow the heart are also useful.

SYSTOLIC AND DIASTOLIC DYSFUNCTION

Much of what we have learned about long-term therapy in heart failure since the 1980s is based on large clinical trials of patients with systolic dysfunction; in fact, most of these trials excluded patients with diastolic dysfunction. By far the most important reason for this selection bias is that systolic dysfunction is reliably diagnosed and quantified by measurements of ejection fraction, which is, by definition, depressed in these patients. As noted, it is much more difficult both to diagnose diastolic dysfunction and to "stage" its severity, because ejection fraction can be normal, or only modestly depressed. This selection bias is quite important because systolic and diastolic dysfunction are so different that they can almost be viewed as different conditions (Table 9-1).

Diastolic dysfunction is common in elderly women, aged 70 years and older, whereas systolic dysfunction in more often seen in men whose average age (based on data from clinical trials) is about 60 years (Lindenfeld et al., 1997). Survival rate is better in patients with diastolic dysfunction than in those with systolic dysfunction, and in women than in men (Ho et al., 1993; Vasan et al., 1995, 1996; Adams et al., 1998). However, because diastolic dysfunction predominates in women and has different etiologies than systolic dysfunction, a direct causal relationship between ventricular architecture and survival cannot be stated with certainty.

It is customary to develop treatment plans for patients with diastolic dysfunction that are based on data from studies of systolic dysfunction. Up to a point this is not unreasonable and seems logical in dealing with the neurohumoral response and circulatory abnormalities. However, different stimuli activate different signal transduction cascades in generating the different cardiac myocyte phenotypes seen in systolic and diastolic dysfunction. This raises the possibility that a greater understanding of the signaling pathways that mediate these different growth responses will lead to specific therapies for systolic and diastolic dysfunction. It appears that increased left ventricular afterload plays a greater role in causing diastolic dysfunction, resulting both from the high peripheral resistance in patients with hypertension and the greater aortic impedance caused by aortic arteriosclerosis in the elderly. For this reason, it is probably especially important to lower blood pressure in these patients. It is clear, therefore, that the data available from clinical trials of systolic dysfunction should be used with some caution in treating diastolic dysfunction in the many patients, mostly elderly women, with that condition. Trials using elderly women as study patients are badly needed.

TABLE 9-1. *Diastolic and systolic dysfunction*

Characteristic	Diastolic dysfunction	Systolic dysfunction
Age	Younger (approx. 60 years)	Older (>70 years)
Gender	Commonly male	Commonly female
Etiology	>50%: ischemic heart disease	Often hypertension
Comorbidity	Uncommon	Common

AN OVERVIEW OF THERAPEUTIC STRATEGY

Developing a rational therapeutic strategy for the management of heart failure is aided by several therapeutic guidelines (Table 9-2). These general principles suggest strategies that can be useful in most patients with this syndrome, regardless of the etiology, but they are not equally relevant in all patients. In the first place, therapy based on these guidelines generally has both beneficial and deleterious effects. More significant, the value of many interventions differs when evaluated in terms of short-term symptomatic improvement and long-term survival. Furthermore, the goals of therapy are not the same in all patients. In early heart failure, a major objective is to slow deterioration, whereas the primary goal in end-stage heart failure is generally to relieve suffering. For this reason, drugs that prolong life expectancy in patients with mild or moderate symptoms may, because of short-term deleterious effects, be contraindicated in more severely symptomatic patients; whereas in the latter, drugs may be needed to alleviate symptoms despite the possibility that they might shorten survival. These caveats notwithstanding, the principles outlined in Table 9-2 are useful in identifying the potential benefit and harm of most therapeutic interventions.

An overarching consideration in managing heart failure is the distinction between therapy directed to correct abnormalities in the peripheral circulation, in the heart, and in the myocardial cell. Most treatments modify all three, but often in different directions. This means that efforts to correct one abnormality can worsen another. Inotropic agents, for example, strengthen the heart and are helpful in correcting circulatory abnormalities, but over the long term they injure cardiac myocytes and so shorten survival. In contrast, β-adrenergic blockers initially worsen hemodynamic symptoms, but prolong survival, most likely because of their energy-sparing effects and ability to inhibit maladaptive growth of failing cardiac myocytes. Optimal management of heart failure, therefore, requires an understanding of the many different problems that can be encountered in these patients, how these problems interact with one another, and how each responds to a given therapeutic strategy.

One value of using the principles listed in Table 9-2 as a guide to therapy is that they serve as a reminder to distinguish between the effects of a drug on the circulation, on the heart, and on the myocardial cell. Correcting a circulatory abnormality, such as fluid retention or vasoconstriction, is generally quite simple—the hemodynamic response to most drugs is easily predicted, and the problems caused by "too much" and "too little" can thereby be minimized. Too much diuresis, while reducing preload, can decrease cardiac output so much as to lower blood pressure, and too much vasodilatation, although reducing afterload, can cause an excessive decrease in blood pressure. These extremes are

---

TABLE 9-2. *General principles of therapy*

Viewed from the circulation
  Match preload to the lusitropic state: diuretics
  Match afterload to the inotropic state: vasodilators
  Minimize maladaptive neurohumoral responses: neurohumoral blockers
Viewed from the heart
  Match inotropy to afterload: positive inotropic agents
  Match lusitropy to preload: positive lusitropic agents
  Optimize chronotropy: negative chronotropic agents
Viewed from the cardiac myocyte
  Spare energy
  Preserve viability
  Prevent maladaptive growth

readily avoided in the less severely ill patient, although in end-stage heart failure the treating physician must walk the razor's edge. In giving diuretics, for example, the choice can come down to leaving the patient "too wet" or "too dry." Much less obvious, of course, are the effects of therapy on cardiac myocytes. Yet, as noted by MacKenzie (1908) at the beginning of the 20th century:

> The more I study the symptoms of heart failure, and the more I reflect on the part played by the heart muscle, the more convinced am I that the explanation of heart failure can be summed up in the general statement that heart failure is due to the exhaustion of the reserve force of the heart muscle as a whole, or of one or more of its functions. This statement may seem so self-evident as scarcely to need amplification, but as a matter of fact, this, the essential principle on which diagnosis, prognosis and treatment should be based, is often practically ignored.

The challenge, which is central to this text, is to define this reserve force, and to prevent it from being exhausted.

A major problem often caused by drugs given to correct the circulatory abnormalities in heart failure is that this therapy generally triggers the hemodynamic defense reaction. This is especially important in patients given short-acting vasodilators, because by lowering blood pressure, these drugs evoke a maladaptive sympathetic response that damages the heart (Packer, 1990). Diuretic therapy, as noted in Chapter 4, also has deleterious effects in that reduced blood volume is a major activator of the renin-angiotensin system (Francis et al., 1990).

The consequences of modifying the neurohumoral response in heart failure are less clear than those of diuresis and vasodilatation. The reason is that the hemodynamic defense reaction has both deleterious and beneficial effects, which means that altering this response can do both good and harm. Administration of a β-adrenergic receptor blocker to minimize the myocardial damage caused by norepinephrine, can, if not done carefully, cause circulatory collapse by weakening the failing heart. Conversely, it is surprisingly dangerous to strengthen contraction of the myocytes in the failing heart. This has been made clear by clinical trials of inotropic agents, most of which show that increasing myocardial contractility, while of short-term benefit, has adverse long-term consequences. Less is known about efforts to improve lusitropic function, but it is probably a good idea to view any effort to improve the pump performance of a failing heart as entering "enemy territory."

Prevention of the deterioration of failing cardiac myocytes (see Table 9-2) is highly desirable. The problem is that we do not really know how to do this; in fact, virtually all that we know about prolonging survival has been learned by accident, from unexpected results of clinical trials. This goal, therefore, remains largely a desirable result, rather than a concrete therapeutic strategy. Much like the mice in Aesop's fable, who know that it is desirable to put a bell on the cat, we agree on a worthy goal, but we are not sure how to do this safely. Yet this field is moving ahead rapidly, and we have already stumbled onto several "bells" that prolong survival in these patients.

THERAPY DIRECTED TO THE CIRCULATION

Until the 1980s, virtually all drugs used to treat heart failure, with the important exception of digitalis, had their primary effects on the circulation and not the heart. Most prominent were the diuretics, the first class of drugs listed in Table 9-2, whose potential value had been recognized since ancient times. In the 1960s, when safe, powerful diuretics came on the market, the natural history of heart failure changed dramatically; no longer were hospitals filled with suffering, edematous patients. In effect, these drugs took the "congestive" out of congestive heart failure (CHF). The second major advance in circulatory therapy for heart failure occurred in the 1970s, when recognition of the maladaptive effects of vasoconstriction led to the use of vasodilators to "unload" the failing heart (Cohn and Franciosa, 1977). It has only been since the early 1980s that the value of neurohumoral blockade (Francis et al., 1984), the third approach listed in Table 9-2, has been recognized. That so many revolutionary changes in the therapy of heart failure have occurred within a quarter of a century provides ample testimony to the practical value of the partnership between basic biomedical research and evidence-based medicine.

Diuretics

Calomel (mercurous chloride) had been used to treat dropsy since the end of the 18th century, but the unpredictable effects of this toxic drug made its use quite dangerous. The first safe diuretics were the organic mercurials, whose benefits in heart failure were discovered accidentally when Saxl and Heilig (1920) observed a dramatic diuresis when these heavy metal compounds were given to patients with syphilitic heart disease. Although the organic mercurials were useful, they had to be given by injection and, more important, when given more than twice weekly, they lost their effectiveness. A major advance was provided by oral diuretics, the thiazides, which act at the distal tubule. Shortly after these agents were introduced in the late 1950s, potassium-sparing aldosterone antagonists and powerful loop diuretics, which act at the loop of Henle, became available. These three classes of diuretic, which have different mechanisms of action that potentiate one another (for review, see Brater, 1998), allow fluid retention (backward failure) to be relieved in virtually every patient with heart failure. As is true of all of the drugs used to treat heart failure, there is a potential hazard. In the case of the diuretics, this is excessive volume depletion (Fig. 9-1). Although volume depletion improves backward failure, it reduces preload (end-diastolic volume), which by the operation of Starling's Law of the Heart decreases ejection. In addition to worsening forward failure, the reduced cardiac output activates the hemodynamic defense reaction, which stimulates the kidneys to retain sodium, which increases the tendency to retain fluid. This, in turn, increases the need for additional diuretic therapy, which establishes the vicious cycle shown in Fig. 9-1, in which increasing amounts of diuretics are required to manage increasing fluid retention, but at the price of worsening forward failure.

The vicious cycle described in Fig. 9-1 represents a terrible dilemma in managing patients with end-stage heart failure because using diuretics to alleviate backward failure worsens forward failure. From a practical standpoint, this vicious cycle is especially troublesome because worsening failure—which is the natural history of this syndrome— itself causes a progressive decrease in cardiac output. Another problem caused by diuretics, especially thiazides and loop diuretics, is potassium and magnesium depletion. The former problem was once managed by giving potassium supplements or an additional potassium-sparing diuretic, but this complication is less common because virtually all heart failure patients are receiving angiotensin-converting enzyme (ACE) inhibitors, which inhibit potassium excretion.

Despite their potential to worsen forward failure and cause electrolyte depletion, the diuretics remain a keystone of therapy for heart failure because salt and water retention are seen in almost all of these patients. Largely because of the effectiveness of modern diuretics, the horrible suffering once caused by fluid overloading is rarely seen.

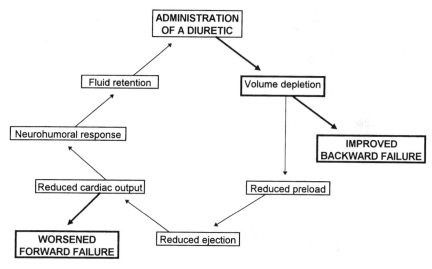

FIG. 9-1. Diuretics reduce extracellular fluid volume and so are effective in treating backward failure. These drugs, however, also reduce preload, which according to Starling's Law of the Heart reduces ejection and so can worsen forward failure. Because the neurohumoral response to the decrease in cardiac output causes further fluid retention by the kidneys, this can establish a vicious cycle that increases the need for diuretics.

Vasodilators

The maladaptive features of the vasoconstrictor response in heart failure (Fig. 9-2) led in the late 1970s to the introduction of vasodilator therapy. Although these drugs initially improve both symptoms and objective measurements of ventricular performance, their ability to prolong survival has been disappointing. Worsened long-term prognosis is seen with a variety of vasodilators, including minoxidil (Franciosa et al., 1984), nifedipine

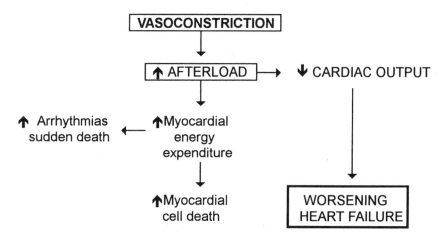

FIG. 9-2. Vasoconstriction, by increasing left ventricular afterload, reduces cardiac output and so worsens heart failure. The increased afterload also increases myocardial energy expenditure, which can be arrhythmogenic and cause myocyte necrosis.

TABLE 9-3. *Long-term effects of vasodilator therapy on survival*

Class of vasodilator	Long-term effect
Converting enzyme inhibitors	++
Nitrates + hydralazine	+
AT₁ Receptor blockers	?
Long-acting L-type calcium channel blockers	
Amlodipine	0
Felodipine	0
Alpha-adrenergic blockers	—
Mibefradil (T-type calcium channel blocker)	—
Short-acting L-type calcium channel blockers	— —
Monoxidine	— —
Minoxidil	— — —
Prostacyclin	— — —
Ibopamine	— — —
Flosequinan	— — —
Phosphodiesterase inhibitors	— — —

++: Significant improvement; +: some improvement; 0: no effect; ?: not known; —: some worsening; — —: significant worsening; — — —: contraindicated.

(Elkayam et al., 1990), diltiazem (Goldstein et al., 1991), flosequinan (Packer et al., 1993), prazosin (Cohn, 1993), ibopamine (Hampton, 1997), prostacyclin (Califf et al., 1997), and mibefradil (Elkayam, 1998) (Table 9-3). As discussed later, the phosphodiesterase inhibitors, which by increasing cyclic adenosine monophosphate (AMP) levels in the heart have positive inotropic as well as vasodilator effects, also increase mortality.

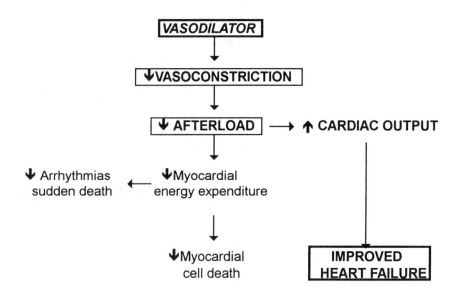

HEMODYNAMIC RESPONSE TO VASODILATOR THERAPY

FIG. 9-3. The hemodynamic response to a vasodilator, by reducing the harmful effects of vasoconstriction illustrated in Fig. 9-2, would be expected to be beneficial in managing patients with heart failure.

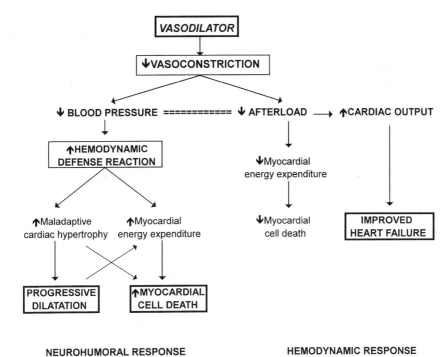

FIG. 9-4. Vasodilator therapy, in addition to providing the beneficial effects shown in Fig. 9-3, lowers blood pressure and so activates the hemodynamic defense reaction. Because most mediators of this neurohumoral response increase myocardial energy expenditure and evoke maladaptive growth, vasodilator therapy can cause myocyte necrosis and accelerate dilatation (remodeling) in the failing heart.

The dramatic differences between the short-term and long-term effects of vasodilators can be explained by the ability of most of these drugs to evoke the neurohumoral response discussed in Chapter 4. The initial decrease in blood pressure alleviates the deleterious effects of vasoconstriction and so is beneficial (Fig. 9-3). For this reason, vasodilators provide a logical short-term solution to some of the problems caused by neurohumoral activation. As shown in Fig. 9-4, excessive, or overly rapid lowering of blood pressure causes vasodilators to activate the hemodynamic defense reaction. This effect is especially marked when short-acting drugs are used, in which a rapid decrease in blood pressure activates baroreceptor responses that amplify the signals generated by the reduced cardiac output. Among the immediate results are tachycardia, increased myocardial contractility, and accelerated relaxation, all of which increase myocardial energy expenditure. In addition, most mediators of this neurohumoral response stimulate maladaptive hypertrophy, which, as discussed throughout this text, can cause both progressive dilatation (remodeling) and programmed cell death in the failing heart.

Neurohumoral Blockade

The first reports that therapy could prolong survival in heart failure came from clinical trials of drugs that were chosen because of their vasodilator activity (Cohn et al., 1986; CONSENSUS Trial Study Group, 1987). Although it had been hoped that the energy-sparing effects of afterload reduction might improve prognosis, thoughtful consideration of these early trials indicated that the beneficial long-term results could not be explained simply on the basis of the reduced peripheral resistance. In V-HeFT-1 (Cohn et al., 1986), which examined two vasodilator regimens designed to lower both preload and afterload, only the combination of isosorbide dinitrate and hydralazine showed a survival benefit; prazocin, an α-adrenergic blocker appeared initially to have no effect, and a later follow-up showed a trend to reduced survival (Cohn, 1993). The results of CONSENSUS 1, which showed that the ACE inhibitor enalapril almost doubled 50% survival time in end-stage heart failure (from 6 to 12 months), was initially greeted with disbelief. I well remember the first presentation of these data, at a meeting in Oslo in 1986, when several in the audience questioned the decision of the Data and Safety Monitoring Board to stop the trial prematurely; one individual at this meeting said, in effect, that the magnitude of the observed reduction in mortality rate was not credible because this benefit had not been seen with other vasodilators. It turns out that this observation was absolutely correct; virtually no other vasodilator causes the marked reduction in mortality rate seen with the ACE inhibitors (see Table 9-3). Instead, these survival benefits, like those of the nitrates, are probably due to the ability of ACE inhibitors to blunt the neurohumoral response. This can be understood by examining Fig. 9-4, in which a vasodilator that also blocks the hemodynamic defense reaction can retain the benefits of the hemodynamic response (see Fig. 9-4, right) without the price of the maladaptive neurohumoral response caused by a decrease in blood pressure (see Fig. 9-4, left).

In the following discussion, it is assumed that the beneficial long-term effects of the combination of nitrates and hydralazine are due exclusively to the former. This assumption is not proven because in the long-term trials using nitrates, these drugs were given in combination with hydralazine, a direct-acting vasodilator. This combination was chosen because, when these trials were designed, combining a drug whose effect was mainly to dilate arterioles (hydralazine) with a drug that mainly dilates veins (nitrates) was judged to be advantageous. Two reasons that many attribute the beneficial effects of the nitrate-hydralazine combination to the nitrates, rather than to hydralazine, is that nitrates alone inhibit remodeling in animal models of heart failure (McDonald et al., 1993) and that other direct-acting vasodilators are associated with a poor long-term response (see Table 9-3).

Nitrates

Nitrates, in combination with hydralazine, have been shown in two large trials to reduce mortality rate in heart failure (Cohn et al., 1986, 1991). Nitrates, which generate nitric oxide (NO) (Elkayam, 1996), also inhibit progressive cardiac dilatation (McDonald et al., 1993; for review, see Judgett, 1996). It is not clear, however, whether improved survival rate is due to inhibition of left ventricular remodeling and, if so, whether progressive dilatation is slowed simply by the reduced preload and afterload or by a growth-inhibitory effect of NO. Because most other vasodilators do not prolong survival, it is tempting to attribute the apparent long-term benefit of nitrates to counterregulatory actions of NO.

In addition to serving as a physiologic vasodilator, NO activates phosphodiesterase inhibitors that increase cyclic GMP levels and blunt the response to sympathetic stimulation. Cyclic GMP itself has antiproliferative effects that may be due in part to inhibition of MAP kinase pathways (Yu et al., 1997). Although inhibition of maladaptive cell growth represents an attractive explanation for the long-term benefits of nitrates in heart failure, effects on connective tissue, such as increased collagen deposition caused by improved perfusion or the inflammatory effects of this free radical gas, are also possibilities.

ACE Inhibitors

The converting enzyme inhibitors (generally referred to as ACE inhibitors) have been conclusively shown to improve long-term prognosis in heart failure, a benefit that is seen with all members of this class of drugs. Improved survival rate is seen in very sick patients (CONSENSUS Trial Study Group, 1987) and in patients with milder but significant symptoms. The magnitude of the effect, estimated by metaanalysis of 32 trials, is to reduce mortality rate by about 23% (for review, see Garg et al., 1995). The extent of the reduction in mortality rate is similar for several subgroups, including age, sex, and presumed etiology (ischemic and nonischemic): overall, sicker patients seem to gain the most benefit. These trials also suggest that ACE inhibitors slow progressive deterioration of the failing heart more than they prevent sudden death, but distinguishing patients who died of progressive heart failure from those who had a lethal arrhythmia is not very precise.

The ability of ACE inhibitors to reduce hospitalization rates for heart failure patients supports the view that these drugs slow progression of the Cardiomyopathy of Overload. An important implication of this interpretation is that these drugs should be used early in the course of the disease (see Fig. 8-1). There are few survival data in patients with left ventricular dysfunction and either mild or no symptoms, but studies of these less ill patients indicate that ACE inhibitors do delay the development of more severe heart failure (The SOLVD Investigators, 1992; Pfeffer et al., 1992; The Acute Infarction Ramipril Efficacy Study Investigators, 1993; Kober et al., 1995). When large populations are screened for heart failure, which, as noted earlier, will soon be feasible, many individuals with mild left ventricular dysfunction will be identified. The possibility that most of these individuals would benefit from an ACE inhibitor has enormous public health and economic implications.

The mechanism for the beneficial effects of the ACE inhibitors is far from clear. As already noted, although these drugs were introduced for the treatment of heart failure because they are vasodilators, their ability to prolong survival is almost unique among this class of drugs. However, it has become clear that blocking angiotensin II formation also inhibits maladaptive growth (Linz et al., 1989; Katz, 1990a; Sadoshima and Izumo, 1993; Yamazaki et al., 1995). These effects, are mediated by heptahelical receptors that are coupled to $G_{\alpha q}$ (Sadoshima et al., 1995) and stimulate JAK/STAT-controlled MAP kinase pathways that are also activated by the enzyme-linked cytokine receptors discussed in Chapter 5 (Marrero et al., 1995; Pan et al., 1997; Dostal et al., 1997). In the failing heart, a major consequence of this mitogenic signaling is almost certainly worsening of the Cardiomyopathy of Overload (Katz, 1994).

ACE inhibitors also block proteases other than the angiotensin-converting enzyme. Most important is the enzyme that catalyzes bradykinin breakdown. This means that ACE inhibitors, in addition to reducing the levels of angiotensin II (which has both vasoconstrictor and mitogenic actions) increase the levels of bradykinin (which has both vasodilator and growth-inhibitory actions) (Fig. 9-5). It is not yet clear which of these synergistic effects is most important in patients with heart failure. A major side effect of the ACE inhibitors, a dry cough, is generally caused by the increased bradykinin.

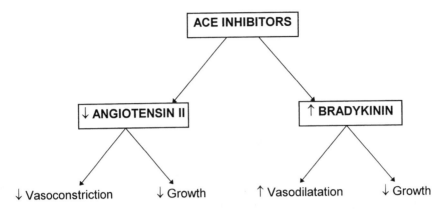

FIG. 9-5. In addition to blocking the production of angiotensin, converting enzyme inhibitors (ACE inhibitors) also inhibit bradykinin breakdown. The result is a coordinated response that reduces the levels of a vasoconstrictor and growth promoter, and increases the levels of a vasodilator and growth inhibitor.

AT_1 Receptor Blockers

The existence of several classes of angiotensin receptor adds another level of complexity to the story of the ACE inhibitors. As discussed in Chapter 4, there are both "regulatory" and "counterregulatory" receptors, called AT_1 and AT_2, respectively, and specific blockers for each of these receptor classes are available. It is likely that the benefits of ACE inhibitors, which block angiotensin II formation, are due to reduced activation of the regulatory AT_1 receptors, an interpretation that has led to clinical trials using drugs that inhibit angiotensin II-binding to AT_1 receptors. Even though early evaluations of the effects of AT_1 receptor blockers in heart failure are promising (Pitt et al., 1997), it has not yet been established that these drugs are as effective as the ACE inhibitors (McKelvie et al., 1998; for review, see Packer and Cohn, 1999). One potential concern is that the AT_1 receptor blockers elevate serum angiotensin II levels, which, because the AT_2 receptors are not blocked, can increase the counterregulatory actions of AT_2 receptor activation. Pending the results of additional trials that are underway, it is not certain that the beneficial effects of the ACE inhibitors will be seen with the AT_1 receptor blockers, so that this class of drugs should be reserved for patients who cannot tolerate an ACE inhibitor because of bradykinin-induced cough or other side effects.

Aldosterone Blockers

Spironolactone, which blocks aldosterone-binding to its intracellular receptors, has been used for many years as a potassium-sparing diuretic. As noted, however, the problem of diuretic-induced hypokalemia is seen much less commonly than in the past because most heart failure patients are given ACE inhibitors. It came as a surprise, therefore, when a recent trial that randomized patients to aldosterone or placebo was stopped by the Data Safety and Monitoring Committee because of a highly significant 27% decrease in all-cause mortality rate, which was the primary end-point of this study (Pitt, 1998). One can only guess at the mechanism for this effect, which is currently available as a preliminary, unconfirmed report. As noted in Chapter 7, binding of steroid hormones to their intracellular receptors forms transcription factors that exert mitogenic effects on the heart. This makes it tempting to attribute the beneficial long-term effects of spironolactone to a growth-inhibitory response; such an interpretation is speculative so that until additional data become available it must remain tentative.

Other Blockers of the Neurohumoral and Inflammatory Responses

Several additional agents that block neurohumoral and inflammatory pathways are currently being examined for possible beneficial effects in patients with heart failure (Table 9-4). Many of these have been tested in animals, but experimental findings do not always predict the clinical value of a drug. This is seen in the case of *mibefradil*, a selective T-type calcium channel blocker that has growth-inhibitory effects (for review, see Katz, 1996). Although this drug inhibits ventricular remodeling and improves survival in a rat model of heart failure (Mulder et al., 1997), unexpected adverse interactions with other drugs and lack of survival benefit led the manufacturers to withdraw this T-type calcium channel blocker from clinical use (Po and Zhang, 1998). Blockade of the regulatory endothelin (ET-1) receptors has likewise been shown to inhibit remodeling in rat models of heart failure (Sakai et al., 1996; Oie et al., 1998) so that clinical trials of these drugs are now underway. Studies are also in progress to examine the effects of central α_2-adrenergic and imidazoline stimulation, which activates these counterregulatory pathways to cause vasodilatation. Unfortunately, a trial of *monoxidine,* which blocks central imidazoline-mediative signaling, was recently stopped because of adverse effects.

Other drugs being studied in heart failure include cyclooxygenase blockers, whose potential value is suggested by damaging effects of some of the prostaglandins generated by these enzymes. Recognition of the deleterious effects of cytokines in heart failure, has led to the initiation of clinical trials examining a possible role for cytokine blockers in these patients (Deswaletal, 1999). Short-term benefits of growth hormone (Fazio et al., 1996), a peptide growth factor that is a member of the cytokine family, have led to studies of a possible long-term benefit of this agent in heart failure. These and other investigational approaches to therapy, many of which are listed in Table 9-4, are in early stages of development, and it is unlikely that many drug classes on this list will ever reach the clinic. However, this field has seen many surprises, so that some of the agents listed in Table 9-4, as well as additional drugs not on this list, may well become standard therapy in the future. It is likely, therefore, that, within a few years, patients with heart failure may

TABLE 9-4. *Some new, experimental therapies for heart failure*

Aldosterone blockers
AT_1 receptor blockers
Endothelin (ET-1) receptor blockade
Central α_2-adrenergic and imidazoline receptor stimulation
Natriuretic peptides (ANP and BNP)
Bradykinin and related peptides
T-type calcium channel blockade
Parasympathetic and puringeric mechanisms
G Protein-coupled receptor modifiers (e.g., βARK inhibitors)
Thyroid hormone
Intracellular signal transduction pathway modification
Cyclooxygenase inhibition
Cytokine blockade
Cytokines and other peptide growth factors (e.g., growth hormone)
Inhibitors of apoptosis

benefit from new approaches that can modify neurohumoral and inflammatory responses. The practical implications—and challenges—posed by the availability of so many different treatments for heart failure are discussed in Chapter 10.

THERAPY DIRECTED TO THE HEART

A second general approach to managing heart failure (see Table 9-2) is to improve the pump performance of the failing heart. As recently as a decade ago, when heart failure was generally agreed to be due largely to depressed myocardial contractility, inotropic agents were viewed as holding the key to managing this syndrome. The logic then was that the stronger the inotrope, the better would be the outcome. As has come to be widely known, exactly the opposite has been found in clinical trials, results that again demonstrate the validity of a generalization often repeated in this text: that in heart failure, what is obvious is often not important, and what is important is often not obvious.

Inotropic Therapy

Three classes of inotropic drugs have been studied extensively in patients with heart failure. Two act by increasing cyclic AMP levels in the heart; these are the β-adrenergic and dopaminergic agonists, which increase cyclic AMP production, and the phosphodiesterase inhibitors, which decrease cyclic AMP breakdown. The third class of drugs are the cardiac glycosides, whose actions and effects in heart failure are discussed separately. A few additional inotropic agents are mentioned briefly at the end of this section.

Drugs That Increase Cyclic AMP Levels

The β-agonists and phosphodiesterase inhibitors are discussed together because both have the same biochemical effect—to increase cyclic AMP levels. These drugs also have the same overall effect on the natural history of heart failure: an initial but short-lived improvement caused by increased contractility (and in the case of the phosphodiesterase inhibitors, also by vasodilatation), followed by an accelerated mortality rate resulting largely from a greater frequency of sudden death. The adverse effects of β agonists are so marked that only a few large trials have been reported (e.g., The Xamoterol in Severe Heart Failure Group, 1990). A metaanalysis of nine trials of therapy with β agonists, which reviewed 1,234 randomized patients (Yusef and Teo, 1990), found a doubling of mortality rate in those receiving the active drug (odds ratio: 2.07; 95% CI 1.23–3.49). More recently, a long-term trial of ibopamine, a dopaminergic agonist that at higher concentrations stimulates β receptors, was stopped prematurely because of a significant 26% increase in mortality rate (Hampton et al., 1997). Overall, these results are so dismal that, with the exception of intermittent dobutamine (see later text), chronic use of this class of drugs has been abandoned.

It took much longer for investigators to appreciate the hazards of the phosphodiesterase inhibitors, mainly because their adverse effects are less dramatic. It is interesting, however, that in the mid-1980s, Packer and Leier (1987) published data showing that the 1-year mortality rate in heart failure trials in which patients were given vasodilators ranged between 35% and 55%, whereas in studies in which similar patients were given phosphodiesterase inhibitors, the 1-year mortality rate ranged between 50% and 95%. Although these data did not come from trials designed to compare these two treatments, a subsequent metaanalysis of several small, properly designed trials by Yusef and Teo

(1990) found a 58% increase in mortality rate in patients given phosphodiesterase inhibitors (odds ratio: 1.58; 95% CI 1.04–2.41). This adverse effect was subsequently confirmed in several large randomized clinical trials, which make it clear that these agents cause a significant increase in mortality rate (Packer et al., 1991; Cowley and Skene, 1994; Lubsen et al., 1996; Cohn et al., 1998). Although there remains some question as to whether it is appropriate to exchange a transient improvement in symptoms for a worsened long-term survival rate, it is generally agreed that this tradeoff is to be avoided in patients with mild symptoms, in whom the goal is to prolong survival, and in whom alternative forms of treatment are both effective and safe. It is less clear, however, whether inotropic therapy is always contraindicated in more severely ill patients, in whom relief of symptoms can be more important than adding a few weeks, or even months, to life expectancy. Intermittent administration of dobutamine in end-stage heart failure, for example, is recommended by some, even though this drug appears eventually to increase mortality rate (Dies et al., 1986; Elis et al., 1998). The reason is that the goals in therapy for end-stage heart failure emphasize quality of life and relief of suffering, rather than prolongation of survival, which in most of these patients is very short. For this reason, even though long-term administration of inotropic agents should be avoided in mild-moderate heart failure (Packer and Cohn, 1999), intermittent, short-term use for the relief of intolerable symptoms may be justified in selected patients (see Chapter 10).

The mechanisms for the adverse long-term effects of drugs that increase cyclic AMP levels are not fully understood, but the excess mortality rate in the aforementioned trials appears to be due to an increased incidence of sudden death, mainly in sicker patients. These deaths are undoubtedly related to the well-known proarrhythmic effects of cyclic AMP (Podzuweit et al., 1976), which increases the susceptibility to ventricular fibrillation (Lubbe et al., 1978). Potential causes for these arrhythmogenic effects include accelerated automaticity and increased dispersion of refractoriness. The latter is caused by inhomogeneous effects on the many repolarizing potassium currents in the heart. Cyclic AMP also promotes calcium overload and worsens the state of energy starvation in the failing heart (Katz, 1986), which, together with its proarrhythmic effects, adequately explains the adverse effects of both β agonists and phosphodiesterase inhibitors in the failing heart.

Cardiac Glycosides (Digitalis)

Withering, who toward the end of the 18th century discovered that digitalis is effective for the treatment of dropsy, noted the ability of this drug to cause a diuresis and to slow the heart. Almost 200 years were to pass, however, before these actions were explained, and even longer before the long-term effects of digitalis in patients with heart failure could be properly evaluated. This plant alkaloid has many effects, however, so that even modern scientists are not sure of the mechanisms responsible for the responses to this drug in patients with heart failure.

Early digitalis preparations were simply the dried leaf of the purple foxglove, *Digitalis purpura*, which contained several active substances. "Digitalis leaf" was among the last pills to be used in the United States. (By definition, a pill is a small, round object, hardly an ideal way to dispense a medication because when dropped, pills easily roll out of sight.) A more important disadvantage of digitalis leaf was its variable potency, as was evident in the various shades of green found in these pills that depended on the time of year that the leaves were picked, dried, and rolled. The availability of several pure cardiac glycosides by the middle of the 20th century led to a debate as to which alkaloid had the best therapeutic-to-toxic ratio. This was not a trivial question because, until powerful diuretics became available, cardiac glycosides were the mainstay of therapy for heart failure, so that as these patients worsened, doses were increased to—and often beyond—levels that produced severe toxicity. This explains why, until the mid-1980s, almost half of the pages in standard textbook chapters on the treatment of heart failure were devoted to digitalis (Katz, 1987). Debates as to which cardiac glycoside was the safest came to an end when it was realized that the same mechanisms that caused the toxic effects of these drugs were also responsible for their therapeutic benefits. As a result, virtually all patients in the United States who currently take digitalis receive a single preparation—digoxin.

Cardiac glycosides have both central effects and effects on the heart and circulation. The latter include a vasoconstrictor response and the well-known positive inotropic effect, which occur when sodium pump inhibition leads to an increase in cytosolic sodium, which reduces calcium efflux via the sodium/calcium exchanger. The resulting increase in cellular calcium stores increases vascular tone and myocardial contractility. Sodium pump inhibition also causes a decrease in intracellular potassium that depolarizes the resting heart by reducing the potassium gradient across the plasma membrane. The decrease in resting potential inactivates depolarizing currents, which, along with the increase in intracellular calcium, accounts for most of the prominent arrhythmogenic effects of these drugs.

In addition to their effects on the heart and blood vessels, cardiac glycosides have important, centrally mediated effects. The latter, which are counterregulatory, include stimulation of vagal centers in the brain stem that increases parasympathetic tone and inhibits sympathetic outflow. These responses slow both the sinus node pacemaker and atrioventricular conduction, and cause reflex vasodilatation. The balance between the peripheral and central effects of digitalis is altered in the patient with heart failure. Whereas cardiac glycosides cause vasoconstriction in normal individuals, the opposite is seen in patients with heart failure (Mason and Braunwald, 1964). The latter effect was subsequently shown to be due to reduced sympathetic efferent activity (Ferguson et al., 1989). The sympatholytic effect of digitalis, as discussed later, means that this drug can be viewed as having centrally mediated α- and β-adrenergic blocking effects.

In the era when rheumatic valvular disease was the major cause of heart failure, rapid atrial fibrillation developed in most of these patients. Because the vagomimetic effects of digitalis inhibit atrioventricular conduction, cardiac glycosides were very effective in slowing the rapid heart rates, an effect that accounted for much of their unequivocal benefit. Until recently, however, it was not clear whether digitalis could help patients with heart failure who remained in normal (sinus) rhythm. This question was recently addressed in a large clinical trial (The Digitalis Investigation Group, 1997), some of whose results are summarized in Table 9-5. Digoxin was found to have no effect on either overall or cardiovascular mortality rate, but the drug did reduce the number of heart failure deaths. This benefit, however, was offset by an increased number of arrhythmogenic deaths and deaths from coronary heart disease. Digoxin also reduced the number of hospitalizations for cardiovascular disease, including an almost 25% reduction in the number of admissions for worsening heart failure. A somewhat fanciful interpretation of these findings is that the central effects of digoxin, which in some ways resemble those of the β blockers, slow heart failure progression, whereas the inotropic effects of the drug increase the number of sudden deaths. This interpretation, although having some intellectual appeal, is overly simplistic and goes far beyond the available data.

TABLE 9-5. *Long-term effects of digoxin in heart failure**

	Digoxin	Placebo	Risk ratio
Number of patients	3397	3403	
Total mortality	1181	1194	0.99 (0.93–1.07)
Cardiovascular deaths	1016	1190	1.01 (0.91–1.10)
Heart failure deaths	394	449	0.88 (0.71–1.01)*
Other cardiac death (arrhythmia, coronary disease, cardiac surgery)	508	444	1.14 (1.01–1 30)
Total hospitalizations	6356	6777	
Cardiovascular	1694	1850	0.87 (0.81–0.93)†
Worsening failure	910	1180	0.72 (0.66–0.79)†

*p=.06
†*p*<.001
Data from the Digitalis Investigation Group (1997)

When digitalis is given to heart failure patients in sinus rhythm, it generally causes a short-term improvement in symptoms (for review, see Packer and Cohn, 1999; Hauptman and Kelly, 1999). However, once these drugs are started, they appear to be dangerous to stop. This was shown in two large trials in which digoxin withdrawal was associated with worsening symptoms (Packer et al., 1993; Uretsky et al., 1993). This indicates that cardiac glycosides, while able to improve symptoms, cannot be expected to modify overall survival in heart failure patients with sinus rhythm. The controversies that have swirled around this drug for centuries have not ended. Many believe that the improvement in symptoms and reduction in hospitalizations make the cardiac glycosides a useful adjunct in treating heart failure, whereas others view these drugs as overly toxic. Recent evidence suggests that most of the clinical benefits of digoxin are seen at low doses (Gheorghiade et al., 1995; Slatton et al., 1997). A final judgment regarding the use of cardiac glycosides in patients with heart failure and sinus rhythm may therefore be that, once symptoms become significant, the benefits of low doses of these drugs exceed their hazards.

Other Inotropic Agents

Several novel mechanisms by which myocardial contractility can be increased are listed in Table 9-6. One mechanism is to stimulate sodium channel opening, which can increase intracellular calcium when the increased cytosolic sodium competes for efflux via the sodium/calcium exchanger—this is similar to the mechanism of the inotropic effect of the cardiac glycosides. Cellular calcium stores can also be increased by drugs, called "calcium agonists," that act directly to open L-type calcium channels and by agents that decrease the normal ability of phospholamban to inhibit calcium transport into the sarcoplasmic reticulum. Other drugs have been developed to prolong the action potential by inhibiting the development of repolarizing potassium currents, which increases calcium entry by delaying the voltage-dependent inactivation of the L-type calcium channels. All of these inotropic mechanisms, however, have theoretic hazards. Increasing cytosolic calcium, for example, is likely to worsen the state of energy starvation in the failing heart, whereas drugs that prolong the action potential, like other conditions that prolong the Q-T interval, are potentially arrhythmogenic. There is also a tendency of drugs that increase contractility to impair relaxation. Until these approaches are thoroughly tested, attempts to increase contractility should be viewed with an open (but skeptical) mind.

TABLE 9-6. *Some new, experimental approaches to increasing contractility and improving relaxation in failing hearts*

Inotropic agents
  Sodium channel activators: drugs that increase cellular sodium by increasing sodium channel opening
  Potassium channel blockers: drugs that prolong the action potential by decreasing potassium channel opening
  Calcium "agonists": drugs that increase the opening of L-type calcium channels
  Calcium "sensitizers": drugs that increase the calcium sensitivity of the contractile proteins
  Phospholamban inhibitors: drugs that prevent phospholamban from increasing calcium uptake into the sarcoplasmic reticulum
Lusitropic agents
  Inhibit phospholamban dephosphorylation or otherwise promote calcium uptake by the sarcoplasmic reticulum
  Decrease the calcium sensitivity of the contractile proteins
  Inhibit calcium entry into the cytosol
  Reduce contractility

Lusitropic Therapy

Recognition of the importance of relaxation abnormalities in the failing heart has led to a search for means to stimulate the calcium pump of the sarcoplasmic reticulum, the major determinant of the rate and extent of relaxation. Inhibitors of phospholamban dephosphorylation, for example, might be useful in diastolic dysfunction, but as pointed out in Chapter 3, this action also would be expected also to increase contractility, which is not desirable in these patients. Another way to facilitate relaxation would be to reduce the calcium sensitivity of the myofilaments, but this would also have a negative inotropic effect. Inhibiting calcium entry into the cytosol would reduce the amount of calcium that must be removed from the cytosol to relax the heart but would also decrease contractility. Clinically useful means to stimulate relaxation seem rather far from clinical application at this time.

Optimize Heart Rate

Optimizing heart rate is a mechanism that is mentioned briefly mainly for the sake of completeness (see Table 9-2). The problems caused by excessive slowing of the heart, generally caused by atrioventricular block, are readily corrected by the use of electronic pacemakers. More difficult are the rare cases of incessant tachycardia, which require expert management by arrhythmia experts who can perform ablation therapy, or, when this is not possible, who can prescribe the difficult and dangerous antiarrhythmic drugs needed to treat these tachycardias. The more common challenge posed by the sinus tachycardia commonly seen in heart failure, which contributes to the state of energy starvation, can be managed with β blockers (and perhaps, as was once customary, with digitalis).

Arrhythmias

The problem of serious arrhythmias is mentioned briefly here, but for appropriately detailed discussions of this important topic, refer to standard texts. About half of the deaths in heart failure are "sudden" or unexpected, although it is usually difficult to determine how many of these deaths are due to a primary arrhythmia. As many as one fourth of documented arrhythmic deaths appear to be due to bradyarrhythmias (sinus slowing and atrioventricular block) (Luu et al., 1982), whereas the majority are caused by ventricular tachycardia and fibrillation (for review, see Uretsky and Sheahan, 1997; Gill and Camm, 1997; Packer and Cohn, 1999).

The approach to arrhythmia prevention in heart failure has undergone a true Kuhnian paradigm shift since 1989, when a large trial of antiarrhythmic drugs was stopped prematurely because of an excess of sudden deaths (The Cardiac Arrhythmia Suppression Trial [CAST] Investigators, 1989). Even though the drugs examined in this trial reduced the frequency of the nonlethal ventricular ectopy long recognized as heralding sudden cardiac death, the same drugs *increased* the frequency of lethal arrhythmias, once again illustrating the precept that what is obvious is often not important and what is important is not often obvious. A likely explanation for "proarrhythmic" effects of "antiarrhythmic" drugs is that these agents, which suppress the nonlethal arrhythmias by depressing conduction in regions of the heart that generate the "warning" arrhythmias, increase the likelihood of more dangerous arrhythmias by depressing conduction throughout in the heart. Abolishing these warning arrhythmias is like shooting a a scout from a nearby army— the sound of the shot can attract a horde of heavily armed soldiers.

One drug that appears not to share the hazards of antiarrhythmic therapy is amiodarone, which has emerged as the drug of choice for these patients. Implantable cardioverter-defibrillators are also quite effective in preventing lethal arrhythmias, but they have less effect in prolonging survival. Furthermore, these devices are expensive and, in some patients with end-stage heart failure, only prolong the final stages of dying. Whether amiodarone or an implanted device provides the best means to prevent sudden death in heart failure remains controversial (Uretsky and Sheahan, 1997; Gill and Camm, 1997; Packer and Cohn, 1999).

THERAPY DIRECTED TO THE CARDIAC MYOCYTE

The major lesson that has been learned from the past decade of clinical trials is the importance of slowing the progressive deterioration of the failing heart. The failure of most vasodilators to improve long-term prognosis (see Table 9-3) along with the adverse effects of the inotropes have demonstrated that effective treatment for the circulatory and cardiac abnormalities in heart failure patients does not mean that survival will be prolonged. Yet largely by accident, ACE inhibitors, nitrates, and β blockers have been found to improve prognosis, and there is preliminary evidence that this property is shared by an aldosterone antagonist (Table 9-7). Two of these classes of drugs, the *nitrates* and *ACE inhibitors*, were introduced as vasodilators, but as has already been discussed, their ability to prolong survival appears to be due in part to inhibition of remodeling. A survival benefit of *aldosterone antagonists* has so far been demonstrated in only one trial in which, according to preliminary data, treatment of patients with severe ischemic and idiopathic dilated cardiomyopathy with spironolactone is associated with a 27% reduction in mortality rate and a 36% decrease in hospitalization rate for heart failure (Pitt, 1998).

TABLE 9-7. *Drugs that improve survival in patients with heart failure*

Established benefit
Angiotensin-converting enzyme inhibitors
β-Adrenergic blockers
Nitrates (in combination with hydralazine)
Possible benefit
Aldosterone blockers (one trial only)

Although the underlying mechanism for this putative benefit is not yet known, it is tempting to speculate that inhibition of the growth-promoting effects of aldosterone plays a role. Solid evidence for interpretation, however, must await further research. The following discussion highlights a fourth class of drug, whose ability to prolong survival in heart failure has only recently been shown; these drugs are the β-adrenergic receptor blockers.

β-Adrenergic Receptor Blockers

The possibility that β blockade might benefit patients with chronic heart failure was suggested in the mid-1970s both by clinical observations (Waagstein et al., 1975) and by theoretic considerations (Katz, 1973). However, because of enthusiasm for the new inotropic drugs then being developed, these early reports were generally ignored. It was not until the late 1980s, when the hazards of inotropic therapy were becoming clear, that serious consideration was given to the possibility that negative inotropic agents might be of value in the treatment of heart failure. Despite promising data from controlled trials that showed a striking long-term improvement in left ventricular function (e.g., Gilbert et al., 1990), confirmation by two metaanalyses (Hjalmarson and Waagstein, 1991; Eichhorn 1992) and a growing theoretic basis for using these drugs (Katz, 1992), the short-term hazards of β blockers made it difficult to enroll patients in long-term survival trials (Waagstein et al., 1993). Resistance to use of β blockers in heart failure began to crumble with the publication of data from the United States (Packer et

Effects of Therapy on Heart Failure Mortality

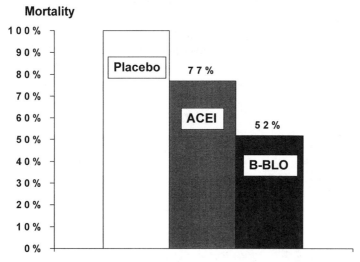

FIG. 9-6. Survival benefits of ACE inhibitors alone (ACEI) and with the addition of a β-blocker (B-BLO) compared to patients treated with placebo. The benefit of ACE inhibitors is based on a metaanalysis of trials comparing placebo and ACEI (Garg and Yusef 1995), that for β blockers are based on the metaanalysis of LeChat and colleagues (1998). The latter, which has been confirmed in trials using bisoprolol (CIBIS II) and metoprolol (MERIT), indicates that, when used together, these two classes of drug can reduce mortality rate by almost 50%.

TABLE 9-8. *Possible mechanisms by which β-adrenergic blockers improve survival in patients with heart failure*

Inhibit necrosis: energy sparing effects
    Slowing of heart rate
    Negative inotropic effect
Inhibit maladaptive growth
    Block cAMP-activated growth factors
    Block formation of the β-receptor–β-arrestin complex
Inhibit apoptosis

al., 1996) and Australia/New Zealand (Australia/New Zealand Heart Failure Research Collaborative Group, 1997) carvedilol trials. A metaanalysis of all survival trials through 1997 (LeChat et al., 1998), which indicated that β blockers reduce mortality rates by 30% to 35%, was soon followed by the announcement of almost identical results in trials of bisoprolol, a nonselective β blocker (CIBIS-II Investigators and Committees, 1999), and the β_1 selective blocker metoprolol (MERIT-HF Investigators, 1998). These results demonstrate that the benefits are a "class effect" of β-adrenergic blockade. The significance of the benefits of β blockade is highlighted by the fact that these trials were carried out in patients who were already receiving ACE inhibitors, which themselves reduce mortality rate by about 27% (Garg et al., 1995). The combined benefit of these two classes of drugs, therefore, is to reduce mortality rate by about 50% (Fig. 9-6).

The mechanism for the ability of β blockers to prolong survival and reduce hospitalization for progressive heart failure is not yet established (Table 9-8). A few years ago, the most attractive explanation for a long-term benefit of these drugs were their energy-sparing effects (Katz, 1973, 1992), which could inhibit necrosis. The more recent recognition that β-adrenergic stimulation can cause apoptosis (see Chapter 6) provides another plausible explanation for this benefit. Another potential mechanism, that these drugs inhibit maladaptive growth of the failing heart (Katz 1989, 1990b), is suggested by the data of Hall and colleagues (1995), which indicate that although metoprolol initially reduces ejection fraction, this deleterious effect is followed by a large increase in ejection fraction along with decreases in both left ventricular volume and mass (Table 9-9). Although the long-term data in Table 9-9 are uncontrolled, because

TABLE 9-9. *Long-term effects of metoprolol on ventricular volume and mass in patients with heart failure*

Therapy	LV EDV (ml)	LV ESV (ml)	SV (ml)	EF (%)	LV mass (g)
Placebo					
Baseline	288	219	69	24	303
3 months	263	204	59	25	318
Metoprolol					
Baseline	252	192	60	24	327
3 months	237	162	75	33	327
18 months	177	100	77	44	269

LV, left ventricular; EDV, end diastolic volume; ESV, end-systolic volume; SV, stroke volume; EF, ejection fraction
Data from Hall et al., 1995

the randomization in this trial ended after 3 months, similar decreases in left ventricular volume have been found in several other studies of long-term β blocker use (Sabbah et al., 1994; Gilbert et al., 1996; Doughty et al., 1997). Available data, therefore, are consistent with the view that β blockade inhibits remodeling and that the resulting decrease in end-diastolic volume, perhaps even more than an increase in stroke volume, accounts for the increased ejection fraction that is seen in all long-term studies with these agents (Hjalmarson and Waagstein, 1991; Eichhorn, 1992). These putative growth-inhibitory effects, as discussed earlier in this text, could be due to the ability of β blockade to inhibit the activation of growth factors, such as CREB; to prevent the activation of MAP kinases that are activated by ligand-bound β receptors; or to reduce the formation of the β-receptor–β-arrestin complex that serves as a platform for tyrosine-kinase activated growth. It is possible, and I believe likely, that *all* of these effects, along with reduced energy utilization and inhibition of apoptosis, contribute to the survival benefits described earlier.

It is important to appreciate the hazards of a "rebound" that often occurs when β-blocker therapy is stopped suddenly (for review, see Eichhorn, 1999). Because prolonged β blockade allows downregulated receptors to be reactivated, a potentially dangerous situation is created by abrupt β-blocker withdrawal in heart failure patients, whose circulating catecholamine levels can be very high. In ischemic heart disease, it is well known that sudden withdrawal of these drugs can cause fatal myocardial infarction or sudden death in as many as 50% of patients (Alderman et al., 1974; Miller et al., 1975).

ANTICOAGULATION

It has long been known that patients with heart failure are vulnerable to embolism, especially those with atrial fibrillation. Even in patients with sinus rhythm, sluggish blood flow provides a substrate for intravascular clotting that has been estimated to occur in about 2% of these patients each year (see Packer and Cohn, 1999). Although there have been no adequate randomized controlled trials, retrospective analyses indicate that warfarin anticoagulation provides a significant benefit to these patients, both in terms of prolonging survival and reducing morbidity (Al-Khadra et al., 1998).

SURGICAL THERAPY, HEART TRANSPLANTATION, THE ARTIFICIAL HEART, AND LEFT VENTRICULAR ASSIST DEVICES

The need for coronary revascularization in patients with hibernating myocardium has already been discussed, as has the necessity to correct, as far as possible, such structural abnormalities as intracardiac shunts and valve disorders. The value of correcting mitral insufficiency caused by marked left ventricular dilatation has also been mentioned in the context of ventriculectomy, in which a large portion of the left ventricle is removed to reduce wall stress. The lzatter operation, however, is controversial. Whereas the value of replacing a leaky mitral valve is well established, excision of a wedge of the left ventricular wall has potential long-term deleterious effects that may outweigh any advantage to be gained by the immediate reduction in wall tension (for review, see Kass, 1998). In addition to the obvious problems caused by removal of a substantial fraction of the heart's limited number of terminally differentiated myocytes, ventriculectomy must be viewed as a mutilating operation that disrupts the intricate architecture of the ventricular wall, which is made up of overlapping layers of spiral bundles. Cardiomyoplasty, another surgical approach to heart failure in which the *latissimus dorsi* (a skeletal muscle) is wrapped around a failing ventricle and stimulated with an electronic pacemaker, has some theoretic advantages. However, data from appropriate long-term trials are not yet available (Kass, 1998). In evaluating early reports of possible benefits of these and other surgical treatments for heart failure, it must be remembered that, as is true for most therapy of this syndrome, there may be major discrepancies between short-term and long-term results.

There is no question that heart transplantation, when performed in appropriate patients, provides remarkable benefits. The problem with this solution to the growing population with heart failure, in addition to the obvious hazards of rejection and need for immunosuppression, is simply that there are not enough donor hearts; only about 2,500 annually (Evans et al., 1986). This procedure, therefore, cannot help more than a fraction of the hundreds of thousands who die each year of heart failure.

Another solution to the problem of heart failure would be to implant a "permanent" mechanical heart. Efforts to develop an artificial heart have been underway at least since the 1960s. Enthusiasm, which has waxed and waned over the past 30 years, remains high in some places, but many technical problems still remain to be worked out. Although it seems that widespread use of a permanent artificial heart is not on the horizon, there is growing, generally favorable experience with implantable *left ventricular assist devices* (*LVADs*), which were originally developed as a "bridge to transplant," that is, devices to maintain a dying patient until heart transplant became possible (for review, see Goldstein et al., 1998). Temporary placement of these devices has been reported to reverse many of the maladaptive features of overload-induced hypertrophy (Muller et al., 1997; Zafeiridis et al., 1998), although significant improvement is not always seen (Mancini et al., 1998). Furthermore, the ability of a short course of therapy to reverse maladaptive changes in cardiac myocyte phenotype does not demonstrate that this approach can provide significant and sustained clinical improvement (Katz, 1998). In the last analysis, therefore, heart failure must be viewed as a "medical" and not a "surgical" disorder, which means that the most promising approaches for the future lie in improved means to slow, and hopefully reverse, the molecular disorders described in this text.

CONCLUSION

In concluding this discussion of the management of heart failure, it is useful to refer to the horse analogy that has been useful in my earlier discussions of this subject (Fig. 9-7). This somewhat fanciful analogy still has some relevance, especially because it is clear that the "ideal" solution, to heal the horse, while difficult, lies within our grasp. A major limitation of this model is that it does not depict the need to use several approaches simultaneously, a challenge that is considered further in Chapter 10. A better analogy, perhaps, is to view the therapeutic tools available for treating heart failure as musical instruments. When *"integrated into a sound rationale of therapy"* (Silber and Katz, 1975), they yield a harmonious and pleasing symphony; whereas the same instruments, if poorly orchestrated, cause a cacophony.

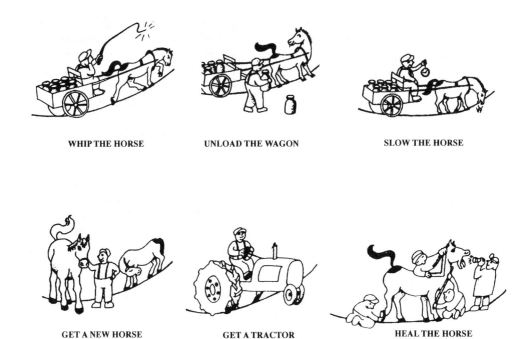

FIG. 9-7. View of the failing heart as a sick, tired horse pulling a wagon up a steep hill. Although application of the whip (inotropes) encourages the horse to move faster, this can kill the animal. Unloading the wagon (vasodilators) would seem to be advantageous, but in heart failure, this approach can harm the horse by activating harmful neurohumoral responses. Slowing the horse (β blockers), while delaying the journey, can be beneficial, especially if this also helps to heal the horse. Replacing the horse (cardiac transplantation) is useful as long as there are enough spare horses, and getting a tractor is a solution only if reliable machines are available. The ideal solution, of course, is to learn what ails the animal and to use this information to heal the horse.

BIBLIOGRAPHY

Braunwald EH, ed (1997). *Heart Disease. A Textbook of Cardiovascular Medicine,* 5th ed. WB Saunders, Philadelphia.

Cohn JN, ed (1988). *Drug Treatment of Heart Failure*. ATC, Secaucus, NJ.

Hosenpud JD, Greenberg BH, eds (1994). *Congestive Heart Failure. Pathophysiology, Diagnosis, and Comprehensive Approach to Management.* Springer, NY. 1994.

McCall D, Rahimtoola SH, eds (1995). *Heart Failure.* Chapman & Hall, NY.

Poole-Wilson PA, Colucci WS, Massie BM, Chatterjee K, Coats AS, eds (1997). *Heart Failure. Scientific Principles and Clinical Practice.* Churchill Livingstone, New York.

Rose EA, Stevenson LW, eds (1998). *Management of End-Stage Heart Disease.* Lippincott-Raven, Philadelphia.

Schlant RC, Alexander RW, O'Rourke RA, Roberts R, Sonnenblick EH eds (1994). *Hurst's The Heart,* 8th ed. McGraw-Hill, New York.

Topol E, ed (1997). *Textbook of Cardiovascular Medicine.* Lippincott-Raven, Philadelphia.

Willerson JT, Cohn JN, eds (1995). *Cardiovascular Medicine.* Churchill Livingstone, New York.

REFERENCES

The Acute Infarction Ramipril Efficacy (AIRE) Study Investigators (1993). Effect of ramipril on mortality and morbidity of survivors of acute myocardial infarction with clinical evidence of heart failure. *Lancet* 342:821–828.

Adams KF, Dunlap SH, Sueta CA, Clarke SW, Patterson JH, Blauwet MB, Jensen LR, Tomasko L, Koch G (1998).

Relation between gender, etiology and survival in patients with symptomatic heart failure. *J Am Coll Cardiol* 28:1781–1788.

Alderman EL, Coltart J, Wettach GE, Harrison DC (1974). Coronary artery syndromes after sudden propranolol withdrawal. *Ann Intern Med* 81:625–627.

Al-Khada AS, Salem DN, Rand WM, Udelson JE, Smith JJ, Konstam MA (1998). Warfarin anticoagulation and survival: a cohort analysis from the Studies of Left Ventricular Dysfunction. *J Am Coll Cardiol* 31:749–753.

Australia/New Zealand Heart Failure Research Collaborative Group (1997). Randomised, placebo-controlled trial of carvedilol in patients with congestive heart failure due to ischemic heart disease. *Lancet* 349:375–380.

Benge W, Litchfield RL, Marcus ML (1980). Exercise capacity in patients with severe heart failure. *Circulation* 61:955-959.

Brater DC (1998). Diuretic therapy. *N Engl J Med* 339:387–395.

Califf RM, Gheorghiade M, eds (1998). Managing the patient with advanced heart failure. *Am Heart J* 135(Suppl): S201–S326.

Califf RM, Adams KF, Armstrong PW, McKenna WJ, Gheorgiade M, Urestsky BF, McNulty SE, Darius H, Chulkman K, Zannad F, Handberg-Thurmond E, Harrell FE Jr, Wheeler W, Soler-Soler J, Swedberg K (1997). A randomized controlled trial of epoprostenol therapy for severe heart failure: the Flolan International Randomized Survival Trial (FIRST). *Am Heart J* 134:44–54.

The Cardiac Arrhythmia Suppression Trial [CAST] Investigators. (1989). Effects of encainide and flecainide, imipramine and moricizine on mortality in a randomize trial of arrhythmia suppression after myocardial infarction. *N Engl J Med* 321:406–410.

CIBIS-II Investigators and Committees (1999). The cardiac insufficiency bisoprolol study II (CIBIS-II): a randomised trial. *Lancet* 353:9–13.

Clerico A, Iervasi G, Del Chicca MG, Emdin M, Maffei S, Nannipieri M, Sabatino L, Forini F, Manfredi C, Donato L (1998). Circulating levels of cardiac natriuretic peptides (ANP and BNP) measured by highly sensitive and specific immunoradiometric assays in normal subjects and in patients with different degrees of heart failure. *J Endocrinol Invest* 21:170–179.

Cohn JN (1993). Introduction. The Vasodilator-Heart Failure Trials (V-HeFT). Mechanistic studies from the VA cooperative studies. *Circulation* 87(Suppl):VI-1–VI-4.

Cohn JN (1996). Treatment of heart failure. *N Engl J Med* 335:490–498.

Cohn JN, Franciosa JA (1977). Vasodilator therapy of cardiac failure. *N Engl J Med* 297:27–31, 254–257.

Cohn JN, Archibald DG, Ziesche S, Franciosa JA, Harston WE, Tristani FE, Dunkman WB, Jacobs W, Francis GS, Cobb FR, Shah PM, Saunders R, Fletcher RD, Loeb HS, Hughes VC, Baker B (1986). Effect of vasodilator therapy on mortality in chronic congestive heart failure. Results of a Veterans Administration cooperative study (V-HeFT). *N Engl J Med* 314:1547–1552.

Cohn JN, Johnson G, Ziesche S, Cobb F, Francis G, Tristani F, Smith R, Dunkman WB, Loeb H, Wong M, Bhat G, Goldman S Fletcher RD, Doherty J, Hughes CV, Carson P, Cintron G, Shabetai R, Haakenson C (1991). A comparison of enalapril with hydralazine-isosorbide dinitrate in the treatment of chronic congestive heart failure. *N Engl J Med* 325:303–310.

Cohn JN, Goldstein SO, Greenberg BH, Lorell BH, Bourge RC, Jaski BE, Gottleib SO, McGrew F, DeMets D, White BG (1998). A dose-dependent increase in mortality with vesnarinone among patients with severe heart failure. *N Engl J Med* 339:1810–1816.

CONSENSUS Trial Study Group (1987). Effects of enalapril on mortality in severe congestive heart failure: Results of the Cooperative North Scandinavian Enalapril Survival Study (CONSENSUS). *N Engl J Med* 316:1429–1435.

Cowley AJ, Skene AM (1994). Treatment of severe heart failure: quantity or quality of life? A trial of enoximone. Enoximone Investigators. *Br Heart J* 72:226–230.

Deswal A, Bozhurt B, Seta Y, et al. (1999). Safety and efficacy of a soluble P75 tumor necrosis factor receptor (Enbrel, etanercept) in patients with advanced heart failure. *Circulation* 99:3224–3226.

Dies F, Krell MJ, Whitlow P, Liang C-S, Goldenberg I, Applefield MM, Gilbert EM (1986). Intermittent dobutamine in ambulatory outpatients with chronic cardiac failure (Abstract). *Circulation* 74:II-38.

The Digitalis Investigation Group (1997). The effect of digoxin on mortality and morbidity in patients with heart failure. *N Engl J Med* 336:525–533.

Doughty RN, Whalley GA, Gamble G, MacMahon S, Sharpe N on behalf of the Australia/New Zealand Heart Failure Research Collaborative Group (1997). Left ventricular remodeling with carvedilol in patients with congestive heart failure due to ischemic heart disease. *Am J Cardiol* 29:1060–1066.

Dostal DE, Hunt RA, Kule CE, Bhat GJ, Karoor V, McWhinney CD, Baker KM (1997). Molecular mechanisms of angiotensin II in modulating cardiac function: intracardiac effects and signal transduction pathways. *J Mol Cell Cardiol* 29:2893–2901.

Eichhorn EJ (1992). The paradox of β-adrenergic blockade for the management of congestive heart failure. *Am J Med* 92:527–538.

Eichhorn EJ (1999). Beta-blocker withdrawal: the song of Orpheus. *Am Heart J.* In press.

Eichhorn EJ, Bristow MR (1996). Medical therapy can improve the biological properties of the chronically failing heart. *Circulation* 94:2285–2296.

Elis A, Bental T, Kimchi O, Ravid M, Lishner M (1998). Intermittent dobutamine treatment in patients with chronic refractory congestive heart failure: a randomized, double-blind, placebo-controlled study. *Clin Pharmacol Ther* 63:682–685.

Elkayam U (1996). Nitrates in the treatment of congestive heart failure. *Am J Cardiol* 77:41C–51C.

Elkayam U (1998). Results of the MACH-1 Trial. Presented at the XXI Congress of the European Society of Cardiology. 25 August, 1998, Vienna, Austria.

Elkayam U, Amin J, Mehra A, Vasquez J, Weber L, Rahimtoola SH (1990). A prospective, randomized, double-blind, crossover study to compare the efficacy and safety of chronic nifedipine therapy with that of isosorbide dinitrate and their combination in the treatment of congestive heart failure. *Circulation* 82:1954–1961.

Evans RW, Manninen DL, Garrison LP Jr, Maier AM (1986). Donor availability as the primary determinant of the future of heart transplantation. *JAMA* 255:1892–1898.

Fazio S, Sabatini D, Capaldo B, Vigorito C, Giordano A, Guida R, Pardo F, Biondi B, Sacca L, (1996). A preliminary study of growth hormone in the treatment of dilated cardiomyopathy. *N Engl J Med* 334:809–814

Ferguson DW, Berg WJ, Sanders JS, Roach PJ, Kempf JS, Kienzle MG (1989). Sympathoinhibitory responses to digitalis glycosides in heart failure patients: direct evidence from sympathetic neural recordings *Circulation* 80:65–77.

Francis GS, Benedict C, Johnstone DE, Kirlin PC, Nicklas J, Liang C-s, Kubo SH, Rudin-Toretsky E, Yusef S (1990). Comparison of neuroendocrine activation in patient with left ventricular dysfunction with and without congestive heart failure. A substudy of the studies of left ventricular dysfunction (SOLVD). *Circulation* 82:1724–1729.

Franciosa JA, Park M, Levine TB (1981). Lack of correlation between exercise capacity and indexes of resting left ventricular performance in heart failure. *Am J Cardiol* 47:33–39.

Franciosa JA, Jordon RA, Wilen MM, Leddy CL (1984). Minoxidil in patients with chronic left heart failure. Contrasting hemodynamic and clinical effects in a controlled trial. *Circulation* 70:63–68.

Francis GS, Goldsmith SR, Levine TB, Olivari MT, Cohn JN (1984). The neurohumoral axis in congestive heart failure. *Ann Intern Med* 101:370–377.

Frazier OH, Benedict CR, Radovancevic B, Bick RJ, Capek P, Springer W, Macris MP, Delgado R, Buja LM (1996). Improved left ventricular function after chronic left ventricular unloading. *Ann Thorac Surg* 58:1515–1520.

Garg R, Yusef S, for the Collaborative Group on ACE inhibitor trials. Overview of randomized trials of angiotensin-converting enzyme inhibitors on mortality and morbidity of patients with heart failure. *JAMA* 273:1450–1456.

Gheorghiade M, Hall VB, Jacobsen G, Alam M, Rosman H, Goldstein S (1995). Effects of increasing maintenance dose of digoxin on left ventricular function and neurohormones in patients with chronic heart failure treated with diuretics and angiotensin-converting enzyme inhibitors. *Circulation* 92:1801–1807.

Gilbert EM, Anderson JL, Deitchman D, Yanowitz FG, O'Connell JB, Renlund JB, Bartholomew M, Mealy PC, Larabee P, Bristow MR (1990). Long-term β-blocker vasodilator therapy improves cardiac function in idiopathic dilated cardiomyopathy: a double-blind, randomized study of bucindolol versus placebo. *Am J Med* 88:223–229.

Gilbert EM, Abraham WT, Olsen S, Hattler B, White M, Mealy P, Larabee P, Bristow MR (1996). Comparative hemodynamic, left ventricular functional and antiadrenergic effects of chronic treatment with metoprolol versus carvedilol in the failing heart. *Circulation* 94:2817–2825.

Gill JS, Camm AJ (1997). Management of arrhythmias in patients with heart failure: evaluation and treatment with drugs and devices. In Poole-Wilson PA, Colucci WS, Massie BM, Chatterjee K, Coats AS, eds. *Heart failure. Scientific Principles and Clinical Practice.* Churchill Livingstone, New York, pp 747–758.

Goldstein DJ, Oz MC, Rose EA (1998). Implantable left ventricular assist devices. *N Engl J Med* 339:1522–1533.

Goldstein RE, Boccuzzi SJ, Cruess D, Nattel S, the Adverse Experience Committee, and the Multicenter Diltiazem Postinfarction Research Group (1991). Diltiazem increases late-onset congestive heart failure in postinfarction patients with early reduction in ejection fraction. *Circulation* 83:52–60.

Gradman A, Deedwania P, Cody R, Massie B, Packer M, Pitt B, Goldstein S (1989). Predictors of total mortality and sudden death in mild to moderate heart failure. *J Am Coll Cardiol* 14:564–570.

Hall SA, Cigarroa CG, Marcoux L, Risser RC, Grayburn PA, Eichhorn EJ (1995). Time course of improvement in left ventricular function, mass and geometry in patients with congestive heart failure treated with beta-adrenergic blockade. *J Am Coll Cardiol* 25:1154–1161.

Hampton JR, van Veldhuisen DJ, Kleber FX, Cowley AJ, Ardia A, Block P, Cortina A, Cserhalmi L, Follath F, Jensen G, Kayanakis J, Lie KI, Mancia G, Skene AM for the Second Prospective Randomised Study of Ibopamine on Mortality and Efficacy (PRIME II) Investigators (1997). Randomised study of the effects of ibopamine on survival in patients with advanced severe heart failure. *Lancet* 349:971–977.

Hauptman PT, Kelly RA (1999). Digitalis. *Circulation* 99:1265–1270.

Heusch G (1998). Hibernating myocardium. *Physiol Rev* 78:1055–1085.

Hjalmarson Å, Waagstein F (1991). New therapeutic strategies in chronic heart failure: challenge of long-term beta-blockade. *Eur Heart J* 12(Suppl F):63–69

Ho KKL, Pinsky JL, Kannel WB, Levy D (1993). The epidemiology of congestive heart failure: The Framingham Study. *J Am Coll Cardiol* 22(Suppl A):6A–13A.

Judgett BI (1996). Effect of nitrates on myocardial remodeling after acute myocardial infarction. *Am J Cardiol* 77:17C–23C.

Kass DA (1998). Surgical approaches to arresting or reversing chronic remodeling of the failing heart. *J Cardiac Failure* 4:57–66.

Katz AM (1973). Biochemical "defect" in the hypertrophied and failing heart. Deleterious or compensatory? *Circulation* 47:1076–1079.

Katz AM (1986). Potential deleterious effects of inotropic agents in the therapy of chronic heart failure. *Circulation* 73(Suppl III):184–188.

Katz AM (1987). Role of the basic sciences in the practice of cardiology. *J Mol Cell Cardiol* 19:3–17.

Katz AM (1989). Changing strategies in the management of congestive heart failure. *J Am Coll Cardiol* 13:512–523.

Katz AM (1990a). Angiotensin II: hemodynamic regulator or growth factor? *J Mol Cell Cardiol* 22:739–747.

Katz AM (1990b). Cardiomyopathy of Overload. A major determinant of prognosis in congestive heart failure. *N Engl J Med* 322:100–110.

Katz AM (1992). Heart failure in 2001: a Prophesy. *Am J Cardiol* 70:126C–131C.

Katz AM (1994). The cardiomyopathy of Overload: an unnatural growth response in the hypertrophied heart. *Ann Intern Med* 121:363–371.

Katz AM (1996). Calcium channel diversity in the cardiovascular system. *J Am Coll Cardiol* 28:522–529.

Katz AM (1998). Regression of left ventricular hypertrophy: new hope for dying hearts. *Circulation* 98:623–624.

Kober L, Torp-Pedersen C, Carlson JE, Bagger H, Eliasen P, Lyngborg K, Videbaek J, Cole DS, Auclert L, Pauly NC, Aliot E, Persson S, Camm AJ, for the Trandolapril Cardiac Evaluation (TRACE) Study Group (1995). A clinical trial of the angiotensin-converting-enzyme inhibitor trandolapril in patients with left ventricular dysfunction after myocardial infarction. *N Engl J Med* 333:1670–1676.

LeChat P, Packer M, Chalon S, Cucherat M, Arab T, Boissel J-P (1998). Clinical effects of β-adrenergic blockade in chronic heart failure. *Circulation* 98:1184–1191.

Lindenfeld J, Krause-Steinrauf H, Salerno J (1997). Where are all the women with heart failure? *J Am Coll Cardiol* 30:1417–1419.

Linz W, Schölkens BA, Ganten D (1989). Converting enzyme inhibition specifically prevents the development and induces regression of cardiac hypertrophy in rats. *Clin Exp Hypertens Theory Practice* A11:1325–1350.

Lipkin DP, Poole-Wilson PA (1986). Symptoms limiting exercise capacity in chronic heart failure. *BMJ* 292:653–655.

Lubbe WF, Podzweit T, Daries PS, Opie LH (1978). The role of cyclic adenosine monophosphate in adrenergic effects on ventricular vulnerability to fibrillation in the isolated perfused heart. *J Clin Invest* 61:1260–1269.

Lubsen J, Just H, Hjalmarson AC, La Framboise D, Remme WJ, Heinrich-Nols J, Dumont JM, Seed P (1996). Effect of pimobendan on exercise capacity in patients with heart failure: main results from the Pimobendan in Congestive Heart Failure (PICO) trial. *Heart* 76:223–231.

Luu M, Stevenson LW, Brunken RC, Drinkwater DC, Schelbert HR, Tillisch JH (1989). Diverse mechanisms of unexpected cardiac arrest in advanced heart failure. *Circulation* 80:1675–1680.

MacKenzie J (1908). *Diseases of the Heart,* Oxford University Press, London.

Maeda K, Tsutamoto T, Wada A, Hisanaga T, Kinoshita M (1998). Plasma brain natriuretic peptide as a biochemical marker of high left ventricular end-diastolic pressure in patients with symptomatic left ventricular dysfunction. *Am Heart J* 135:825–832.

Mancini DM, Beniaminovitz A, Levin H, Catanese K, Flannery M, DiTullio M, Savin S, Cordisco E, Rose E, Oz M (1998). Low incidence of myocardial recovery after left ventricular assist device implantation in patients with chronic heart failure. *Circulation* 98:2383–2389.

Marrero MB, Schieffer B, Paxton WG, Heerdt L, Berk BC, Delafontaine P, Bernstein KE (1997). Direct stimulation of Jak/STAT by the angiotensin II AT$_1$ receptor. *Nature* 375:247–249.

Mason DT, Braunwald E (1964). Studies on digitalis: X. Effects of ouabain on forearm resistance and venous tone in normal individuals and in patients with heart failure. *J Clin Invest* 43:532–543.

McDonagh TA, Robb SD, Murdoch DR, Morton JJ, Ford I, Morrison CE, Tunstall-Pedoe H, McMurray JJ. Dargie HJ (1998). Biochemical detection of left-ventricular systolic dysfunction. *Lancet* 351:9–13.

McDonald KM, Francis GS, Matthews J, Hunter D, Cohn JN (1993). Long-term oral nitrate therapy prevents chronic ventricular remodeling in the dog. *J Am Coll Cardiol* 21:514–521.

McKelvie R, Yusef S, Pericak D, Lindgren E, Held P. For the RESOLVD Investigators (1998). Comparison of candesartan, enalapril, and the combination in congestive heart failure; randomized evaluation of strategies for left ventricular dysfunction (RESOLVD Pilot Study). *Eur Heart J* 19(Suppl):133.

MERIT-HF Investigators (1998). Communication with Gottleib SS, Goldstein S, Wedel H concerning the results of the MERIT-HF Trial. (Cited by Packer and Cohn, 1999).

Miller RR, Olson HG, Amsterdam EA, Mason DT (1975). Propranolol-withdrawal rebound phenomenon: exacerbation of coronary events after abrupt cessation of antianginal therapy. *N Engl J Med* 293:416–418.

Mulder P, Richard V, Compagnon P, Henry J-P, Lallemand F, Clozel J-P, Koen R, Macè B, Thuillez C (1997). Increased survival after long-term treatment with mibefradil, a selective T-channel calcium antagonist, in heart failure. *J Am Coll Cardiol* 29:416–421.

Muller J, Wallukat G, Weng Y, Dandel M, Spiegelsberger S, Semrau S, Brandes K, Theodoridis V, Loebe M, Meyer R, Hetzer R (1997). Weaning from mechanical support in patients with dilated cardiomyopathy. *Circulation* 96:542–549.

Oie E, Bjoneheim R, Grogaard HK, Kongshaug H, Smiseth OA, Attramadal H (1998). ET-receptor antagonism, myocardial gene expression, and ventricular remodeling during CHF in rats. *Am J Physiol* 275:H868–H877.

Packer M (1990). Calcium channel blockers in chronic heart failure. The risks of "physiologically rational" therapy. *Circulation* 82:2254–2257.

Packer M, Cohn JN (1999). Consensus recommendations for the management of heart failure. *Am J Cardiol* 83(Suppl 2a):1A–38A.

Packer M, Leier CV (1987). Survival in congestive heart failure during treatment with drugs with positive inotropic actions. *Circulation* 75(Suppl IV):55–63.

Packer M, Carver, JR, Rodeheffer RJ, Ivanhoe, RJ, DiBianco R, Zeldis SM, Hendrix GH, Bommer WJ, Elkayam U, Kukin ML, Mallis GI, Sollano JA, Shannon J, Tandon PK, DeMets DL (1991). Effect of oral milrinone on mortality in severe heart failure. *N Engl J Med* 325:1468–1475.

Packer M, Rouleau J, Swedberg K, Pitt B, Fisher L, Klepper M and the PROFILE Investigators and Coordinators (1993). Effect of flosequinan on survival in chronic heart failure: preliminary results of the PROFILE study. *Circulation* 88(Suppl I):301.

Packer M, Gheorghiade M, Young JB, Constanti PJ, Adams KF, Cody RJ, Smith LK, Van Vorhees L, Gouley LA, Jolly MK, for the RADIANCE Study (1993). Withdrawal of digoxin from patients with chronic heart failure treated with angiotensin converting enzymes inhibitor. *N Engl J Med* 329:1–7.

Packer M, Bristow MR, Cohn JN, Colucci WS, Fowler MB, Gilbert EM, Shusterman NH for the US Carvedilol Heart Failure Study Group (1996). The effect of carvedilol on morbidity and mortality in patients with chronic heart failure. *N Engl J Med* 334:1349–1355.

Pan J, Fukuda K, Kodama H, Makino S, Takahashi T, Sano M, Hori S, Ogawa S (1997). Role of angiotensin II in activation of the JAK/STAT pathway induced by acute pressure overload in the rat heart. *Circ Res* 81:611–617.

Pfeffer MA, Braunwald E, Moyé LA, Basta L, Brown EJ Jr, Cuddy TE, Davis BR, Geltman EM, Goldman S, Flaker CG, Klein M, Lamas GA, PAcker M, Rouleau J, Rouleau JL, Rutherford J, Wertheimer JH, Hawkins CM on behalf of the SAVE Investigators (1992). Effect of captopril on mortality and morbidity in patients with left ventricular dysfunction after myocardial infarction. Results of the survival and ventricular enlargement trial. *N Engl J Med* 327:669–677.

Pitt B, Segal R, Martinez FA, Meurers G, Cowley AJ, Thomas I, Deedwania PC, Net DE, Snavely DB, Chang PI, on behalf of ELITE Study Investigators (1997). Randomized trial of losartan versus captopril in patients over 65 with heart failure (Evaluation of Losartan in the Elderly Study, ELITE). *Lancet* 349:747–752.

Pitt B (1998). Presentation of the RALES Trial at the 71st Scientific Sessions of the American Heart Association. (Reported in *Clin Cardiol* 22:47, 1999).

Po AL, Zhang WY (1998). What lessons can be learned from withdrawal of mibefradil from the market. *Lancet* 351:1829–1830.

Podzuweit T, Lubbe WF, Opie LH (1976). Cyclic adenosine monophosphate, ventricular fibrillation, and antiarrhythmic drugs *Lancet* 1:341–342.

Rahimtoola SH (1989). The hibernating myocardium. *Am Heart J* 117:211–221.

Rahimtoola SH (1997). Importance of diagnosing hibernating myocardium: How and in whom? *J Am Coll Cardiol* 30:1701–1706.

Remme WJ for The Task Force of the Working Group on Heart Failure of the European Society of Cardiology (1997). The treatment of heart failure. *Eur Heart J* 18:736–753.

Sabbah HN, Shimoyama H, Kono T, Gupta RC, Sharov VG, Scicili G, Levine TB, Goldstein S (1994). Effects of long-term monotherapy with enalapril, metoprolol, and digoxin on the progression of left ventricular dysfunction and dilatation in dogs with reduced ejection fraction. *Circulation* 89:2852–2859.

Sadoshima J, Izumo S (1993). Molecular characterization of angiotensin II-induced hypertrophy of cardiac myocytes and hyperplasia of cardiac fibroblasts: a critical role of the AT_1 receptor subtype. *Circ Res* 73:413–423.

Sadoshima J, Qiu Z, Morgan JP, Izumo S (1995). Angiotensin II and other hypertrophic stimuli mediated by G protein-coupled receptors activate tyrosine kinase, mitogen-activated protein kinase, and 90-kD S6 kinase in cardiac myocytes. The critical role of Ca^{2+}-dependent signaling. *Circ Res* 76:1–15.

Sakai S, Miyauchi T, Kobayashi M, Yamaguchi I, Goto K, Sugishita Y (1996). Inhibition of myocardial endothelin pathway improves long-term survival in heart failure. *Nature* 384:353–355.

Saxl P, Heilig R (1920). Über die diuretiche Wirkung von Novasurol und anderen Quecksilberinjektionen. *Wein klin Wochenschr* 33:943.

Silber EN, Katz LN (1975). *Heart Disease.* Macmillan, New York.

Slatton ML, Irani WN, Hall SA, Marcoux LG, Pae RL, Grayburn PA, Eichhorn EJ (1997). Does digoxin provide additional hemodynamic and autonomic benefit at higher doses in patients with mild to moderate heart failure and normal sinus rhythm? *J Am Coll Cardiol* 29:1206–1213.

The SOLVD Investigators (1992). Effect of enalapril on mortality and the development of heart failure in asymptomatic patients with reduced left ventricular ejection fraction. *N Engl J Med* 327:685–691.

Stevenson LW, Massie BM, Francis GS (1998). Optimizing therapy for complex or refractory heart failure: a management problem. *Am Heart J* 135:S293–S309.

Uretsky BF, Sheahan RG (1997). Primary prevention of sudden cardiac death in heart failure: will the solution be shocking? *J Am Coll Cardiol* 30:1589–1597.

Uretsky BF, Young JB, Shahidi FE, Yellen LG, Harrison MC, Jolly MK, on behalf of the PROVED Investigative Group (1993). Randomized study assessing the effect of digoxin withdrawal in patients with mild to moderate chronic congestive heart failure; results of the PROVED Trial. *J Am Coll Cardiol* 22:955–962.

Vasan RS, Benjamin EJ, Levy D (1995). Prevalence, clinical features and prognosis of diastolic heart failure. An epidemiologic perspective. *J Am Coll Cardiol* 26:1565–1574.

Vasan RS, Benjamin EJ, Evans JC, Larson MG, Reiss CK, Levy D (1996). Prognosis of diastolic heart failure: Framingham Heart Study. (Abstract). *Circulation* 92(Suppl I):665.

Volterrani M, Clark AJ, Ludman PF, Swan JW, Adamopoulos S, Piepoli M, Coats AJS (1994). Predictors of exercise capacity in chronic heart failure. *Eur Heart J* 15:801–809.

Waagstein F, Hjalmarson Å, Varnauskas E, Wallentin I (1975). Effect of chronic beta-adrenergic blockade in congestive cardiomyopathy. *Br Heart J* 37:1022–1036.

Waagstein F, Bristow MR, Swedberg K, Camerini F, Fowler MB, Silver MA, Gilbert EM, Johnson MR, Gross FG, Hjalmarson Å, for the Metoprolol in Dilated Cardiomyopathy (MDC) Trial Study Group (1993). Beneficial effects of metoprolol in idiopathic dilated cardiomyopathy. *Lancet* 342:1441–1446.

Wijns W, Vatner SF, Camici PG (1998). Hibernating myocardium. *N Engl J Med* 339:173–181.

The Xamoterol in Severe Heart Failure Group (1990). Xamoterol in severe heart failure. *Lancet* ii:1–6.

Yamazaki T, Komuro I, Kudoh S, Zou Y, Shiojima I, Mizuno T, Takano H, Hiroi Y, Ueki K, Tobe K, Kadowaki T, Nagai R, Yazaki Y (1995). Angiotensin II partly mediates mechanical stress-induced cardiac hypertrophy. *Circ Res* 77:258–265.

Yu S-M, Hung L-M, Lin C-C (1997). cGMP-elevating agents suppress proliferation of vascular smooth muscle by inhibiting the activation of epidermal growth factor signaling pathway. *Circulation* 95:1269–1277.

Yusef S, Teo K (1990). Inotropic agents increase mortality in patients with congestive heart failure. (Abstract). *Circulation* 82:III-673.

Zafeiridis A, Jeevanandam V, Houser SR, Margulies KB (1998). Regression of left ventricular hypertrophy following left ventricular assist device support. *Circulation* 98:656–662.

10

Care of the Heart Failure Patient

Someone may think that to know the Ideal Good may be desirable as an aid to achieving those goods which are practicable and attainable: having the Ideal Good as a pattern we shall more easily know what things are good for us, and knowing them, obtain them. Now it is true that this argument has a certain plausibility; but it does not seem to square with the actual procedure of the sciences . . . it is not easy to see . . . how anybody will be a better physician or general for having contemplated the absolute Idea. In fact, it does not appear that the physician studies even health in the abstract: he studies the health of the human being—or rather of some particular human being, for it is individuals that he has to cure.

Aristotle, *Nicomachean Ethics* I.vi.14-16

One of the essential qualities of the clinician is interest in humanity, for the secret of the care of a patient is in caring for the patient.

Peabody FW, *The Care of the Patient*

We must continually remind ourselves that we practice medicine on single patients and we seek an individual response that may not match the mean effect of an intervention in a large trial. The challenge to the physician is to combine the data from these trials with other therapeutic and patient-related insights to form a rational approach to managing the care of a single person.

JN Cohn, *N Engl J Med* (1999); 340:1512

Much of this text, indeed virtually all that has filled the pages up to this point, deals with the pathophysiology of heart failure and its relationship to current therapeutic strategies. This reflects my view that knowledge of the hemodynamic, biochemical, and molecular features of this syndrome is essential for optimal patient management. The rapid advances in modern understanding of this syndrome have been made possible by a remarkable interplay between the basic sciences, which are uncovering key features of the mechanisms responsible for this syndrome, and clinical trials that are telling what "works" (and what "does not work") in selected populations. This interplay has provided the basis for new therapies for heart failure that are meeting the goals of effective treatment: they prolong survival, reduce suffering and, at the same time, lower health care costs. Current treatment of this syndrome, however, is far from ideal in that not everyone is managed according to modern standards. Many patients with damaged hearts are not identified sufficiently early in the course of their illness to benefit fully from the drugs that are known to prolong survival. Others who receive the correct diagnosis are not given optimal therapy, and patients frequently fail to do what is recommended. This final chapter, therefore, moves from basic and clinical science to deal with another key aspect of heart failure, ensuring an optimal level of care for the individual patient.

TABLE 10-1. *What the health care provider should know to prove optimal management of the patient with heart failure*

1. Pathophysiology of the underlying disease
2. Mechanisms of action of therapy
3. Response of the individual patient

The challenge posed by the growing population with heart failure must be met at several levels (Table 10-1). Cost-effective screening is needed to identify patients with early heart failure. This topic is considered in Chapter 8, which examines growing evidence that a significant fraction of heart failure is familial in origin, and in Chapter 9, in which the potential use of such "markers" as BNP (brain natriuretic peptide) levels is discussed. The importance of early diagnosis is highlighted by evidence that treatment of asymptomatic patients can slow progression and so improve outcome. Another challenge is to develop treatment plans that are appropriate for each individual patient, a task which is becoming increasingly difficult as more is learned of the many factors that play a role in this syndrome. A final challenge, which is turning out to be more difficult than many had appreciated, is to ensure that each patient follows through on the recommended treatment plan. One approach to meeting these challenges is through an integrated health care delivery mechanism that in the following pages is referred to as a *Heart Failure Program*.

THE HEART FAILURE PROGRAM

Traditional management of heart failure focuses most responsibility on one individual; in developed countries, this is almost always a physician. These individuals can be primary care practitioners, internists, cardiologists, and, in a few cases, "heart failure experts" who have limited their practices to this syndrome. Considerable debate has recently emerged as to which of these classes of practitioners do "best" at managing these patients. This debate is avoided in this chapter, because it is becoming clear that heart failure management can be optimized using a team approach (reviewed by Philbin, 1999).

Growing understanding of the pathophysiologic mechanisms that operate in heart failure, many of which are described in the present text, is making it increasingly difficult for most practitioners who work alone to remain up to date in this field. Yet current information in this rapidly changing field is essential in defining the goals of therapy in each patient, and in establishing treatment plans by which these goals can be achieved. These challenges are compounded by a rapid broadening of the scope of services that, when properly used, greatly improve the quality of care. Unfortunately, an occasional face-to-face visit with a practitioner, generally ending with the patient receiving some advice and a few prescriptions, falls far short of what is best for this condition. The reason is that heart failure management requires ongoing communication between each patient and members of a health care team that can include physicians, physician's assistants, nurses, dietitians, social service personnel, home health agencies, and pharmacists; participating physicians can be primary care practitioners, internists, geriatricians, cardiologists, and heart failure experts.

In addition to dispensing medical information and prescriptions, members of such teams can provide the support and encouragement that patients need to cope with their deadly illness and to follow the complex therapeutic regimens that are so common. These programs can also help give the emotional support that is invaluable in achieving a favorable outcome (Krumholz et al., 1998a). Communication with heart failure patients must be a "two-way street" because optimal care requires ongoing input from the patient to those responsible for his or her care. Especially for the more severely ill, those who manage this syndrome have to be kept abreast of changing symptoms, weight gain, and potential side effects of the many drugs given to these patients. Several considerations that underlie the need for comprehensive heart failure management programs are detailed in the following paragraphs.

Complexity

Optimal management of the heart failure patient is far more complex than was taught even a few years ago. The once conventional approach to patient management, in which therapy is directed to alleviating such hemodynamic abnormalities as fluid retention and pulmonary congestion, is clearly inadequate in most cases. Patients with mild to moderate symptoms must also be managed mainly to slow progression; however, therapeutic strategies that prolong survival are changing rapidly and often run counter to the teachings of even a few years ago. Furthermore, defining the end-points of therapy is far from obvious. Problems arise because drugs that prolong long-term survival can make patients feel worse temporarily, and when given to the wrong patient or in the wrong dose, can be dangerous, sometimes lethal. Conversely, drugs that improve symptoms over the short term often worsen prognosis. These considerations add enormously to the difficulties in defining goals for these patients and in evaluating the effects of therapy.

The increasing number of effective drugs that can be used to treat heart failure represents both a challenge and an opportunity. It is clear that not all drugs can be given to every patient, nor can all patients be expected to react to a given drug in a similar manner. Selection among the many effective drugs is especially challenging because, as we have learned from clinical trials, there is benefit in adding new drugs to therapy that is already known to be of value. We are, in a way, beginning to suffer an "embarrassment of riches" in the management of heart failure. Even though the growing list of effective drugs improves the opportunity to target therapy to the pathophysiology that operates in each patient, the availability of so many potent therapeutic agents also increases the risk of error.

Another corollary to the increasing complexity of treatment is that assessment of clinical response is becoming more difficult. Unless end-points are thoughtfully defined and carefully followed, many benefits of therapy can be lost, and harm can result from missed opportunities and errors. To administer the right drugs, each in its correct dose, health care providers must understand the complex pathophysiology that operates in each patient and how available treatment options can modify that pathophysiology. The difficulties in this complex and often counterintuitive field will almost certainly increase over the next decade because additional classes of drugs are likely to become available (see Tables 9-4 and 9-6).

Cooperation among the various health care professionals who work in the setting of a Heart Failure Program can help in processing the new and important information about heart failure that is being generated at many levels. The steady flow of new discoveries regarding the molecular mechanisms that cause the failing heart to deteriorate represents the foundation for optimal care. Application of this knowledge is facilitated by the results of ongoing clinical trials and such practical information as how best to maintain contact with patients, and how to encourage them to follow the increasingly difficult programs for managing this syndrome. Exchange of information among the members of a heart failure team represents one of the most effective means to address the increasing complexity in managing these patients.

Individualized Patient Management

The value of the many clinical trials in heart failure carried out since the mid-1980s is undeniable, but it must be remembered that these trials concern populations and not individuals. As Aristotle noted, physicians treat individuals and not health in the abstract. One corollary to this ancient observation is that the principles of therapy described in this text must be tailored to meet the needs of each individual who suffers from heart failure. Several limitations of randomized clinical trials make this an especially important caveat. These include the obvious but sometimes overlooked fact that, as noted by Hampton (1998), "the results of a clinical trial apply only to the patients who are actually included." As discussed in Chapter 9, however, virtually every randomized trial in heart failure has excluded patients with diastolic dysfunction. In addition, clinical trials generally exclude individuals who are not likely to follow instructions (Mant, 1999). Thus, while heart failure trials have provided invaluable information about both underlying pathophysiology and treatment, the results are only a guide to therapy. In the last analysis, it is the response of the individual patient, and not a published result, that matters most in treating this— and any—human disease.

Tailoring of therapy to the individual patient must be based on information, such as changing symptoms, that can be obtained only from the patient. This requires frequent communication with an informed patient, who is at the "front line" in assessing progression of the underlying heart disease and responses to treatment. Patients must be made aware of the importance of a gain in weight, an increase in abdominal girth, or worsening dyspnea. Monitoring of such changes is especially important because appropriate adjustments in medication can both alleviate these signs and symptoms, and avoid expensive hospitalizations.

Heart failure patients need to be monitored frequently, in person or by telephone, especially as this syndrome moves into its final stages. To minimize hospitalization when heart failure progresses, contacts must be made increasingly often, and in more advanced cases, even daily. This is done most efficiently in the setting of a Heart Failure Program, in which specially trained nurses and physician's assistants can carry out these evaluations. Nurses and physician's assistants, working as members of an organized team, can enjoy considerable autonomy in carrying out their focused evaluations and making needed adjustments in therapy. These and other health care professionals are especially valuable because emphasis in training, as well as daily practice, is on the bedside clinical evaluation that is central to managing this syndrome. A few pounds of weight gain, increasing rales, or a slight increase in jugular venous pressure, for example, are among the best predictors of impending decompensation. When heeded, such simple steps as adjustment in diuretic or vasodilator dosage can alleviate suffering and avoid hospitalization.

The careful monitoring needed to manage heart failure requires that the data be evaluated by individuals who understand both the syndrome and the therapy. Attention must be paid to clues regarding the almost inevitable hemodynamic deterioration caused by progression of the Cardiomyopathy of Overload. This is a difficult task because evidence for progression is often obfuscated by the undesired side effects of treatment. Virtually every drug that makes these patients better can also make them worse. Evaluation of the individual patient, therefore, is central to the management of this syndrome. Such evaluations require that the clinical and hemodynamic data provided by each patient be integrated with the physiologic, biochemical, and molecular concepts reviewed in this text.

Exercise

It is becoming increasingly apparent that exercise can help many patients with heart failure. Whereas rest was commonly recommended only a few years ago, it has become clear that inactivity can worsen the skeletal muscle myopathy in these patients. Instead, it appears that a carefully monitored exercise program can improve both functional capacity (Belardinelli et al., 1999) and left ventricular function (Giuanuzzi et al., 1997). Management of these programs is among the responsibilities that can be discharged effectively by a Heart Failure Program.

Diet

The importance of diet, which was a mainstay of therapy in the era before modern diuretics, is often overlooked. Even though the unpalatable 200-mg sodium diets of the past are rarely needed, dietary instruction remains an important element of heart failure management. There remains no doubt, for example, that excessive dietary intake of sodium can worsen symptoms, so that patients need to be made aware of such simple dietary precautions as avoiding prepared foods, which are generally loaded with salt. Adequate nutrition is also important in minimizing the effects of the skeletal muscle myopathy. In addition, dietary supplements like coenzyme Q10 (Soja and Mortensen, 1997) and antioxidants (McMurray et al., 1993; Keith et al., 1998) are still under active investigation and may be found to play a role in ameliorating this syndrome. The role of diet in prevention of atherosclerosis must not be overlooked in the large number of patients in whom the underlying cause of heart failure is coronary artery disease.

End-of-Life Care

The terrible prognosis in heart failure, which has been emphasized throughout this text, means that most patients can be expected to die within a few years after their heart disease becomes symptomatic. In about half of these patients, death is sudden and unexpected. The other half experience a slow, progressive deterioration that, while not as dreadful as described in Chapter 1, requires thoughtful and compassionate end-of-life care and appropriate utilization of such resources as a hospice.

One emerging problem is that prolongation of life by "heroic" measures may not always be a desirable goal in end-stage heart failure (Krumholz et al., 1998b). The issue of resuscitation is compounded by the availability of devices, such as the implantable defibrillator, that can prevent lethal arrhythmias, but at the expense of replacing sudden death with a more protracted final course. When to use such devices and whether to inactivate implanted devices in end-stage heart failure are becoming important issues (Stevenson, 1998). These and other issues, which involve ethical as well as "medical" considerations, are probably best addressed by a team that has both training and experience in the management of end-stage heart failure.

Patient Education and Compliance

Efforts to reduce morbidity, prolong survival, and control costs in heart failure require patient education and cooperation (Dunbar, 1998). Engaging patients in their care is an art; to expect a patient to take medications that have side effects and often produce little obvious symptomatic improvement requires knowledge and incentives. Finding means to interest patients in their illness and to inform them about the goals of therapy is especially important in prescribing β blockers, which can temporarily worsen symptoms. A Heart Failure Program can provide the resources needed to teach patients how to avoid complications of therapy and help supply the knowledge and motivation that patients need to follow the complex therapeutic regimens described in this text.

Conventional practice models, when analyzed in the early 1990s, had a poor record in this regard; for example, many heart failure patients were not taking the correct dose of ACE inhibitors at a time when these drugs were universally accepted as effective therapy for this condition (Bourassa et al., 1993; Raijfer, 1993; Baker et al., 1994). This problem can be traced partly to physicians who do not prescribe these drugs, or if they do, prescribe them at suboptimal doses. Even when correct prescriptions are written, as many as half of the patients stop taking these drugs after a year for reasons that include cost, lack of the education and motivation needed to follow a rigorous therapeutic regimen, and the side effects of therapy. This problem will almost certainly worsen as more patients take β blockers, whose overall benefits concerning long-term survival are comparable to those patients taking ACE inhibitors. The fact that β blockers often produce side effects that discourage patient compliance highlights the importance of patient education and appropriate motivational incentives.

Involving patients in a program managed by individuals trained in patient education is one of the best ways to ensure patient compliance. This is a realistic goal because compliance is uniformly excellent in clinical trials, in which monitoring is generally assured by a team not unlike that in a Heart Failure Program. For this reason, the clinical research teams that operate these trial centers represent useful models for Heart Failure Programs that are being developed throughout the world.

These and other considerations explain why the interdisciplinary approach provided by a Heart Failure Program is emerging as the most effective way to manage this syndrome (Rich et al., 1995; Fonarow et al., 1997; Hanamanthu et al., 1997; West et al., 1997).

THE CHALLENGES AND PITFALLS OF "POLYPHARMACY"

The final topic to be considered in this text is that of "polypharmacy," a generally pejorative term that refers to the concurrent use of several drugs in a single patient. Polypharmacy is sometimes used as an example of poor clinical management, as when a hurried physician moves patients through a busy office by writing a different prescription for each complaint. The excessive costs and ghastly problems caused by the drug-drug interactions that can result from such a practice led to a commonly held belief that the fewer remedies prescribed, the better the clinical management. Another common teaching is that it is better to administer a high dose of a single drug than to give lower doses of several drugs. Neither of these generalizations is always true in managing heart failure.

In many settings, the concurrent use of several drugs to achieve a therapeutic goal is widely accepted. The value of combination therapy in treating infections and of several classes of antitumor drugs in treating malignant disease is clearly established. Recent clinical trials in heart failure have also demonstrated, and I believe convincingly, that the concurrent use of several drugs improves the clinical outcome in heart failure.

How then are we to think about the polypharmacy that is emerging in the management of heart failure? Where will this practice end? How many drugs must be given concurrently to prolong life, relieve symptoms, and reduce costs? In addressing these questions, it is helpful to realize that most heart failure drugs are not "chemicals" whose benefits are due to unnatural mechanisms, and which cause adverse effects by "poisoning" patients. Instead, most effective therapeutic agents act by modifying known (or postulated) physiologic, biochemical, or molecular processes. When used correctly, these agents stimulate adaptive mechanisms or block maladaptive responses, and so help to restore normal homeostasis. This is clearly the appropriate way to view nitrates, whose symptomatic benefit and safety are well established in patients with angina pectoris. These drugs generate nitric oxide (NO), a natural vasodilator that relieves the chest pain syndrome caused by ischemic heart disease by improving blood flow to the myocardium. This view also applies to the growing number of agents that have been found to benefit patients with heart failure.

A major theme of this text is the complexity of signal transduction in the human body. Chapters 4 through 8 review many signaling pathways that can harm patients with heart failure. One important feature of this physiologic signaling is the redundancy that facilitates survival when one or more vital regulatory systems is impaired. This normal redundancy is a problem for those who work with transgenic mice, in which "knockout" of a gene judged to be essential for survival often has little or no effect because these animals have many ways to compensate for a missing receptor, signal mediator, or enzyme. An analogous situation is seen in the modern airplane, which is built with many "backup" systems that, in the event of an equipment failure, allow the damaged plane to reach an airport and land safely. This safety is made possible by a design that allows a four-engine jet to fly on one engine, which not only requires that a single functioning engine provide enough power to keep the plane in the air but also that each engine be able to distribute hydraulic pressure to all control systems needed to fly the airplane.

A fanciful example of signal redundancy is provided in Fig. 10-1, which shows a four-engine jet with four independent hydraulic systems, each powered by one of the engines. Although each system has its own primary effectors, interconnections among the four systems allow all control systems to be operated in the event that any three of the engines fail. A similar redundancy is seen in the vastly more complex human body, wherein layers of signaling mechanisms can maintain life when one or more vital systems becomes impaired or inoperative. This organizational plan is ideal when the desired result is survival during a short-term emergency. As highlighted in Chapter 4, however, the same signaling systems that provide short-term benefit in an emergency can do considerable harm when called upon for long periods in chronic disease. Managing the redundancy in maladaptive signaling, which is a major problem in heart failure, therefore represents one of the most important problems in managing these patients. To overcome these deleterious effects completely, it is probably necessary to block *all* of the pathways that carry the maladaptive signals. This requires the concurrent use of many different drugs.

Most modern treatment of heart failure, as pointed out throughout this text, disables or otherwise blunts maladaptive signaling. This principle is seen in the case of the diuretics, which remove the excessive fluid accumulated by the kidneys as the result of the hemodynamic defense reaction. More recently, the same principle has been used to explain the unexpected benefits of β-adrenergic blockade in heart failure. As modern understanding of this syndrome advances, however, therapeutic targets are becoming less obvious. We can, for example, anticipate that therapy will move into the cell to target maladaptive growth responses. It seems likely that new drugs will soon be available to inhibit signaling pathways responsible for such deleterious responses as calcium overload, progressive cell elongation, and apoptosis. The redundancy of the signaling pathways that control

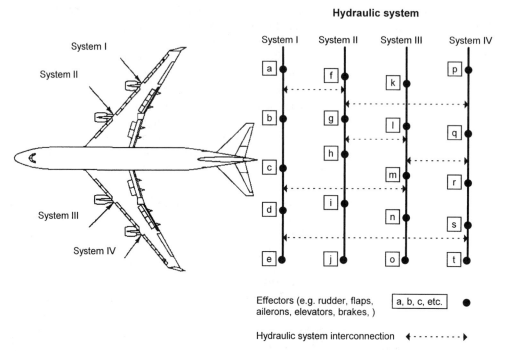

FIG. 10-1. Fanciful diagram of the hydraulic system of a four-engine jet, in which each of four independent hydraulic systems is powered by one of the engines. Each system controls its own primary effectors (a, b, c, and so on). However, interconnections among the hydraulic systems (*dotted lines*) allow all of the effectors to be controlled by another hydraulic system if an engine fails.

these processes, however, makes it difficult to completely inhibit these and other maladaptive response. As many interventions are needed to disable all of the hydraulic systems shown in Fig. 10-1, so are many different drugs required to inactivate the redundant systems responsible for maladaptive signaling in patients with heart failure. It therefore seems inevitable that "polypharmacy" will become increasingly important in managing this syndrome. Success in blocking the many vicious cycles that operate in these patients will require additional classes of drugs. As already noted, however, not all drugs can (or should) be given to all patients. Selection and use of these drugs in each patient with heart failure is best done by a team of health care professionals who combine a thorough knowledge of this syndrome and its therapy with a compassionate understanding of each patient.

BIBLIOGRAPHY

See Bibliography for Chapter 9.

REFERENCES

Baker DW, Konstam MA, Bottorff M, Pitt B (1994). Management of heart failure I. Pharmacologic treatment. *JAMA* 272:1361–1366.
Bellardinelli R, Georgiou D, Cianci G, Purcaro A (1999). Randomized, controlled trial of long-term moderate exer-

cise training in chronic heart failure. Effects on functional capacity, quality of life and clinical outcome. *Circulation* 99:1173–1182.

Bourasssa MG, Gurné O, Bangdiwala SI, Ghali JK, Young JB, Rousseau M, Johnstone DE, Yusef S for the SOLVD Investigators. Natural history and patterns of current practice in heart failure. *J Am Coll Cardiol* 22(Suppl A):14–19.

Dunbar SB, Jacobson LH, Deaton C (1998). Heart failure: strategies to enhance patient self-management. *AACN Clinical Issues* 9:244–256.

Fonarow GC, Stevenson LW, Walden JA, Livingston NA, Steimle AE, Hamilton MA, Moriguchi J, Tillisch JH, Woo MA (1997). Impact of a comprehensive heart failure management program on hospital readmission and functional status of patients with advanced heart failure. *J Am Coll Cardiol* 30:725–732.

Giannuzzi P, Temporelli PL, Corrà U, Gattone M, Giordano A, Tavazzi L, for the ELVD Study Group (1997). Attenuation of unfavorable remodeling by exercise training in postinfarction patients with left ventricular dysfunction. Results of the Exercise in Left Ventricular Dysfunction (ELVD) Trial. *Circulation* 96:1790–1796.

Hampton JR (1998). The limits of evidence-based cardiovascular therapy. *Cardiovasc Drugs Ther* 12:487–491.

Hanamanthu S, Butler J, Chomsky D, Davis S, Wilson JR (1997). Effect of a heart failure program on hospitalization frequency and exercise tolerance. *Circulation* 96:2842–2848.

Keith M, Geranmayegan A, Sole MJ, Kurian R, Robinson A, Omran AS, Jeejeebhoy KN (1998). Increased oxidative stress in patients with congestive heart failure. *J Am Coll Cardiol* 31:1352–1356.

Krumholz HM, Butler J, Miller J, Vaccarino V, Williams CS, Medes de Leon CF, Seeman TE, Kasl SV, Berkman LF (1998a). Prognostic importance of emotional support for elderly patients hospitalized with heart failure. *Circulation* 97:958–964.

Krumholz HM, Philips RS, Hamel MB, Teno JM, Bellamy , Broste SK, Califf RM, Vidaillet H, Davis RB, Muhlbaier LH, Connors AF Jr, Lynn K, Goldman L for the SUPPORT Investigators (1998b). Resuscitation preferences among patients with severe congestive heart failure. Results form the SUPPORT Project. *Circulation* 98:648–655.

Mant D (1999). Can randomised trials inform clinical decisions about individual patients. *Lancet* 353:743–746.

McMurray J, Chopra M, Abdullah I, Smith E, Dargie JH (1993). Evidence of oxidative stress in chronic heart failure in humans. *Eur Heart J* 14:1493–1498.

Philbin EF (1999). Comprehensive multidisciplinary programs for the management of patients with congestive heart failure. *J Gen Int Med* 14:130–135.

Rajfer SI (1993). Perspective of the pharmaceutical industry on the development of new drugs for heart failure. *J Am Coll Cardiol* 22(Suppl A):198–200.

Rich MW, Beckham V, Wittenberg C, Leven CL, Freedland KE, Carney RM (1995). A multidisciplinary intervention to prevent the readmission of elderly patients with congestive heart failure. *N Engl J Med* 333:1190–1195.

Soja AM, Mortensen SA (1997). Treatment of congestive heart failure with coenzyme Q10 illuminated by meta-analysis of clinical trials. *Mol Aspects Med* 18(S):S159–S168.

Stevenson LW (1998). Rites and responsibility for resuscitation in heart failure. Tread gently on the thin places. *Circulation* 98:619–622.

West JA, Miller NH, Parker KM, Senneca D, Ghandour G, Clark M, Greenwald G, Heller RS, Fowler MB, DeBusk RF (1997). A comprehensive management system for heart failure improves clinical outcomes and reduces medical resource utilization. *Am J Cardiol* 79:58–63.

Subject Index

Page numbers followed by *t* and *f* indicate tables and figures, respectively.